T0281552

Nursing's Greatest Leaders

David Anthony Forrester, PhD, RN, ANEF, FAAN, is professor, Division of Nursing Science, School of Nursing, Rutgers University, Newark, New Jersey. Dr. Forrester graduated with a BSN from the University of Texas System School of Nursing, with an MSN from the University of Texas at Arlington, and with a PhD in research and theory development in nursing from New York University. Dr. Forrester is a widely known scholar who serves as a peer reviewer for a number of professional/scholarly nursing journals; he has published extensively on a wide range of topics, including HIV/AIDS; critical care family needs; aggressiveness of nursing care at the end of life; gender-related health, including health of minority men and women; falls risk assessment and prevention in the acute care setting; nursing leadership; and nursing history. He is a fellow of the National League for Nursing's Academy of Nursing Education and the American Academy of Nursing. He is an active member of a number of professional and scholarly associations, including the American Nurses Association, New Jersey State Nurses Association, National League for Nursing, New Jersey League for Nursing, and Sigma Theta Tau International (STTI). Dr. Forrester served as the leader for the international faculty of the STTI Nurse Faculty Leadership Academy.

Nursing's Greatest Leaders

A History of Activism

David Anthony Forrester, PhD, RN, ANEF, FAAN

Editor

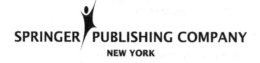

SPRINGER PUBLISHING COMPANY
NEW YORK

Springer Publishing Company, LLC
11 West 42nd Street
New York, NY 10036
www.springerpub.com

Acquisitions Editor: Joseph Morita
Production Editor: Kris Parrish
Composition: Exeter Premedia Services Private Ltd.

ISBN: 978-0-8261-3007-5
e-book ISBN: 978-0-8261-3008-2

16 17 18 19 20 / 5 4 3 2 1

The author and the publisher of this Work have made every effort to use sources believed to be reliable to provide information that is accurate and compatible with the standards generally accepted at the time of publication. The author and publisher shall not be liable for any special, consequential, or exemplary damages resulting, in whole or in part, from the readers' use of, or reliance on, the information contained in this book. The publisher has no responsibility for the persistence or accuracy of URLs for external or third-party Internet websites referred to in this publication and does not guarantee that any content on such websites is, or will remain, accurate or appropriate.

Library of Congress Cataloging-in-Publication Data

Nursing's greatest leaders : a history of activism / [edited by] David Anthony Forrester.
   p. ; cm.
 ISBN 978-0-8261-3007-5—ISBN 978-0-8261-3008-2 (eBook)
 I. Forrester, David Anthony, editor.
 [DNLM: 1. Nurses—Biography. 2. History of Nursing. 3. History, 19th Century. 4. History, 20th Century. 5. Leadership—Biography. WZ 112.5.N8]
 RT37.N5
 610.73092'2—dc23

             2015036221

Printed in the United States of America by McNaughton & Gunn.

*This book is dedicated to my loving husband, Kevin,
who makes me a better person, and to all nurses
everywhere who choose to be leaders.*

—DAF

Contents

Contributors   *xiii*
Foreword   Susan B. Hassmiller, PhD, RN, FAAN   *xv*
Preface   *xvii*
Acknowledgments   *xix*

Part I: Introduction

1.   Exemplary Nursing Leadership   3
      David Anthony Forrester

      Why Study Exemplary Nursing Leadership Within the Context of
          Nursing History?   3
      What Is *Leadership* and What Is *Exemplary Nursing Leadership?*   5
      What Is the Difference Between *Nursing Leadership* and *Nursing
          Management?*   5
      What Are the Essential Traits or Characteristics of Exemplary Nurse
          Leaders?   6
      Five Practices of Exemplary Nursing Leadership   7
      Summary   17

Part II: Modeling the Way

2.   Florence Nightingale: Where Most Work Is Wanted   *21*
      Frances Ward

      Radicalization   *23*
      Modeling the Way in Practice   *26*
      Modeling the Way in War   *29*
      Modeling the Way in Peace   *34*
      The End of Empire   *37*
      An Improving Woman   *40*
      Demystification   *46*
      Timeline   *49*
      Questions for Discussion   *50*

Part III: Inspiring a Shared Vision

3. Mother Mary Aikenhead: A Life of Vision   57
   Deborah Cleeter
   Childhood   58
   The Novitiate   60
   Inspiring a Shared Vision   60
   Foundress, Congregation of Irish Sisters of Charity   62
   Ministries for Prisons, Schools, and Orphanages   63
   Hospitals, Nursing, and Hospice   63
   Leading in the Face of Personal Struggle   65
   Global Legacy   65
   Journey Toward Canonization   66
   Exemplary Leadership   66
   Timeline   67
   Questions for Discussion   68

4. Clara Barton: Angel of the Battlefield   71
   Karen Egenes and Frances Vlasses
   Early Efforts to Inspire a Shared Vision   74
   Developing the Tools to Inspire a Shared Vision   77
   Role Models for Inspiring a Shared Vision—Clara Barton in
       Europe   77
   Inspiring a Shared Vision—Developing New Strategies   81
   Inspiring a Shared Vision on a Local Level   83
   Inspiring a Shared Vision Abroad—International Relief Efforts   86
   Inspiring a Shared Vision—In Time of War   88
   Attainment of the Vision   92
   Clara Barton's Leadership Legacy   95
   Timeline   100
   Questions for Discussion   102

Part IV: Challenging the Process

5. Margaret Higgins Sanger: The Law Shall Be Broken   107
   Patricia K. Hindin
   The Law Shall Be Broken   108
   Early Years   108
   The Making of Margaret Sanger   112
   Public Service and Progress in Birth Control   118
   Major Accomplishments   120
   Timeline   123
   Questions for Discussion   125

6.   Sister Elizabeth Kenny: Conviction and Controversy   127
Mary Kamienski

Nature Versus Nurture   128
The Vision   130
Commitment to the Vision   131
Beyond Polio   132
Societal Values   133
Not a Nurse   134
The Reality of Polio   134
The American Frontier   138
The War Rages On   140
Timeline   143
Questions for Discussion   144

7.   Clara Louise Maass: Servant Leader Undaunted   147
Carol Emerson Winters

Spending Childhood as an Adult   149
Training School for Nurses   149
The Spanish–American War   150
Nursing Soldiers With Yellow Fever   152
Nursing American Troops in the Philippine Islands   154
Annulment of Nursing Contract and Return Home to
    New Jersey   156
The Yellow Fever Commission Is Established in Cuba   158
Returning to Cuba to Nurse Yellow Fever Patients   160
Clara Maass Volunteers to Be Bitten by Infected Mosquitoes   161
Clara Maass Develops Yellow Fever   162
Posthumous Honors   164
Modeling the Way   167
Challenging the Process   168
Timeline   168
Questions for Discussion   170

Part V: Enabling Others to Act

8.   Dorothea Lynde Dix: Privilege, Passion, and Reform   175
Barbara Ann Caldwell

Setting the Stage: The Influence of Family   176
Enacting Nontraditional Female Roles: Educator and Writer   178
Finding Mentors: Religious and Educational Commitment   179
Political Leadership and the Moral Movement   182
Developing Leadership Expertise and Campaigning for
    Change   184

Prisoners' Letters and Expansion of Leadership   *186*
Transition to National Leadership   *186*
International Leadership and Recognition   *188*
Caught in a Power Struggle   *189*
Timeline   *191*
Questions for Discussion   *192*

9.   Lillian D. Wald: Pioneer of Public Health   *195*
     Mary Ann Christopher, Regina Hawkey, and Mary Christine Jared
     An Age of Transformation   *196*
     Early Life   *197*
     Building on the Public Health and Settlement Movements   *199*
     Empowering Communities to Help Themselves   *203*
     Mobilizing Social Institutions to Improve the Health of
          Communities   *206*
     Enlisting Philanthropic and Business Interests to Promote the
          Public's Health   *209*
     Exemplary Leadership in Action: The Spanish Flu Pandemic of
          1918–1919   *211*
     Lillian Wald's Legacy as a Leader—Alive and Well Today   *215*
     A Community in Crisis: VNSNY's Response to
          Superstorm Sandy   *216*
     Timeline   *219*
     Questions for Discussion   *220*

10. Mary Breckinridge: Angel on Horseback   *223*
     Denise M. Tate
     Nursing Leadership   *224*
     Family and Early Life   *225*
     Later Life   *228*
     Challenging the Process   *230*
     Inspiring a Shared Vision   *233*
     Attention! Nurse Graduates   *234*
     The Creation of Wendover   *234*
     Encouraging the Heart   *236*
     Enabling Others to Act   *237*
     Modeling the Way   *238*
     The Passing of Mary Breckinridge   *238*
     Mary Breckinridge Hospital   *239*
     Breckinridge Honored   *239*
     Mary Breckinridge's Leadership Legacy   *240*
     Timeline   *241*
     Questions for Discussion   *242*

Part VI: Encouraging the Heart

11. Edith Louisa Cavell: Courage in the Face of Duty 247
Barbara J. Patterson

Assuming Her Duty to Humanity 249
Encouraging the Heart: Changing Nursing in Belgium 252
Encouraging the Heart: The Matron 254
Leadership Lessons From Edith Cavell and World War I 258
Edith Cavell's Leadership Legacy 260
Timeline 262
Questions for Discussion 264

Part VII: The Future

12. Nurses Leading Change: The Time Is Now! 269
Susan W. Salmond and David Anthony Forrester

An Unsustainable U.S. Health System: High Cost Without High
    Return in Health Outcomes 270
Re-Visioning Health Care 272
A New Context: The Time Is Now for Nursing and Nurse
    Leaders 277
The Future of Nursing: Leading Change, Advancing Health 279
Preparing Nurse Leaders for a New Future 282
Questions for Discussion 284

Index 287

Contributors

Barbara Ann Caldwell, PhD, APN-BC, is professor, Division of Advanced Nursing Practice, and specialty director, Psychiatric–Mental Health Program, School of Nursing, Rutgers University, Newark, New Jersey.

Mary Ann Christopher, MSN, RN, FAAN, is president, Strategic Transformation in Health (STH) Consulting, Avon, New Jersey.

Deborah Cleeter, MSN, EdD, RN, is chief executive officer of the Sawgrass Leadership Institute, Ponte Vedra Beach, Florida.

Karen Egenes, EdD, RN, CNE, is associate professor and chair, Health Promotion Department, Marcella Niehoff School of Nursing, Loyola University, Chicago, Illinois.

David Anthony Forrester, PhD, RN, ANEF, FAAN, is professor, Division of Nursing Science, School of Nursing, Rutgers University, Newark, New Jersey.

Regina Hawkey, MPA, RN, NE-BC, is senior vice president and chief of provider services, Visiting Nurse Service of New York, New York, New York.

Patricia K. Hindin, PhD, CNM, CLC, is assistant professor, Division of Advanced Nursing Practice, School of Nursing, Rutgers University, Newark, New Jersey.

Mary Christine Jared, MS, RN, PMHNP-BC, is a nurse executive and a board-certified psychiatric–mental health nurse practitioner, Visiting Nurse Service of New York, New York, New York.

Mary Kamienski, PhD, APRN, FAEN, FAAN, is professor, Division of Advanced Nursing Practice, and specialty director, Family Nurse Practitioner and Family Nurse Practitioner in Emergency Care Programs, School of Nursing, Rutgers University, Newark, New Jersey.

Barbara J. Patterson, PhD, RN, ANEF, is professor, associate dean for scholarship and inquiry, and director of the PhD Program, School of Nursing, and chair of the Institutional Review Board, Widener University, Chester, Pennsylvania.

Susan W. Salmond, EdD, RN, ANEF, FAAN, is professor, Division of Nursing Science, executive vice dean, School of Nursing, and codirector of the Northeast Institute for Evidence Synthesis and Translation, School of Nursing, Rutgers University, Newark, New Jersey.

Denise M. Tate, EdD, APRN-BC, is associate dean, Undergraduate Nursing Programs, W. Cary Edwards School of Nursing, Thomas Edison State College, Trenton, New Jersey.

Frances Vlasses, PhD, RN, NEA-BC, ANEF, FAAN, is professor and chair, Health Systems, Leadership, and Policy Department, and codirector, Institute for Transformative Interprofessional Education, Marcella Niehoff School of Nursing, Loyola University, Chicago, Illinois.

Frances Ward, PhD, RN, CRNP, is professor emerita of nursing, Temple University, Philadelphia, Pennsylvania.

Carol Emerson Winters, PhD, RN, CNE, is professor and director, Nursing Education Concentration, MSN program, College of Nursing, East Carolina University, Greenville, North Carolina.

Foreword

In 2010, I served as study director for the Institute of Medicine (IOM) report, *The Future of Nursing: Leading Change, Advancing Health* (IOM, 2011). The committee and I had spent months crafting a report that described the changes needed to prepare the nursing workforce to provide exceptional care in the 21st century. We poured our lifeblood into the report and we had great expectations. We wanted to galvanize nurses and other stakeholders to first understand how nurses could best be used to improve health and then take action to change the face of health and health care. We intended for the report to serve as a blueprint for the transformation of health and the health system.

To shape the future, I turned to the past—to Florence Nightingale, the inventor of modern nursing. The summer before the report was released, my husband, Bob, and I set off for London and Embley Park, England, and Scutari, Turkey, to literally follow in Florence Nightingale's footsteps. I sought to learn all I could from the woman who shaped a movement to improve sanitation, improve quality patient care, and embark on large-scale prevention efforts. As early as 1894, Nightingale connected the importance of good childcare to building health. "Money would be better spent in maintaining health in infancy and childhood than in building hospitals to alleviate disease. It is much cheaper to promote health than to maintain people in sickness," she wrote (Lundy, Janes, & Hartman, 2001, p. 4).

Retracing Florence Nightingale's life changed me forever. It broadened the scope of what I thought was possible to inspire change for patients, families, and communities, and it gave me the courage to embark on a movement—The Future of Nursing: Campaign for Action, a joint initiative of the Robert Wood Johnson Foundation and AARP—that implements the IOM report recommendations. The campaign uses many of the skills that Nightingale perfected: a reliance on evidence, using networks and soliciting partners to elicit change, and speaking and writing often on the importance of using nursing to improve health.

But Florence Nightingale is just the first of many visionary nurse leaders who inspire me each day. Many of nursing's heroes are included in *Nursing's Greatest Leaders: A History of Activism*. I found myself captivated by the stories of the extraordinary women contained in these pages, from Clara Barton's steadfastness in establishing the American Red Cross, to Edith Louisa Cavell's courage in helping 200 Allied soldiers escape from German-occupied Belgium during World War I, for which she was executed.

This book is perfect for men and women who aspire to lead nursing and society into a better future. It will equally benefit undergraduate students enrolled in leadership courses, graduate students preparing for leadership roles, and nurses already established in leadership roles. *Nursing's Greatest Leaders: A History of Activism* deepened my love for nursing and reinforced why nursing is repeatedly ranked the most trusted profession (Riffkin, 2014). I hope readers will be motivated, as I was, by these incredible nurse leaders, and that more nurses will follow in their footsteps.

Susan B. Hassmiller, PhD, RN, FAAN
Robert Wood Johnson Foundation, Senior Adviser
for Nursing, and Director, Campaign for Action

REFERENCES

Institute of Medicine (IOM). (2011). *The future of nursing: Leading change, advancing health.* Washington, DC: National Academies Press.

Lundy, K. S., Janes, S., & Hartman, S. (2001). Opening the door to health care in the community. In K.S. Lundy, & S. Janes (Eds.), *Community health nursing: Caring for the public's health* (pp. 4–29). Burlington, MA: Jones & Bartlett Learning.

Riffkin, R. (2014, December 18). Americans rank nurses highest on honesty, ethical standards. *Gallup Poll; Social Issues.* Retrieved from http://www.gallup.com/poll/180260/americans-rate-nurses-highest-honesty-ethical-standards.aspx

Preface

This book shares the life stories of some of the most revered leaders in nursing. It reports the distinguished history of nursing leadership, activism, and impact. First and foremost, this book is about leadership—nursing leadership. But it is also a book about history—nursing history within the context of an ever-evolving society.

This is a scholarly historical report with fidelity to the vision, intelligence, resourcefulness, and political awareness of nurse leaders committed to advancing the discipline and meeting the increasingly complex needs of society. In the aggregate, this is a compelling history not only of events and people within the context of their times but also of the contributions of so many visionary women who had the sheer courage, tenacity, and passion to move the nursing profession into the future—to the betterment of society around the world.

What is special about this book—why we wrote it—is that it provides an easily accessible one-stop reference on nursing leadership and nursing history. By telling the stories of some of the nursing discipline's most prominent leaders, this book fills an educational gap for many nursing students and nurses regarding nursing, nursing leadership, nursing history, and nursing's impact on society.

This book will be of interest to readers around the world, including anyone who has an interest in the leadership and history of nursing, medical/health-related professions, women's studies, or an actual or potential interest in the nursing profession. This book will be of great benefit to undergraduate nursing students enrolled in leadership courses and to graduate nursing students (in both master's and doctoral degree programs) who are preparing for leadership roles in nursing practice, advanced practice nursing, nursing administration, and nursing education and research. Finally, this book will benefit any nurse who is currently in a leadership position and wishes to increase her or his leadership capacity by learning more about the practices of exemplary nursing leadership, and how nurses might participate in leading the nursing profession and society into the future.

Although many of the fascinating life stories of the nurse leaders included in this volume were lived out long ago and far away, they are just as relevant today as when they occurred. These nurses' stories tell of the evolution of nursing and society over the centuries and around the world. Their stories will facilitate an exploration of the very nature of leadership. Using the five practices of exemplary leadership described by Kouzes and Posner (2012) as a framework, the contributing authors examine these nurse leaders' behaviors in the following categories: modeling the way, inspiring a shared vision, challenging the process, enabling others to act, and encouraging the heart.

The criteria used to select the nurse leaders for inclusion in this book were quite simple. Nurse leaders were chosen who have had a significant and enduring impact on the nursing profession, health, health care, and society. These nurses were selected because they exemplified courage, bravery, fearlessness, open-mindedness, and innovation. No judgments were made in placing one nurse leader's story before or after another. The nurse leader biographies appear according to the exemplary leadership practice the contributing authors thought they best illustrated:

- *Modeling the Way*—Florence Nightingale (British; 1820–1910), considered to be the founder of "modern nursing."
- *Inspiring a Shared Vision*—Mother Mary Aikenhead (Irish; 1787–1858), arguably the first visiting nurse in the world; and Clara Barton (American; 1821–1912), humanitarian and founder of the American Red Cross.
- *Challenging the Process*—Margaret Higgins Sanger (American; 1879–1966), who was a birth control activist and sex educator, opened the first birth control clinic in the United States, and established Planned Parenthood; Elizabeth Kenny (Australian; 1880–1952), who challenged conventional wisdom and promoted a controversial new treatment approach for poliomyelitis; and Clara Louise Maass (American; 1876–1901), who sacrificed her life in the fight against yellow fever.
- *Enabling Others to Act*—Dorothea Lynde Dix (American; 1802–1887), widely known as a pioneer crusader for the mentally ill; Lillian D. Wald (American; 1867–1940), who founded the Henry Street Settlement, which evolved into the Visiting Nurse Service of New York; and Mary Breckinridge (American; 1881–1965), who established the Frontier Nursing Service (FNS) to provide health care in the Appalachian Mountains of eastern Kentucky.
- *Encouraging the Heart*—Edith Louisa Cavell (British; 1865–1915), a World War I nurse heroine who faced a firing squad.

This book is intended to be an educational, entertaining series of biographies of some of nursing's most important leaders as activist agents of change. It offers a comprehensive, interesting, and readable text, written with the purpose of educating and inspiring its readers to lead nursing, health, health care, and society into a better future.

David Anthony (Tony) Forrester

REFERENCE

Kouzes, J. M., & Posner, B. Z. (2012). *The leadership challenge* (5th ed.). San Francisco, CA: Jossey-Bass.

Acknowledgments

The photographs are by Thomas DiStefano. The autograph, philatelic, and numismatic materials are from the editor's private collection.

The editor wishes to acknowledge the excellent editorial and production team that brought this book to fruition. Particular gratitude is expressed for the encouragement and support of Joseph Morita, senior acquisitions editor; Jenna Vaccaro, assistant editor; Kris Parrish, production editor at Springer Publishing Company; and Exeter Premedia Services Private Ltd.

Nursing's Greatest Leaders

PART I

Introduction

Exemplary Nursing Leadership

David Anthony Forrester

No one leads alone.
—*Joel Kurtzman*

This book is first and foremost about nursing leadership. But it is also a book about nursing's distinguished history of activism and its impact on society. It is a collection of biographies of some of nursing's most revered leaders. By sharing their stories, the contributing authors are inviting you to learn leadership by example from the exemplary leadership practices and behaviors of these nurses.

Today, more than ever, we need nurse leaders. One of the key messages of the Institute of Medicine's (IOM's) report *The Future of Nursing: Leading Change, Advancing Health* (IOM, 2011) is, "Nurses should be full partners, with physicians, and other health professionals, in redesigning health care in the United States" (p. 8). Whether on the front lines of nursing practice, administration, education, research, or policy making, nurse leaders are needed to transform the health care system and, therefore, advance the health of society. In the health policy arena, nurses must reconceptualize their roles to be policy makers and have a visible and vocal presence on advisory committees, commissions, and boards. Only then will nurses be full partners in advancing the nation's health systems and improving patient care (IOM, 2011).

WHY STUDY EXEMPLARY NURSING LEADERSHIP WITHIN THE CONTEXT OF NURSING HISTORY?

History can often help individuals to deal more effectively with persistent issues and conflicts by throwing light on their origins, and by indicating long-term trends that show the general direction in which things are moving.

—*Isabel M. Stewart*

Why not study nursing leadership within the context of nursing's history? Nursing history is replete with examples of extraordinary achievements accomplished by nurse leaders who were oftentimes confronted by the most challenging of circumstances, and yet, not only did they manage to persevere, they actually succeeded beyond all reasonable expectations. Their lived experiences have value for us in that they advanced nursing and society in their times and, therefore, have had a lasting effect on us both as citizens and as nurses in contemporary society. We are, in fact, the "better future" they envisioned and inspired others to work collectively to achieve.

Early leaders in American nursing promoted the study of nursing history and advocated for its inclusion in nursing curricula. Among these early leaders were M. Adelaide Nutting, Lavinia L. Dock, and Isabel M. Stewart. They all became noted authorities on nursing history through their classic publications on the subject: *A History of Nursing: The Evolution of Nursing Systems from the Earliest Times to the Foundations of the First English and American Training Schools for Nurses* (Nutting & Dock, 1907), *A History of Nursing: From the Earliest Times to the Present Day with Special Reference to the Work of the Past Thirty Years* (Dock, 1912), *A Short History of Nursing* (Dock & Stewart, 1925, 1938), and *The Education of Nurses* (Stewart, 1943). They dedicated themselves to fostering a greater understanding of, and respect for, nursing's distinguished history and believed that understanding and dealing with problems and trends in nursing practice and education requires nurses to be familiar with their history (Donahue, 1985).

If the study of history is necessary for our education to be effective citizens, then the study of nursing history is worthwhile and necessary for effective nurses who are, or wish to become, exemplary leaders. Historical knowledge of nursing's leaders, even though they may have lived long ago and far away, constitutes a carefully and critically constructed collective memory for nursing. The way things are now in nursing and society descended from the way things were before.

Our history is our "collective memory" and by studying our collective memory in nursing, we have the potential of developing insight and, even perhaps, wisdom. It is this learned insight and wisdom that may permit us to better achieve our intended goals of advancing nursing, health, health care, and, ultimately, society. To achieve these goals, we must study our history and the leadership practices and behaviors of those who led us to where we are today.

There is one more reason to study nursing leadership within the context of nursing history—it is fun. By studying nursing history, we are given the opportunity to not only confront and make sense of complex leadership challenges encountered by nursing leaders long ago but also learn from them, their experiences, and the exemplary leadership practices and behaviors that helped them persevere and succeed.

WHAT IS *LEADERSHIP* AND WHAT IS *EXEMPLARY NURSING LEADERSHIP?*

Leadership, itself, is a topic about which much is written but little is actually known with any degree of certainty. We have difficulty actually defining leadership but are usually able to identify leadership when we have observed it or experienced it in our own lives.

The consensus view of the contributing authors of this book is that *leadership* is a set of specific intentional practices and behaviors for the purpose of influencing others and maximizing their efforts in achieving a valued and mutually agreed-upon goal. Key elements of this definition are that leadership (a) is an intentional process; (b) involves specific intentional practices and behaviors; (c) is purposeful in influencing others; (d) requires the active participation of others; and (e) includes a valued and mutually agreed-upon goal, not simply influence with no important or intended outcome. *Exemplary nursing leadership* is active, future oriented, and produces change. Exemplary nurse leaders are, therefore, activist agents of change who strive for a better future for nursing, health, health care, and society.

Assumptions About Leadership

In writing this book, the contributing authors made certain specific assumptions about the nature of leadership. These assumptions include the following:

- Whether leadership itself can be taught is uncertain.
- Leadership practices and behaviors can, however, be learned and enhanced through coaching and mentoring.
- Leadership does not require or rely on any formal title, authority, power, or position within any particular hierarchy.
- Because situations requiring leadership vary, leadership requirements vary.
- There may or may not be certain identifiable personal traits or characteristics that predispose one to being an excellent leader.
- Leadership is not management. Typically, leaders lead *people*; managers manage *things*.

WHAT IS THE DIFFERENCE BETWEEN *NURSING LEADERSHIP* AND *NURSING MANAGEMENT?*

In the nursing literature, there are often references to *leadership* followed by a discussion of *management*. Although *nursing leadership* and *nursing management* are related concepts and have several commonalities, they are not the same. Nursing leadership focuses on people and inspiring trust. Nursing leadership is concerned with identifying and communicating passionately held values and principles, modeling expected goal-directed behavior consistent with those values and principles, inspiring and communicating a shared long-range vision for the future, challenging the status quo through innovation and sometimes rule breaking, and facilitating and celebrating others' successes. Nursing management focuses on organizational systems and structure and relies on control. Nursing management is concerned with a short-range view in accepting and maintaining the status quo through rule following and rule enforcement. Although many of the nurse leaders profiled in this book were also excellent nursing managers, it is through their exemplary leadership and their significant and enduring impact on the nursing profession, health, health care, and society that they are best known.

Included in this book are the life stories of some of the most renowned nurse leaders in history. These women were activist agents of change not only within the nursing discipline but also within our larger society. The many accomplishments and outcomes achieved by these nurse leaders transcend the contexts of time and place. The impact of their many contributions on contemporary nursing and society make their stories as relevant today as when they were actually being lived out so long ago. Not only are they relevant today, these nurse leaders' stories provide us with guidance in imagining the future of the nursing discipline and potentially the future of health, health care, and society.

WHAT ARE THE ESSENTIAL TRAITS OR CHARACTERISTICS OF EXEMPLARY NURSE LEADERS?

Some contemporary leadership theories emphasize the actions of leaders more than their personal traits or characteristics. But at least pondering the notion that some individuals are possessed of certain innate traits/ characteristics that contribute to their success as leaders is irresistible. Underlying the trait/characteristic approach to identifying leaders, or people with leadership potential, is the assumption that some people are "natural" leaders and that they are somehow endowed with certain personal traits/ characteristics not possessed by others. Whether true or not, the contributing authors who wrote the biographies of the nurse leaders profiled in this book all agree that these nurses were all activist agents of change, possessed of certain characteristics essential to exemplary leadership, such as the following:

Visionary	Accessible	Generous
Innovative	Approving	Brave
Honest	Accepting	Fearless
Credible	Open	Risk-takers
Ambitious	Energetic	Helpful

Intelligent	Self-confident	Driven
Trustworthy	Dependable	Forward thinking
Resourceful	Committed	Wise
Passionate	Tenacious	Shrewd
Future oriented	Rule breakers	Motivated
Competent	Inspiring	Caring
Self-aware	Politically aware	Able to seek and accept help

These exemplary leadership characteristics are referenced time and time again throughout this book. Perhaps you will want to add to the list as you learn more about the nurse leaders whose stories are told here.

FIVE PRACTICES OF EXEMPLARY NURSING LEADERSHIP

According to Kouzes and Posner (2012), there are five evidence-based practices of exemplary leadership: (a) modeling the way, (b) inspiring a shared vision, (c) challenging the process, (d) enabling others to act, and (e) encouraging the heart. These practices are evidence based in that they are derived from more than 25 years of research and observations of leadership behaviors by scholars from around the world. Embedded in each of these exemplary leadership practices, there are at least two sets of essential behaviors or actions that leaders must demonstrate in order to lead (Kouzes & Posner, 2012). Kouzes and Posner refer to these behaviors/actions as the "ten commitments of exemplary leadership" (Kouzes & Posner, 2012, p. 28). These five practices and 10 commitments of exemplary leadership serve as a framework for analyzing the leadership practices and behaviors of the nurse leaders included in this book.

Of course, there are inherent risks in using a contemporary leadership model as a framework to analyze the leadership practices and behaviors of nurse leaders who lived long before the model existed. We know that leadership, like all things, occurs within its time and context. But as Kouzes and Posner (2012) note, although the *context* of leadership may change dramatically, the *content* of leadership does not. The fundamental *behaviors* and *actions* of exemplary leaders remain essentially the same— past, present, and future. So, the life stories of the nurses included in this volume are just as relevant today as when they were lived out so many years ago.

Modeling the Way

By "modeling the way," exemplary nurse leaders create and model standards of excellence, thus setting an example for others to follow. Modeling clear values and principles is essential in establishing expectations for the nurse leader and others. Communicating a clear set of values is essential for building a vision for the future and is the basis for everything else an excellent leader will do. Setting the example by actually living one's values and principles is essential in establishing credibility as a nurse leader. Complex change can be overwhelming, and nursing leaders may have to set interim goals so that "small wins" can be achieved while working toward meeting larger objectives—"victories." Exemplary nurse leaders often must unravel bureaucracies when the bureaucracies impede action and progress toward shared aspirations. By modeling shared values and behavioral expectations, they put up "signposts" showing others where to go to achieve a shared vision and how to get there (Kouzes & Posner, 2012).

Exemplary Leadership Commitment 1: Clarifying "Values by Finding Your Voice and Affirming Shared Values" (Kouzes & Posner, 2012, p. 42)

Exemplary nurse leaders provide opportunities for their constituents to hear, observe, and understand their values. A clearly understood and communicated set of values provides a foundation on which a vision of the future can be built. In the process of value clarification, effective nurse leaders must first engage in the introspective process of looking inward and taking the time to identify and prioritize their values. Leaders then create shared values by "finding their own voice" and communicating their guiding values and principles in language and behaviors that can be modeled for others so that they are easily understood. Exemplary nurse leaders ensure that others know what they represent by speaking passionately in their "own voice" (Kouzes & Posner, 2012).

Exemplary Leadership Commitment 2: Setting "the Example by Aligning Actions With Shared Values" (Kouzes & Posner, 2012, p. 42)

Exemplary nurse leaders "live their values," by integrating them into everything they do. To ensure a clear understanding of their values, they engage others through open communication, seeking input by asking and answering questions, providing meaningful feedback, and reflecting on what they learn. Effective nurse leaders continuously refine their values and the manner in which they model them. They model actions consistent with their values simply by doing what they say they will do. Nurse leaders encourage others to share their values and model the way by setting a credible example, sharing stories and examples that illustrate their values, and identifying behaviors and situations that are inconsistent with their shared values (Kouzes & Posner, 2012).

Florence Nightingale (British; 1820–1910)

The most famous nurse leader in nursing's distinguished history, Florence Nightingale (Chapter 2), certainly engaged in the exemplary leadership practice of *modeling the way* and abided by the first two leadership commitments of clarifying values and leading by example. Nightingale came to be acclaimed as the founder of modern nursing. A pioneer as well as celebrated social reformer, Nightingale performed a mission of service to humanity throughout her life. She became prominent for training nurses and providing nursing care to British soldiers during the Crimean War. In fact, her persona as the "lady with the lamp" making nighttime rounds of wounded soldiers made her an icon of Victorian culture. But Nightingale made numerous other contributions, including sanitary reform in India, reform of the military health care system in Great Britain, hospital planning, pioneering work in statistics, and the development of a formal nursing educational program based on sound professional standards. She accomplished all of these things in spite of the strict social restraints placed on women in Victorian England.

> I attribute my success to this—I never gave nor took any excuse.
> —*Florence Nightingale*

Inspiring a Shared Vision

A leadership vision provides a mutually agreed-upon view of a preferred future. A shared vision enhances communication, helps build relationships, enables goal attainment with less frustration, and increases productivity (Kouzes & Posner, 2012).

Exemplary leaders are passionate and believe they can make a difference. They build on a foundation of shared values to instill in others a vision of something that is exciting and better than what currently exists. Exemplary nurse leaders are optimistic, positive about the future, and look forward to the future envisioning the possible—envisioning what can be if everyone works together with shared purpose to meet common goals. To bring their vision to fruition, excellent nurse leaders are expressive and use their energy to communicate hope and optimism about the future they envision. They generate enthusiastic support from others by making strong appeals and through quiet persuasion (Kouzes & Posner, 2012).

Exemplary Leadership Commitment 3: Envisioning "the Future by Imagining Exciting and Ennobling Possibilities" (Kouzes & Posner, 2012, p. 100)
Envisioning the future involves learning from the past and present and creating a vision that is sufficiently flexible so that it is adaptable in a changing environment. A leader's vision should identify a common mutually meaningful purpose and inspire hope, motivate people to become involved, and encourage others to act in order to achieve a better future (Kouzes & Posner, 2012).

Exemplary Leadership Commitment 4: Enlisting "Others in a Common Vision by Appealing to Shared Aspirations" (Kouzes & Posner, 2012, p. 100)
Exemplary nurse leaders communicate their vision by involving others from the very beginning, thus creating greater support. The vision must be passionately authentic—that is, totally believed by the leader and compelling to others. Through positive language and their own personal energy, exemplary leaders communicate a mutually shared vision that is understandable to others by using symbols, graphics, word pictures, stories, examples, metaphors, and analogies. Frequent repetition of a compelling shared vision can be very powerful in increasing understanding. Two-way communication, encouraging feedback, and listening and reflecting on input also increase understanding and buy-in. The better the vision is understood, the easier it is to support it (Kouzes & Posner, 2012).

Mother Mary Aikenhead (Irish; 1787–1858) and Clara Barton (American; 1821–1912)

Two nurse leaders who exemplify the leadership practice of *inspiring a shared vision* were Mother Mary Aikenhead and Clara Barton. Two very different leaders, they both abided by the exemplary leadership commitments of envisioning the future by imagining exciting possibilities and appealing to the shared aspirations of others to achieve their vision of nursing, compassionate health care, and a better society.

Mother Mary Aikenhead (Chapter 3) began her nursing career in 1812 when she attended a convent in York, Ireland. The convent did not require nuns to take vows of enclosure. Sister Mary was, therefore, free to go out on her own to help those in need. She returned home to Dublin and started visiting the sick and dying poor in their homes; she thus initiated hospice care and the role of the visiting nurse. She also volunteered her services in Dublin and Cork during cholera epidemics. In 1816, she founded a secular nursing order, the Irish Sisters of Charity. Upon the return of three of her sisters from a year's study at the Hospital de la Pitie in Paris, her order was given the Georgian Mansion in Dublin. Here, in the newly established St. Vincent's Hospital, the Sisters continued their nursing.

Clara Barton (Chapter 4) was a great humanitarian and founder of the American Red Cross. She is best known, perhaps, for her nursing activities and distribution of supplies to soldiers during the American Civil War. It was during the war that Barton became nationally known as the "Angel of the Battlefield." When the Civil War was over, she went to Washington, DC, to establish and head a bureau of records to aid in the search for missing soldiers. This bureau identified and marked the graves of more than 12,000 dead in the National Cemetery at Andersonville, Georgia. During the Franco–Prussian War, Barton helped organize hospitals for wounded soldiers. In 1870 and 1871, she supervised relief efforts for the poor in Strasbourg (at that time, part of Germany) and Paris. For her services, the German Kaiser decorated Barton with the Iron Cross.

In 1873, Barton returned to the United States and began her efforts to organize the American Red Cross. She was finally successful in 1882. Serving as the first president of the American Red Cross (1882–1904), Barton represented the United States at the International Red Cross conferences: Geneva, 1884; Karlsruhe, 1887; Rome, 1892; Vienna, 1897; and St. Petersburg (Leningrad), 1903. In order to extend the services of the Red Cross beyond the battlefield, Barton proposed an American amendment to the Constitution of the International Red Cross. This amendment now provides for Red Cross relief in such national calamities as earthquakes, tornados, fires, floods, famines, and pestilence.

Barton took charge of relief work during the Florida yellow fever epidemic of 1888 and in the Johnstown flood of 1889, assisted during the Russian and Armenian famines in 1891 and 1896, and was in charge of relief after the Galveston hurricane of 1900. In addition, Barton served her country as a nurse during the Spanish–American War, at times carrying out her duties while under fire. Barton was also instrumental in bringing the United States into the Treaty of Geneva. It is because of her influence that the United States has abided by the Geneva Convention since 1882.

Challenging the Process

Change, whether expected, unexpected, planned, or unplanned, is an inevitable constant of life. Successful positive change requires effective leadership and is best achieved based on a sound foundation of mutually held values and a clear, shared vision of a desired future. Exemplary nurse leaders view change as a quest for adventure and seek out opportunities to change the status quo through innovation, experimentation, and risk taking. These leaders understand that innovation, experimentation, and risk taking may involve mistakes, failures, and disappointments. They accept all of these as opportunities to learn. Exemplary nurse leaders are often activist agents of change both for nursing and for society (Kouzes & Posner, 2012).

Exemplary Leadership Commitment 5: Searching "for Opportunities by Seizing the Initiative and Looking Outward for Innovative Ways to Improve" (Kouzes & Posner, 2012, p. 156)
Exemplary nurse leaders "are dedicated to making extraordinary things happen" and "are open to receiving ideas from anyone and anywhere" (Kouzes & Posner, 2012 p. 182). They proactively search for opportunities to address the organizational and environmental shifts that are constantly occurring. They encourage others to challenge the status quo by speaking up and taking initiative in challenging what they see (Kouzes & Posner, 2012).

Exemplary Leadership Commitment 6: Experimenting and Taking "Risks by Constantly Generating Small Wins and Learning From Experience" (Kouzes & Posner, 2012, p. 156)

Exemplary leaders constantly experiment and learn along the way. They are lifelong learners. Exemplary nursing leaders experiment, take risks, constantly generate small wins, and learn from their experiences (Kouzes & Posner, 2012).

Margaret Higgins Sanger (American; 1879–1966), Sister Elizabeth Kenny (Australian; 1880–1952), and Clara Louise Maass (American; 1876–1901)

Three historic nurse leaders who exemplify the leadership practice of *challenging the process* were Mary Higgins Sanger, Sister Elizabeth Kenny, and Clara Louise Maass. They were very different leaders with very different life stories, but they all faced some of the most compelling challenges in nursing history. They all led by taking the initiative, experimenting, and taking risks in pursuing innovative ways of improving nursing, health care, and society.

Margaret Higgins Sanger (Chapter 5) is widely regarded as the founder of the modern birth control movement. She was a nurse, ardent feminist, birth control activist, sex educator, and author. In 1912, she originated the term *birth control* and, in 1914, was arrested for publishing birth control information and sending it through the U.S. mail, which was, at that time, a violation of the Comstock Act—a federal law later deemed to be unconstitutional. Sanger established the first birth control clinic in the United States in 1916 and, as a result, was arrested just 10 days after it opened its doors to the public in Brooklyn. For this offense, she served 30 days in jail but never wavered in her lifelong commitment to the cause of making birth control supplies and education widely available to women. In 1921, Sanger organized the first American Birth Control Conference in New York City under the auspices of the newly formed American Birth Control League. This organization would later become the Planned Parenthood Federation of America. She was a committed feminist who tirelessly fought for women's rights and for women to know that they could have control over their own bodies. She was a prolific author and used her writing skills to advance her ideas and promote her way of thinking. To this day, Margaret Sanger remains an iconic figure in the American reproductive rights movement.

Sister Elizabeth Kenny (Chapter 6), although never credentialed as a licensed nurse, began an independent nursing practice in rural Australia in 1911. She would ride on horseback to visit those in need. Early on, she encountered children who had poliomyelitis and who exhibited the characteristic signs and symptoms of the disease—muscle fatigue, severe pain, contractures, and eventual paralysis. She challenged conventional wisdom and promoted a controversial new treatment approach for polio. She intuitively treated the children's affected limbs with applications of moist heat and gentle movement. This became known as the Kenny Method. Although her treatment method was largely ignored by the medical community in Australia, her work was celebrated in the United States and the Sister Elizabeth Kenny Institute was established in Minneapolis, Minnesota. The Institute remained in operation following Kenny's retirement to Australia in 1951.

Clara Louise Maass (Chapter 7) was born in New Jersey and graduated from the Newark German Training School for Nurses in 1895. She became a contract nurse with the U.S. Army during the Spanish–American War and worked in the fever-ridden camps of Jacksonville, Florida, Savannah, Georgia, Santiago, Cuba, and a government hospital in Manila Philippines. In the spring of 1901, Maass was in Cuba working with Major William C. Gorgas, who was conducting yellow fever experiments. In June of that year, Maass volunteered to be bitten by a *Stegomyia* mosquito, believing that she would be more valuable as a nurse if she developed immunity against yellow fever. She survived a mild attack of yellow fever and, because she doubted her immunization, again allowed herself to be bitten. She died 10 days after the second bite at the age of 25. Maass was the only woman and the only American to die during the testing, which implicated the *Stegomyia* mosquito as the yellow fever carrier and resulted in the eventual conquering of the disease. She was buried with full military honors in Fairmount Cemetery in Newark, New Jersey. Her epitaph reads, "Greater love hath no man than this, that a man lay down his life for his friends."

Enabling Others to Act

Exemplary leaders are relationship oriented and know the wisdom of actively involving others and investing in partnerships, trustworthy cooperative relationships, and team building. They build cohesive teams, encourage participation in decision making, and inculcate a sense of team ownership of the enterprise. Exemplary leaders recognize the value of building the self-esteem of their constituents and know that successful efforts require mutual respect among team members. They nurture personal strength and self-confidence in others and encourage others in taking initiative and having a sense of responsibility. In short, they strive to create an atmosphere of trust, dignity, and empowerment (Kouzes & Posner, 2012).

Exemplary Leadership Commitment 7: Fostering "Collaboration by Building Trust and Facilitating Relationships" (Kouzes & Posner, 2012, p. 214)
Building trust and facilitating relationships are essential in fostering collaboration. To be trusted, leaders must be the first to trust in others. Exemplary nurse leaders engage in four essential behaviors to build and strengthen a trusting relationship; they are (a) *honest* and speak with *candor*—leaders say what they mean and mean what they say; (b) *accessible* and *open*—leaders

know who they are, are open, and generously share information and resources; (c) *approving* and *accepting*—leaders are easy to talk to because they value the diverse views and perspectives of others and they listen without being judgmental or critical; and (d) *dependable* and *trustworthy*—leaders can be counted on in keeping their promises and doing what they say they will do (Kouzes & Posner, 2010).

Exemplary Leadership Commitment 8: Strengthening "Others by Increasing Self-Determination and Developing Competence" (Kouzes & Posner, 2012, p. 214)
Exemplary nurse leaders turn others into leaders by creating a collaborative atmosphere; treating others with respect; and ensuring that people feel competent, capable, and confident. They strengthen others by ensuring their sense of being in control, by providing choices, and by offering opportunities for making their own decisions. These leadership behaviors foster responsibility and accountability—they compel people to action (Kouzes & Posner, 2012).

Dorothea Lynde Dix (American; 1802–1887), Lillian D. Wald (American; 1867–1940), and Mary Breckinridge (American; 1881–1965)
Three nurse leaders who embraced the leadership practice of *enabling others to act* were Dorothea Lynde Dix, Lillian D. Wald, and Mary Breckinridge. They all led by collaborating with others and facilitating relationships to build trust. They all endeavored to strengthen others by increasing the self-determination and competence of those who shared in their vision. All of them were leaders in improving nursing, health care, and society.

Dorothea Lynde Dix (Chapter 8) was a pioneer crusader for the mentally ill. Although she had no formal education as a nurse, Dix became concerned with the needs of mental patients and imprisoned criminals. She was appalled by the mistreatment and common practices of confining mental patients in cages, closets, and cellars—sometimes chained and naked. In her time, mental patients were thought of as incurable and were classified by law as comparable to criminals. The mentally ill were often housed in jails or almshouses. Dix advocated a system of government-controlled mental hospitals, legal commitment based on medical diagnosis, and the abolition of physical restraint of mental patients.

Dix was 39 years old when she began reform efforts that spanned approximately 20 years. Her efforts elevated the standards of care for the mentally ill in the United States and Canada. Among her many accomplishments, Dix is responsible for the establishment of the first state psychiatric hospital in Trenton, New Jersey, and the eventual construction of more than 30 other psychiatric hospitals throughout the United States.

Because of her outstanding humanitarian efforts in the area of mental health and her extraordinary organizational skills, the secretary of war appointed Dix (age 60) to the post of superintendent of the female nurses of the Union Army. This appointment, which commenced June 10, 1861, did not grant military rank to Dix or the members of her nursing corps. It did, however, authorize Dix to organize hospitals, assign nurses for the care of sick and wounded soldiers, and to oversee the distribution of specially donated supplies to Union troops. With the end of the Civil War, the position of superintendent was abolished. Dix returned to her civilian life of mental health reform work.

Lillian D. Wald (Chapter 9) was a pioneer in public health. She became one of the most respected and influential social reformers of the 20th century. In 1893, witnessing the poverty and hardships of the immigrant population living on the Lower East Side of Manhattan, Wald founded the Henry Street Settlement and began providing nursing care for the medically indigent of the city. The Settlement evolved into the Visiting Nurse Service of New York (VNSNY) and is now the largest home health agency of its kind in the world, providing visiting nursing services throughout New York City. Wald was a humanitarian and civil rights activist who was a founding member of the National Association for the Advancement of Colored People (NAACP). An early advocate for nursing in schools, Wald created the National Children's Bureau in 1912 and was a leader in the fight against the 1918 influenza pandemic in New York City. Throughout her lifelong career as a nurse leader, Wald worked tirelessly to empower communities to help themselves.

Mary Breckinridge (Chapter 10) was a nurse midwife who, in 1925, established the Frontier Nursing Service (FNS) to provide professional health care in the Appalachian Mountains of eastern Kentucky. The service was a decentralized system of nurse-midwives providing home visits to clients, district nursing centers, and a hospital serving an area of 700 square miles. The FNS effectively lowered the maternal mortality rate in Leslie County, Kentucky, from the highest in the country to well below the national average. The FNS served as a model of rural health care delivery for the United States and the rest of the world. Breckinridge established the Frontier Graduate School of Midwifery, which was the first rural-based midwifery school in the United States. In 1970, this school became the first in the country to offer a family nurse practitioner (FNP) program.

Encouraging the Heart

Exemplary nurse leaders inspire others with their courage and hope. They encourage the heart by always expecting the best of people. They know that high expectations often lead to high-quality performance and outcomes. They keep hope and determination alive by recognizing and celebrating individual accomplishments over and above normative expectations. Celebrating and rewarding a job well done by providing people with thoughtful, creative, personalized recognition provides something much more lasting than a simple monetary reward like a raise in salary. The practice of *encouraging the heart* can result in people feeling their contributions are valuable. They feel like heroes, thus experiencing a greater sense of commitment to a shared vision and to the community (Kouzes & Posner, 2012).

Exemplary Leadership Commitment 9: Recognizing "Contributions by Showing Appreciation for Individual Excellence" (Kouzes & Posner, 2012, p. 272)

Remember, exemplary nurse leaders are positive individuals. They have positive expectations of themselves and others. Not only do they expect the best, they set an example and model clear unambiguous vision, values, expectations, and goals. They provide frequent positive feedback and reinforcement and always work with others to create a climate conducive to mutual success. They are spontaneous and provide their constituents with personal congratulations, personal notes and public recognition for excellent accomplishments, performance-based promotions, and awards and gatherings to celebrate individual and team successes. Exemplary leaders recognize the value of just saying "thank you" (Kouzes & Posner, 2012).

Exemplary Leadership Commitment 10: Celebrating "Values and Victories by Creating a Spirit of Community" (Kouzes & Posner, 2012, p. 272)

Exemplary nurse leaders are personally involved and display genuine honest caring for their constituents. They see celebrations as opportunities to reinforce core values, standards, and commitment. Visibly and publicly celebrating individuals' accomplishments helps create a greater sense of community, sustains team spirit, and further illustrates that excellent performance and outcomes are the result of many people's efforts (Kouzes & Posner, 2012).

Edith Louisa Cavell (British; 1865–1915)

Edith Louisa Cavell (Chapter 11) was a nurse leader who displayed the exemplary leadership practice of *encouraging the heart* and modeled her values through genuine honest caring for others. Born the daughter of an Anglican minister, the Reverend John Cavell in Norwich, England, Cavell entered the London Hospital as a probationer in 1895. In 1907, Cavell was appointed the first matron of the Berkendael Medical Institute, and in 1909, she founded a school of nursing; both were in in Brussels, Belgium. With the outbreak of World War I, the institute became a Red Cross hospital where Cavell tended to many French and Belgian as well as German wounded. She courageously refused to leave her post even when the fall of the city was imminent. Cavell was arrested by the Germans on August 5, 1915, on charges of harboring Allied soldiers and organizing their underground escape across the frontier. Despite the efforts of the American ambassador, Brand Whitlock, to obtain a mitigation of her sentence, Cavell was executed before a firing squad at 2:00 a.m. on October 12, 1915. Edith Cavell's heroism continues to inspire nurses and others worldwide. She made a difference for the nursing profession and the soldiers she saved. Her sacrifice was for the betterment of society.

SUMMARY

If history were taught in the form of stories, it would never be forgotten.

—*Rudyard Kipling*

This book is about exemplary nursing leadership practices and behaviors as illustrated by the biographies of the nurse leaders whose stories are told here. Their documented stories, at times full of emotion and drama, offer compelling insights into recognizing crucial opportunities for leadership when and where it is needed most. They also offer indelible examples of exemplary nursing leadership practices and behaviors that are germane to the many leadership challenges confronting nursing in today's complex and rapidly evolving society. This book is written for nurses who will lead nursing, health, health care, and society into the future—a preferred future that will require exemplary nursing leadership (Chapter 12).

REFERENCES

Dock, L. L. (1912). *A history of nursing: From the earliest times to the present day with special reference to the work of the past thirty years* (Vol. 4). New York, NY: G. P. Putnam's Sons.

Dock, L. L., & Stewart, I. M. (1925). *A short history of nursing from the earliest times to the present day* (2nd ed.). New York, NY: G. P. Putnam's Sons.

Dock, L. L., & Stewart, I. M. (1938). *A short history of nursing from the earliest times to the present day* (4th ed.). New York, NY: G. P. Putnam's Sons.

Donahue, M. P. (1985). *Nursing: The finest art*. St. Louis, MO: C. V. Mosby.

Florence Nightingale. (n.d.). *Florence Nightingale quotes*. Retrieved June 11, 2015, from BrainyQuote.com website: http://www.brainyquote.com/quotes/quotes/f/florenceni391864.html

Institute of Medicine (IOM). (2011). *The future of nursing: Leading change, advancing health*. Washington, DC: The National Academies Press.

Kouzes, J. M., & Posner, B. Z. (2010). *The leadership challenge: Activities book*. San Francisco, CA: Jossey-Bass.

Kouzes, J. M., & Posner, B. Z. (2012). *The leadership challenge* (5th ed.). San Francisco, CA: Jossey-Bass.

Kurtzman, J. (2010). *Common purpose: How great leaders get organizations to achieve the extraordinary*. San Francisco, CA: Jossey-Bass.

Nutting, M. A., & Dock, L. L. (1907). *A history of nursing: The evolution of nursing systems from earliest times to the foundations of the first English and American training schools for nurses* (Vol. 1). New York, NY: G. P. Putnam's Sons.

Stewart, I. M. (1943). *The education of nurses: Historical foundations and modern trends*. New York, NY: Macmillan Company.

PART II

Modeling the Way

Florence Nightingale: Where Most Work Is Wanted

Frances Ward

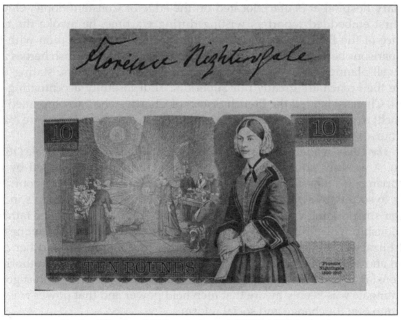

Bank of England £10 note issued 1975–1992 honoring Florence Nightingale.

No sufficient medical preparations have been made for the proper care of the wounded. Not only are there no dressers and nurses—that might be a defect of system for which no one is to blame—but what will be said when it is known that there is not even linen to make bandages for the wounded? The greatest commiseration prevails for the unhappy inmates of Scutari, and every family is giving sheets and old garments to supply their want. But, why could not this clearly foreseen event have been supplied? (Royle, 1999, p. 247)

Thomas Chenery, a graduate of England's Eton College and a diplomatic correspondent for London's *The Times*, reported events of the Crimean War from his post in Istanbul. Often, he reported from the front lines. On October 12, 1854, he shocked Victorian England with his scathing criticism of the abysmal medical services provided to wounded soldiers at the British military hospital at Scutari, located on the edge of Constantinople. One of the first embedded reporters writing during wartime, he awoke the conscience of the British people. He also fueled national humiliation with his comparisons between the exceptionally poor care given to British heroes and the well-planned and executed care given to French soldiers, stating that "here the French are greatly our superiors." Purposefully accentuating his point, Chenery lauded the French Sisters of Charity, who "accompanied the [French] expedition in incredible numbers. These devoted women are excellent nurses" (Royle, 1999, p. 247).

The Times' readers responded, among them Florence Nightingale (1820–1910). A wealthy, educated, deeply rebellious individual frustrated by the Victorian ethos that shaped social customs and mores constraining contributions to society by women, Nightingale played on her countrymen's indignation surrounding events at Scutari hospital. Capitalizing on her father's relationship with Sidney Herbert, the British secretary of war, she requested that Elizabeth Herbert, his wife, influence her husband to support her proposal and to offer introductions for her party to the appropriate authorities at Constantinople. Using whatever means necessary to advance her goals, Nightingale was keenly aware that men held power and that power was the sine quo non for change and social reform.

Concurrently, and independent of Nightingale's approach of Elizabeth Herbert, the secretary of war requested that Nightingale head an official party of nurses to Scutari as a government entourage. Recognizing this as an opportunity to model the way and lead change, Nightingale galvanized 38 women volunteer nurses she had trained, along with 15 Catholic nuns, and sailed to the maelstrom within the Ottoman Empire (Dossey, 1999). While at the military hospital for only a relatively short period—approximately 2 years—as the official superintendent of nurses charged to craft solutions to the debacle that was Scutari, Nightingale was credited with reducing the obscenely high death rate to a much lower figure. Once at Scutari, Nightingale became a national heroine in her early 30s.

Nightingale's launch to celebrity status was propelled by the British public's acclaim for the outcomes of her work at Scutari: decreased death rate, stabilization of the nursing staff, environmental improvements by the Sanitary Commission, and increased order and discipline at the hospital, irrespective of the medical staff's disdainful dismissiveness for the changes she instituted. Her administrative craftsmanship evolved from a complex web of values and behaviors antithetical to women in Victorian England. Significantly, Nightingale occasionally referred to herself as a male. As she noted in an imaginary conversation with her mother in 1851–1852, "I shall go out and look for work. . . . You must look upon me as your son. . . . You must consider me married or a son" (Woodham-Smith, 1983, p. 66).

Enraged at her culture's dismissal of women as vehicles for reproduction and pleasure, Nightingale achieved great social reform, designed hospitals, created medical recording systems, developed statistical approaches for public health management (in wartime as in peacetime), and designed a standardized nursing curriculum eventually used in training schools internationally. Defying categories of gender, Nightingale's public leadership was founded on her desire for a meaningful life, one lived in opposition to the oppressive social code of 19th-century England. In a private note dated March 1852, she wrote:

> Why, oh my God, can I not be satisfied with the life that satisfies
> so many people? I am told that the conversation of all these
> clever men ought to be enough for me. Why am I so starving,
> desperate and diseased on it. . . . My God, what am I to do?

That same year, she wrote: "In my thirty first year I see nothing desirable but death" (Baly, 1991, p. 15). Denying death, yet aware of its presence, that which she did constitutes a leadership narrative of nursing's dark angel.

RADICALIZATION

Florence Nightingale's father, William Edward Shore, acquired great wealth from a relative, Peter Nightingale, on his mother's side of the family, after which he changed his last name to Nightingale (Gill, 2004). Early in life, becoming quite learned by the teachings of her father, Florence was rankled by the purposeless lives expected for women. She had early exposure to influential thinkers and leaders of her era, including politicians, government officers, and educators. One such influence was Adolphe Quetelet, the Belgian statistician, mathematician, and astronomer who applied statistical methods in the social sciences (Diamond & Stone, 1981). Contrary to the upbringing of her older sister, Florence's education, through her father and the influence of those who frequented their home at Embley Park, radicalized her as a woman, providing her skills atypical of ladies of her time. A complex spiritual being, Nightingale was a religious eclectic, influenced primarily by her family's Unitarian views as well as the tenets of the Church of England (Widerquist, 1992). Driven, Nightingale assumed the role of friendly visitor to neighbors requiring assistance (Whelan, 2001; Williamson, 1911, 1914/1999). Rescuing a baby owl, she named her Athena; the pet remained at her side until war broke out in the Crimea (Dossey, 1999). Nightingale's Christian spirituality framed her behaviors toward those in need, shaping her singular focus on improving the care provided to others, including both direct care (nursing care) and indirect care (design of hospital structure, organizational models, medical documentation, and statistical reporting).

Tension between mother and daughter over marriage and work was intense for many years, particularly after Florence announced that God had called her in early 1837 to a life of service to others. She was 16 years old. Believing that service to God meant service to humanity, Nightingale searched for meaningful options. She wrote a friend, Christian von Bunsen, asking "What can an individual do, towards lifting the load of suffering from the helpless and the miserable?" (Calabria, 1997, p. 2). Bunsen advised Nightingale to visit the institution of the deaconesses in Kaiserswerth, Germany, to witness how care was given to ill patients. Forbidden by her mother to become a nurse, Nightingale turned to ill relatives to exercise her calling to care for people. In her early 20s, despondency overwhelmed Nightingale as she became desperately anxious to engage in a meaningful life of service. At a crisis point, she beseeched God to end her life:

> Lord thou knowest the creature which thou has made. Thou knowest that I cannot live—forgive me, God & let me die—this day let me die. It is not for myself that I say this. Thou knowest that I am more afraid to die than to live . . . but I know that by living I shall only heap anxieties on other hearts, which will increase with time. (Calabria, 1997, p. 3)

Determined to live, Nightingale survived this crisis of spirit. Choosing the road less traveled by women in the early 19th century, Nightingale waited until 1844, when she was 24 years old, to announce her intent to become a nurse. Commonly considered as work generally undertaken by drunkards, prostitutes, or criminals in workhouse infirmaries for the indigent, nursing in Great Britain was embodied in Sairey Gamp, the infamous nurse-midwife character imagined by Charles Dickens in *Martin Chuzzlewit* (Dickens, 1844). Rapid growth of cities in the burgeoning modern era driven by exponential industrialization and capitalism, however, demanded a change from the unregulated friendly visiting to systematized care in hospitals. Such care demanded obedient, trained attendants.

Forever proud of his unusual, misfit daughter, William Nightingale supported her from her early childhood, eventually accepting her choice of nursing as a career. William shaped his daughter's values for social reform through his own political career and views drawn from the Liberal wing of the Whig party. Although defeated in 1834 as the Whig candidate for a Parliament seat representing Andover in Hampshire, William Nightingale supported the 1832 Reform Act, legislation aimed at eliminating corruption in the electoral system in England (Gill, 2004). Growing up, Nightingale was immersed in British politics, conversing in her Embley Park drawing room with politicos over social reform. Her activities, successes, and national reputation as a social reformer both during and after her Crimean War efforts were highly correlated with her ability to speak directly with, and thus influence, her network of Parliament friends. Binding these influences to her alliances with popular press journalists, Nightingale succeeded in introducing social reform in England and India. As a woman, she could not hold a seat in Parliament, much to her frustration and chagrin. Nightingale thus labored harder and more painstakingly to use influence to model the way and lead change— a very exhausting process, fraught with political intrigue and lacking in objectivity. Through such processes, Nightingale focused objectively on her goals of social reform, first for British army and military health reform, and then for similar goals in India. When the Liberal wing of the Whig party lost power in Britain in the late 19th century, Nightingale retreated to her home, her bedroom, and continued political influence, albeit in a more indirect manner.

William Nightingale provided Florence with an annual annuity of 500 pounds in 1853, a sum that enabled her to move away from home, travel, and pursue her goals in rooms of her own (Dossey, 1999). Rejecting male suitors and marriage proposals, Nightingale had taken a vow of chastity at age 30, thus freeing herself from the constraints of Victorian life and liberating herself to pursue her goal to become a nurse. Husbandless, educated, and equipped with a generous annual annuity, Nightingale would undertake her own grand tour of Europe, exploring Greece, Germany, and Egypt, conducting medical and hospital tourism while documenting as much as possible about the structure, administration, functions, and personnel in these facilities. In Thebes, she claimed to have conversed with God, responding to his call for her to do good on his behalf, without public knowledge of her efforts (Nightingale, 1849–1850/1987).

When in Germany, Nightingale visited Kaiserswerth, where Theodor Fliedner, a Lutheran minister, had established a hospital and the Lutheran Deaconess Institute for the training of women in theology and nursing. Employing ideas borrowed from the Mennonites, Fliedner planned for young women to learn to care for the sick at the Institute. Nightingale joined the Institute as a student in July 1851; in October 1851, she finished her course of study (Dossey, 1999). Impressed by the steadfast devotion of the deaconesses, Nightingale's German experiences framed her later work both in direct nursing care as well as in administration. In 1850, on return from her first

visit to the Institute and prior to her subsequent 4-month nursing training, Nightingale wrote a 32-page informational pamphlet at the request of
Theodor Fliedner. Recognizing that the written word is a powerful tool for
persuasion, Nightingale used the pamphlet—*The Institution of Kaiserswerth
on the Rhine, for the Practical Training of Deaconesses under the Direction of Rev.
Pastor Fliedner, Embracing the Support and Care of a Hospital, Infant and Industrial Schools, and a Female Penitentiary*—as a vehicle to dismiss a popular myth
that nursing was a Catholic institution, one loyal to Rome (Nightingale, 1851).
Nightingale reviewed the importance of deaconesses, or nurses, in all divisions
of Christianity, existing free from vows prior to the existence of the Sisters of
Mercy in the mid-17th century (O'Brien, 2010). By extension, Nightingale reasoned that women could have a professional nursing career in a nonreligious
institution. Although Nightingale held a spiritual view that nurses served as
handmaids of the Lord, she deeply appreciated the practical necessity of sepa-
rating nursing from religion in England. If viewed as a by-product of Catholic
monasticism, nursing in Protestant England would simply not thrive. Written
anonymously, this pamphlet served as a vehicle for clarification of thought
and realization of the power of publication. Florence keenly sensed this period
as a pivotal point, as her life and her career became one.

Nightingale's training at Kaiserswerth was more than, and quite different from, nursing care of sick patients. She induced best care practices
from individual cases, documenting all the while. She also deduced patterns
of effective administration, noting central administration methods driven
down to hospital units. Voluminous reports on efficient hospital administration, staff motivation and delegation, controls for extraneous factors, and
replicable quality care outcomes were compiled; descriptions of the nursing superintendent, a central control officer, were detailed in Nightingale's
reports. She was learning to turn personal observations onto the page, refine
them, and offer them publically to her peers.

MODELING THE WAY IN PRACTICE

A Kaiserswerth graduate deaconess, Nightingale struggled with self-
definition on her return to England. In a 3-volume, 829-page work entitled
Suggestions for Thought to the Searchers after Religious Truth (1860), Nightingale
undertook a self-exploration on true spiritual experience and the emancipation of women from the dull tyranny of mindless drawing rooms (Poovey,
1993). In her essay *Cassandra*, Nightingale passionately decries the imprisonment of women's minds within trivial pursuits, stating that women needed
meaningful employment or vocations, similar to men. "Why have women
passion, intellect, moral activity—these three—and a place in society where
no one of the three can be exercised?" (O'Malley, 1934, pp. 109–110).

In 1853, Nightingale assumed the role of superintendent of the Institution for the Care of Sick Gentlewomen in Distressed Circumstances in Upper

Harley Street, London. In response to her call from God, she was now free to execute her ideas for compassionate nursing care as well as efficient hospital administration. Equipped with powerful writing abilities, she was free to explore, implement, and publicize her ideas on health care administration and nursing care so carefully culled from her experiences in medical tourism trips throughout Europe, Greece, and Egypt. Respecting only her male role models throughout her life and maintaining what would become her lifelong disdain for women (whom she viewed as not as capable as men), Nightingale executed a plan, *her plan*, the only plan worthy of implementation.

Connections continued to provide opportunity. In the economically stressed years of the 1830s–1840s, there developed an oversupply of governesses. In the 1851 British census, governesses were known as "excess women," with work conditions reflective of a near-slave lifestyle (Neff, 1929/2006). The Institution for the Care of Sick Gentlewomen in Distressed Circumstances managed large numbers of these severely debilitated, chronically ill governesses, an emotionally and physically complex group. As was common in this era of industrialization, urbanization, and poverty, women's groups—usually wives of affluent families—managed care facilities for the poor. Social reform organizations, such as the National Association for the Promotion of Social Science and the International Congress for Charities, Correction, and Philanthropy, boosted women members and focused on solutions for public health, the penal system, and educational problems. At Nightingale's request prior to her coming on board as superintendent, a committee of ladies managed the institution that relocated to No. 1 Upper Harley Street, London.

Consistent with other hospitals of the era, the Institution was very modest, housing only 27 beds in a three-floor building. Nightingale's friend Elizabeth Herbert, the wife of Sidney Herbert, English statesman and the secretary of war from 1845 to 1846, 1852 to 1855, and 1859, had recommended Nightingale for the position of superintendent. In her April 29, 1853, acceptance letter to Lady Canning of the women's committee, Nightingale requested that the committee consider the terms under which "volunteer Nursing Sisters shall be received into the institution, should any such offer themselves" (Dossey, 1999, p. 87). Three months and 2 weeks later—August 12, 1853—she began her career as nursing superintendent. Florence was 33 years old.

By the end of her first day as superintendent, Nightingale knew that she was no longer in Embley Park. With the building still undergoing renovation and chaos being the order of the day, Nightingale wrote to her friend Mary Clarke explaining her decision to leave her Embley Park home to live at Upper Harley Street, despite her mother's and sister's objections:

> Clarkey dear, I will give you a plain answer. I have talked
> matters over ("made a clean breast," as you express it) with
> Parthe [Nightingale's sister], not once but thousands of times.

Years and years have been spent in doing so. It has been,
therefore, with the deepest consideration and with the fullest
advice that I have taken the step of leaving home, and it is a fait
accompli. (Cook, 1914, pp. 138–139)

Chapter one of Nightingale's freedom from home, her emancipation,
had begun.

With incomplete renovations, an operating budget in the red, incompetent staff, and poor environmental conditions, Nightingale developed administrative knowledge from her own meager experiences in nursing, as well as
from her past friendly visiting of ill neighbors and her experiences abroad.
She reorganized patient spaces, insisted on sanitary room and patient conditions, developed nurse teams consisting of one or two probationary pupils
to one nurse, fired drunken or unhygienic nurses and house staff, wrote job
descriptions and daily work assignments, and maintained a clean kitchen
with nutritious food and drink (Goldie, 1987). Air-filled, bright, quiet, and
peaceful spaces conducive to mind and body recovery were mandatory in
what was rapidly becoming Nightingale's Institution.

A superb businesswoman, Nightingale brought change through political prowess. Her technique was self-effacement: Let the Institution's govern-
ing committee and medical staff believe that the best ideas for change were
theirs. Caring more for the success of her vision than for personal attribution,
she worked tirelessly, earning respect from the staff. In a letter to her father,
Nightingale wryly noted:

I perceive that I do all my business by intrigue. I propose in
private to A, B, or C the resolution I think A, B, or C most
capable of carrying in Com'tee & then leave it to them—& I
always win. . . . The opinions of others concerning you depends
not at all, or very little, upon what you are but upon what they
are. Praise and blame are alike—indifferent to me as constituting
an indication of what myself is, tho' very precious as the
indication of the other's feeling. . . . My popularity is too great to
last. (Dossey, 1999, p. 93)

Becoming accustomed to winning, she barreled through religious bias
and swept the facility clean of prejudice when confronted by the committee of
ladies who refused to admit Catholic patients. Risking dismissal, Nightingale
scandalously claimed, "I might take in Jews and their Rabbis to attend them"
(Cook, 1914, pp. 134–135). Her ploy was successful; all religious denomina-
tions were now allowed into the institution. Ever alert to the parodic power of
language, she recalled this tense situation to her friend Mary Clark: "Amen.
From Committee, Charity, and Schism—from the Church of England and all
other deadly sins—from philanthropy and all the deceits of the Devil, Good
Lord, deliver us" (Cook, 1914, p. 135).

Criticized in her early years as being incapable of successfully managing staff, Nightingale matured as a human resource manager with progressive experience (Goldie, 1987). In 1872, in an address to nurses and probationers at St. Thomas Hospital, Nightingale advised these novice students that the

> person in charge every one must see to be just and candid,
> looking at both sides, not moved by entreaties or, by likes
> and dislikes, but only by justice; and always reasonable,
> remembering and not forgetting the wants of those of whom she
> is in change. . . . In a Ward, too, where there is no order there can
> be no "authority"; there must be noise and dispute. (Nightingale,
> 1914, pp. 13–15)

On August 7, 1854, Nightingale completed her first year as the Institution's nursing superintendent. She had not established a training school for nurses, but she summarized in her final quarterly report that "as to good order, good nursing, moral influence and economy, the result has been to me most satisfactory" (Dossey, 1999, p. 95).

In 1854, as Nightingale prepared to leave the Institution, a cholera outbreak occurred in London. Nightingale assumed the nursing superintendent position of cholera patients at Middlesex Hospital in London. There she worked with John Snow, a physician who provided detailed street maps of cholera deaths in 1854. His cholera street cartography pointed to one common source of contamination—the handle of the Broad Street water pump (Hempel, 2007). Nightingale's working relationship with Snow taught her epidemiologic tools that were objective in their power to change health indices of whole populations. She retained this experience and used this new technique of medical disease mapping in future military health challenges during wartime.

MODELING THE WAY IN WAR

By March of 1854, Great Britain had entered the Crimean War. By November, eight Anglican Order sisters accompanied Nightingale to Scutari, including Sarah Anne Terrot. Sarah, a Sellonite sister of the Anglican Order, had cared for patients in a Plymouth cholera epidemic. She was thus considered a valuable, seasoned nurse. Five Catholic nuns were also in Nightingale's nursing party; however, as they had only cared for orphan children in London, they were considered less useful in the care of complex cholera patients. A journal writer, Sarah documented her Scutari experiences, living in the Barrick Hospital alongside Nightingale (Richardson, 1977, p. 85):

> These wards were in a miserable state; there was something
> more sad and depressing than any other part of the Hospital.
> The patients were mostly poor fellows whose constitutions had

early broken down under hardship; many had never reached the Crimea. Very few had seen the Battlefield; and they seemed to feel they were dying without glory. . . . Deaths were more frequent here than elsewhere; it seemed, indeed, as if our daily lives were spent in the valley of the shadow of death.

Sarah reported to Nightingale, a fact that pleased her, since she did not wish to report to a Catholic nun. Nightingale, a focused charge nurse, instructed Sarah and the other nurses to thoroughly clean their rooms, sew sacks of straw together to serve as beds for wounded soldiers, keep a healthy kitchen, and generally maintain a sanitary, uncluttered environment for healing. The filth was overwhelming; most of Nightingale's party invariably fasted rather than become ill from poor, rotten food. Sarah was impressed by Nightingale, stating that while she looked tired, her appearance and manner "impressed me with a sense of goodness and wisdom, of high mental powers highly cultivated and devoted to highest ends" (Richardson, 1977, p. 66).

Nightingale was indeed fatigued, but perhaps as much from political maneuvering as from sickness. The physicians at Scutari did not want, nor had they sought, the services of Nightingale and her party. Despite clashes with medical authorities, Nightingale doggedly aligned with rank-and-file physicians, assisting them with their patients as needed. She also assumed firm control and command of her nursing party. As their advocate, Nightingale jockeyed resources to obtain materials for wound dressings, water basins, clean clothing, and food and fluids for soldiers—and for her nurses. Some nurses vehemently rankled at Nightingale's spartan discipline, lamenting their original decision to join the party. Nightingale ordered nurses to enter wards only on the request of the medical officer of the day. As wounded soldiers increasingly poured into Scutari hospitals, Nightingale realized that deference to physicians—as a strategy to gain access to patients—would inevitably be successful. Nightingale weathered her nurses' dislike of this policy in order to secure the physicians' full capitulation to the obvious need for nurses. She encouraged surgeons to use chloroform as a surgical anesthetic, quite contrary to the orders of Dr. John Hall, inspector-general of hospitals, who preferred no anesthesia: "The smart of a knife is a powerful stimulant, and it is much better to hear a man bawl lustily than to see him sink into the grave" (House of Commons, 1854–1855, p. 56).

As the wounded grew exponentially, Nightingale documented relentlessly. She recorded individual patients' wound status and care, death rates, types of diseases and symptoms managed, availability of supplies and lack of specific supplies, contaminated food and water, and organizational management. She was an early proponent of data-based decision making. Trends in data unveiled patterns, which, as evidence, could sway even the most recalcitrant of physicians or politicians. To effect large-scale change in military care practices, well-documented patterns of data must be thrust onto the public stage, especially to the government. Given her experiences with documentation and Snow's epidemiologic methods of mapping cases, Nightingale appreciated the large public health issues at play at Scutari, equal to her understanding of practical daily details of patient management. Sanitation, to Nightingale, was an obvious solution to the morbidity and mortality experienced at Scutari. Facilitating health by preventing contact with hazardous waste, human and otherwise, was the cornerstone of Nightingale's action plan at Scutari. By November 14, 1854, Nightingale wrote to her friend Dr. William Bowman at the Institution at Upper Harley Street:

> I hope in a few days we shall establish a little cleanliness.
> But we have not a basin nor a towel nor a bit of soap nor a
> broom—I have ordered 300 scrubbing brushes. . . . But one half
> of the Barrack is so sadly out of repair that it is impossible to use
> a drop of water on the stone floors, which are all laid upon rotten
> wood, and would give our men fever in no time. (McDonald,
> 2010, pp. 63–64)

Nightingale dismissed the popular notion of contagion—the belief that disease is passed from one person to another by touch. Sanitation and hygiene were Nightingale's essential pillars of public health. She and her nurses meticulously swept, scrubbed, laundered clothes, made bandages from clean cloth, and managed safe food supplies, as there was, as Snow had argued, no such thing as miasma. Understanding point of contact from Snow, Nightingale championed sanitation, particularly environmental control. As she wrote in *Notes on Nursing: What It Is, and What It Is Not*, Nightingale claimed that the "very first cannon of nursing . . . [is] to keep the air he [the patient] breathes as pure as the external air, without chilling him" (Nightingale, 1860/1969, p. 12).

Nightingale supervised sanitary measures at Scutari as well as the renovations of patient units for maximum light and airflow. Concurrently, she struggled to create a new order of military nurses, women professional in demeanor and skilled in caregiving to those entrusted to them—a radically different orientation from those who cared for ill, impoverished patients in English almshouse infirmaries. Through her efforts in Scutari's military hospitals, Nightingale relentlessly, painstakingly staked out a nursing work culture. In peacetime, her task would have been difficult; in wartime, the spirit of patriotism fueled well-intentioned volunteers. She demanded women who could nurse well—ability, not birth, was her critical criterion. A competent nursing staff was equally essential to a sanitary environment; the former was responsible to ensure the latter.

Unrelenting, Nightingale concurrently nursed patients and administered the entire hospital enterprise. Nightingale's efforts were widely published; she was a ministering angel, the heroine of Scutari. In 1855, Queen Victoria sent Nightingale a brooch designed by Prince Albert as a sign of her appreciation. Depicting a St. George cross, the letters "VR," and the royal cipher, the brooch was inscribed with the following on the back: "To Miss Florence Nightingale, as a mark of esteem and gratitude for her devotion toward the Queen's brave soldiers—from Victoria R, 1855" (Gill, 2004, p. 401). The brooch became known as the Nightingale Jewel.

So popular was Nightingale that Henry Wadsworth Longfellow's 1857 poem "Santa Filomena," published in the *Atlantic Monthly*, referenced the Lady with the Lamp:

> Lo! in that hour of misery
> A lady with a lamp I see
> Pass through the glimmering gloom,
> And flit from room to room. (Longfellow, 1857, pp. 22–23)

In the winter of 1855, a confluence of factors catapulted Nightingale to fame in Britain. Already gifted by Queen Victoria and beloved as the "Lady with the Lamp," a phrase first coined in London's *The Times* to symbolize her practice of moving through rows of patients at the Scutari hospital at night with her lamp swaying at her side, she became known for exposing the government's sluggish response to the inhumane care provided soldiers at the front line. In January 1855, the army numbered 11,000 soldiers; the sick and injured numbered 23,000. Determined to bring order to the hospital system, Nightingale devised a basic triage system for incoming wounded soldiers, demanding that they be thoroughly washed and wounds cleaned and dressed, with each soldier receiving fresh, new bandages. She set up a laundry system, contrary to the common practices on the wards—with resultant resentment from intransigent medical officers. She ordered food to be allocated according to patients' needs, with the sickest receiving broths and extra fluids (Gill, 2004). "Nothing which the '*Times*' has said has been exaggerated of Hardship," Nightingale wrote in her notes (Goldie, 1987, p. 130).

Maneuvering and influencing her political allies behind the scenes, she demanded a government response. Because of family connections, it was to come from the very highest level. Lord Palmerston, who retained a parliamentary seat largely due to the influence of Nightingale's father and other family members, became prime minister in 1855. Noted as a shrewd manager of public opinion through skillful use of the press, Lord Palmerston's first effort was to regain order in the Crimea—and accolades from his public. First, Lord Palmerston constituted a royal Sanitary Commission, comprising two physicians and an engineer. The charge to this Commission, consistent with the nation's growing embrace of sanitation and hygiene, was to immediately improve hospital conditions and thus save lives otherwise at high risk resulting from impure air and preventable sanitary problems. Nightingale applauded the work of the Sanitary Commission, whose flushing of water pipes, unclogging of sewer drains, improved airflow and ventilation in roofs, removal of debris, disinfection of walls, and other improvements cleared the detritus symbolic of death in Scutari (Dossey, 1999). Mortality had begun to decline after Nightingale initiated her sanitary, dietary, and laundry measures; after the efforts of the Sanitary Commission, mortality continued to decline exponentially following aggressive sanitary public health action.

In 1855, Lord Palmerston also created the royal Commissariat Commission, a two-man team led by Sir John McNeill, a surgeon, and Colonel Alexander Tulloch, an army officer trained in law and internal affairs. Both men were passionate about sanitation and public health reform, with Tulloch an advocate of data collection of the health status of soldiers. The Commissariat report emulated Nightingale's reports regarding problems with food, supplies, and hospital and other equipment (Dossey, 1999). Because Lord Palmerston authorized the two commissions with power to act, changes occurred quickly. Deliveries of fresh food began; processes for purchasing and storing of foods were established. For Nightingale, her many letters to her political friend Sidney Herbert and to the press had finally borne fruit—death from poor sanitation and poor hygiene was decreasing. The men in these two royal commissions and Nightingale remained colleagues for years, long after the commissions completed their work and the men involved suffered blocked professional advancement in their fields from jealous colleagues. Her association with these commissioners renewed Nightingale's zeal and passion; she became increasingly determined to heal soldiers, and to do so well.

This same year Nightingale saw an opportunity in war to train a new breed of physicians who would elevate the role to a higher level as a result of improved knowledge to be gained from postmortem examinations and dissections, new therapeutics, and the collection of data and use of statistics. Nightingale saw opportunity for important secondary gains culled from war—new surgical techniques and increasingly intricate knowledge of human anatomy to be learned from the detritus of war. Nightingale appreciated that the morbidity and mortality associated with war offered opportunities to advance anesthetics and surgical techniques. Additionally, regular collection of data illustrated by statistics could provide evidence to document the need for change. Planning to use her own money to renovate a building in Scutari, Nightingale decided in 1855 to begin a medical school, given the large patient population and supply of corpses for dissection (Cook, 1914). Easily able to separate emotion from objectivity, Nightingale was quick to appreciate secondary gains to be accrued from war.

Irrespective of these dramatic improvements, a cholera outbreak subsequently ravaged the hospital, its patients, physicians, and nursing staff. Nightingale fell ill with Crimean fever in May 1855 and only rallied after several months of rest. Encouraged to recuperate at home in Embley Park, Nightingale refused, preferring instead to stay in the Crimea with the soldiers. After several months, Nightingale returned to the bedside, to supervision of care, and documentation of the debacle symbolized by Scutari. She inundated government officials with information from the front, appreciating fully that public sentiment was on her side. Her adoring public lavished

Nightingale with gifts following her illness, as her political colleagues and confidantes in London schemed to create a more permanent testament of their devotion. In November 1855, high-ranking public officials met to create a voluntary national fund, to be called the Nightingale Fund, to support nurses' training in England (Gill, 2004). The resolution drafted by the organizing committee paid tribute to Nightingale's contributions to her country, for which the Fund would serve as a symbol of the public's appreciation:

> 1. The noble exertions of Miss Nightingale in the hospitals of the East demand the grateful recognition of the British people.
> 2. That, while it is known that Miss Nightingale would decline any such recognition merely personal to herself, it is understood that she will accept it in a form that may enable her, on her return to England, to establish a permanent institution for the training, sustenance and protection of nurses to arrange for their proper instruction and employment . . . in hospitals. (Baly, 1986, pp. 8–9)

With flyers announcing it widely distributed throughout England, pledges for the Nightingale Fund poured in. At once, thousands of pounds sterling were received. Prior to the end of the Crimean War, a core endowment was now available to transform Nightingale's dream of a training school for nurses into reality. Sultan Abdulmecid of Turkey also contributed to the Nightingale Fund in 1855, in addition to presenting her with a diamond and carnelian bracelet in appreciation of her services in Turkey (Dossey, 1999).

Believing that her poor health and fragility might hinder her personal oversight and administration of the Fund, Nightingale requested that it be entrusted to several of her male colleagues to make executive decisions on its appropriate use. By June 1856, there was approximately £44,000 in the Fund. Nightingale, financially savvy in banking and business, developed a deed of trust for the Fund for the investment of the contributions. Not willing to spend the money without careful planning, she allowed the funds to accumulate, and only in 1860 was a portion of the funds used to establish a training program for nurses (McDonald, 2009a). The Training School for Nurses at St. Thomas' Hospital enrolled its first students on July 9, 1860, thus inspiring a shared vision for change and solidifying Nightingale's sanitary public health reform values as standard for the education of nurses in England, and eventually in the United States (McDonald, 2009a).

MODELING THE WAY IN PEACE

Russian Czar Nicholas I died in March 1855. His death laid the foundation for peace. On March 30, 1856, the Crimean war ended with the signing of the Treaty of Paris. With the war over, Nightingale stayed until all soldiers in Scutari either died or went home. Almost 4 months later, Nightingale returned to England, entering her family's summer residence at Lea Hurst through the back door.

Considering her war mission a failure, given that no significant changes had been incorporated in the British Army's Medical Department, Nightingale retreated. Awash with war memories of dead and dying soldiers neglected by the highest authorities in the Army, Nightingale once again saw nothing desirable but death. She wrote in her journal in 1857:

> Father, I do not in the least care whether I die or live. I would
> wish to know which it is to be, that I may know what Thou
> wouldest have of me. I do not support that there will be any
> less work for us in any future state of existence (for us, the salt
> of the earth, at least, not till after many future states). Thou wilt
> send us where most work is wanted to be done. Lord, here I am,
> send me. Perhaps when I was sent into this world, it was for this,
> Crimea and all. (Vicinus & Nergaard, 1990, p. 395)

Another opportunity to lead presented itself in 1857 following an invitation by Queen Victoria and Prince Albert to meet them at Balmoral Castle in Scotland to hear what she had learned from her participation in the Crimean War. Nightingale rallied and gathered her support team—including the lead individuals from the Sanitary Commission and the Commissariat Commission, men she valued as essential to the changes instituted in Scutari during the war. Nightingale used her charisma, wit, public acclaim, and religious piety to embed her reform tenets into conversations with the queen and prince. She acted quickly, calmly, and decisively, to persuade the queen to constitute two royal commissions. She positioned her informal cabinet of male allies to support her efforts, with herself acting as core strategist and planner. Before the first commission was constituted, Nightingale was asked for a full report on the Crimean War. Energized by the possibility of making meaningful, permanent changes in the Army's medical system, Nightingale worked tirelessly to produce an 830-page preliminary document—*Notes on Matters Affecting the Health, Efficiency, and Hospital Administration of the British Army: Founded Chiefly on the Experience of the Late War*—that framed the commission's final report. Nightingale's writing—robust with data, statistics, and succinct analyses on the conditions of soldiers and facilities at Scutari—persuaded Lord Panmure, secretary of state for war, to appoint the first commission. Nightingale picked the commissioners and delved into the status of the army in peacetime. Statistically skilled, Nightingale prepared data in pictorial form to impress her audience quickly and without question. Her coxcombs—rose diagrams similar to pie charts or John Snow's earlier dot maps—illustrated death tolls from diseases to be more than the death toll from wounds in the Crimean War (Brasseur, 2005). Trusting only in objective presentation based on data, Nightingale produced her finest work, documenting that the peacetime mortality of soldiers in the army was almost double that of civilians. Friended by physician and medical statistician William Farr, Nightingale learned of data on death and disease in England, information that framed her comparisons of peacetime versus wartime morbidity and mortality statistics.

Nightingale's trusted ally, Sidney Herbert, chaired the royal commission, placing his signature on the final report to lend the male credibility that she thought necessary. Nightingale was the invisible scribe to the report that included proposals for army reform and medical reform, including a uniform system of medical statistics incorporating mortality (rates and causes of death), frequency and types of disease, and types of surgical operations. Nightingale considered statistical data critical to the evaluation of military hospitals' sanitation effectiveness as well as medical–surgical outcomes. Other recommendations, consistent with Nightingale's earlier suggestions, included aggressive sanitation protocols in army barracks, restructuring of the army medical department for efficiency, and establishment of an army medical school. The army medical school, located initially in Chatham, had an especially contentious beginning. *The Lancet*, a prestigious British medical journal founded in 1823, published letters unfavorable to the new medical school in 1858. Nightingale quickly galvanized her resources to avert negative opinions about the new school; on March 14, 1858, she wrote to Dr. William Farr, her physician colleague and medical statistician following the publication of negative letters appearing in *The Lancet*:

> There are three letters in *The Lancet* yesterday against our Army Medical School. They are easily answered, but Mr. Herbert has also received remonstrances from Lord Naas and Lefroy, MP for Dublin. And we want to have the *Lancet* on our side. Would you ask the editor not to commit himself till he has heard our side of the question? You will find Sutherland here tomorrow at 6 o'clock and we will draw up a statement, which we depend upon you to father upon *The Lancet* and make them give a leading article in our favour. (McDonald, 2011, p. 368)

Ultimately, the new school flourished, changing location in 1863 and eventually becoming part of a joint medical school in Millbank, London, with a hospital constructed according to Nightingale's own design specifications.

Once the Commission report was completed, Nightingale made sure the report's recommendations hit the popular press—the British people, her court of public opinion. Accustomed to winning, Nightingale claimed that she would "eat straight through England" to achieve her goal of reforming the British army (Vicinus & Nergaard, 1990, p. 172). The people responded as she anticipated, with a public outcry that overwhelmed the War Office.

Instigating the War Office to change, Nightingale ceaselessly worked in the background to illuminate army medical problems and to propose solutions. Shortly thereafter, the British army medical department was restructured, an army medical school was established, an army statistical department was developed, and military barracks and hospital buildings were redesigned, according to sanitary reforms. Always one to "bite on a fact," Nightingale found statistics "more enlivening than a novel" (Boyd, 1982, p. 209). Nightingale's statistical prowess was rewarded by the Royal Statistical Society—one of the oldest statistical societies in the world—in 1858, when she was elected as the first woman member of the Society (McDonald, 1998).

THE END OF EMPIRE

As Nightingale, Sidney Herbert, and the royal commission on army and military medical reform revolutionized the British Army and military health system using their report as ammunition, India, a key British colony, mutinied. Hundreds were massacred in the bloody 1857 Great Mutiny—the Sepoy Rebellion—in India, the flash point that heralded an end to British paternalism and the beginning of Indian patriotism. The end of the British Raj was within view on the horizon, with the oppressed hungry for control, participation in government, and increasing independence. Although Britain regained control after the Great Mutiny, it had lost credibility and entered a new era of watchfulness. In August 1858, Britain passed the Government of India Act, adding a new member to the British cabinet, the secretary of state for India, who received advice and guidance on internal Indian affairs from the Council of India, with headquarters in Calcutta (Dossey, 1999).

Lord Stanley served as Britain's first secretary of state for India, a man who had dined with Nightingale a year earlier at an introductory meeting arranged by Nightingale's former suitor. Lord Stanley, a contributor to the Nightingale Fund in 1855, deeply understood the need for reform in India; he was also keenly knowledgeable of the many and complex barriers to reform in that British colony. Nightingale, well versed in army and military health issues in India, soon began lobbying Lord Stanley for sanitary reforms in India. Specifically, Nightingale demanded the constitution of the India Sanitary Commission; the goal was sanitation of the army and civilian populations (Dossey, 1999; Gill, 2004).

The royal Sanitation Commission of India was constituted in 1859 with three sanitarians, a statistician, and two members of the India Council. Lord Stanley transferred this Commission to the War Office, given its recent changes aimed at improving overall performance as well as health status of troops. Forever an advocate for timely reform, Nightingale did what she did best, prior to the Commission's establishment. She collected data. Without firsthand knowledge of the health of British soldiers in India or the sanitary state of military bases and the country as a whole, however, Nightingale was incapable of knowing what problems existed in India, and therefore, she was unable to design strategies for improvements. She abhorred stories, narratives of individuals aimed at evoking sympathy. Such stories made her impatient and only fueled her demands for objective data. Having designed a "circular of inquiry"—a questionnaire—to be sent to all military posts in India, Nightingale began to gather baseline data. Data, she knew, was needed to sway opinions of powerful politicians—her target group. She tabulated enough completed questionnaires to fill a room in her house. Additionally, she received copies of regulations regarding sanitation and administration from several hundred military posts throughout the country. Working collaboratively with her colleague, Dr. William Farr, the medical statistician on the Commission, Nightingale completed a commission report that also included an addendum—"Observations by Miss Nightingale." The final report, a two-volume treatise with over 2,000 pages, was published in 1863 (Dossey, 1999).

The report from the Royal India Sanitation Commission report findings paralleled those of the Royal Sanitation Commission (of the British army in England), only with shockingly worse findings. This report documented that the overwhelming majority of British troops in India died from causes associated with poor sanitation. Nightingale publicized the reality that death among British military troops in India was due to preventable illnesses, at an astonishing cost to the Crown. As in the Crimea, morbidity and mortality were correlated with polluted environments. She announced to all who would listen that the three things that decimated the British army in the Crimea were "ignorance, incapacity, and useless rules" (Gill, 2004, p. 420). Her persistence, as well as her influence among powerful political connections, was rewarded. The India Sanitation Commission made broad recommendations for reform, including demanding that British-controlled provinces constitute individual military sanitary commissions. In addition, the previously constituted sanitary commission was expanded to include Indian representatives as full voting members.

Once completed, the report of the Royal India Sanitary Commission was hijacked by a low-level bureaucrat in England, who eliminated all of Nightingale's statistical analyses and other observations—the majority of data required to substantiate the recommendations advocated—and replaced her material with his own executive summary, or "Précis of Evidence" (Dossey, 1999). Nightingale's observations included in the original report were bound in red cloth, becoming referred to as her "little red book." She became enraged at this bureaucratic sabotage. She took immediate action, informing members of Parliament to secure the full report at the appropriate office. Additionally, she offered to use her own financial resources to ensure that the full report would wind its way to her ultimate target audience—the Indian Civil Service. Ultimately, the full report was distributed in 1863, with pressure coming from readers again enraged by articles published in London's

The Times stressing the need for sanitary reform in India. As she had done so often in the past, Nightingale challenged the status quo, and using her influence among both politicians and the public, Nightingale unabashedly deployed all of her available resources to meet her goals. When the secretary of state for war died in April 1863, Nightingale lobbied a journalist for the *Daily News* to "agitate, agitate" for a replacement sympathetic to sanitary reform (Cook, 1914, p. 30). The journalist complied; Nightingale's choice was ultimately named as successor.

For nearly four decades, Nightingale pushed for multiple reform efforts in India, despite the fact that she never visited the country. Her first initiatives in India evolved logically from her successful sanitary reform efforts in the British army. Sanitation was a thread for Nightingale that was woven through all of her Indian efforts. It was her core concept, extending from public health efforts, to engineering work, and to the individual patient cared for by a nurse at the bedside. Her efforts to improve farm irrigation, to curb poverty and famine by introducing land policy, and to extend formal education to women were all accomplished through finding facts, data analysis, and conversations with eminent politicians, members of the royal family, and ordinary people. Once she had the data, she framed the key problems and conceptualized solutions that she documented meticulously—and then distributed to people with powerful influence primarily in politics and the press. While not all of her reforms were instituted, Nightingale remained immersed in Indian sanitary reform for decades; it became, in fact, a lifelong effort (Gourlay, 2003).

Nightingale's efforts in India demonstrate her ability to lead—first, her focus on values that drove her guiding principles, enabling her to model the way for a social reform era within an age of empire. This singular emphasis galvanized her colleagues, parliamentary men in positions of authority, to align with her goals. Nightingale's exemplary ability to reject status quo in favor of *doing the right thing* facilitated dramatic challenges to processes contrary to her values. She captivated both leaders and the public with her passion and behaviors to further her causes, embracing others to join her cause, empowering them to act rather than to be passive spectators. While tenacious in efforts to meet her goals, Nightingale's demeanor, charisma, and drive for excellence softened and warmed the hearts of the British public, endearing them to her work (Kouzes & Posner, 2011). Nightingale led without fanfare, following a road less traveled for women in Victorian England.

Beyond Great Britain and India, Nightingale's technocratic advice—specifically, definition of the urgent problem, preparation of solutions based on data, and efficient implementation—for the management of military hospital design and services extended to the United States and other countries. In fact, at the beginning of the American Civil War, the Union Army used Nightingale's war materials while the Confederate Army reissued her book on field cooking (McDonald, 2001). Two decades later, Nightingale wrote that the Egyptian–Sudan campaign, or the Anglo–Egyptian war of 1882, was a great opportunity to pilot test new ways of implementing nursing services to demonstrate the outcomes of a well-prepared nursing unit on morbidity and mortality among soldiers (McDonald, 2001).

Although shy, almost a recluse in her daily life, Nightingale was never reticent to provide advice regarding military hospital management. Her idealistic admiration for the courage of soldiers, combined with her confidence that sanitary improvements would decrease their morbidity and mortality both in war and in peacetime, framed Nightingale's view that it was her responsibility to inform others—individuals, armies, and nations—of her plan for military health management. Nightingale's sanitation data was undeniable.

AN IMPROVING WOMAN

Between her early idea of instituting a training school for nurses at the Institution for the Care of Sick Gentlewomen in Distressed Circumstances in 1854 and the completion of commission reports in 1858 and 1863, Nightingale had reinvented herself. No longer a woman searching for work meaningful to herself and her God, Nightingale had transformed herself into a highly visible, politically influential social reformer targeting sanitary change, both for wartime as well as peacetime efforts. The darling of Queen Victoria, Nightingale moved offstage as the winds of political change shifted from social reform to a political and social climate of conservatism.

In a changed political environment, Nightingale focused attention on nursing, which she equated with sanitary knowledge. In her immediate post-Scutari life, Nightingale wrote *Notes on Nursing* (Nightingale, 1860/1969). In her preface, Nightingale is stunningly clear that the knowledge of nursing is a knowledge that every woman needed:

> Every woman . . . has, at one time or another of her life, charge
> of the personal health of somebody, whether child or invalid,—
> in other words, every woman is a nurse. Everyday sanitary
> knowledge, or the knowledge of nursing, or in other words, of
> how to put the constitution in such a state as that it will have no
> disease, or that it can recover from disease, takes a higher place.
> . . . If, then, every woman must at some time or another of her
> life, become a nurse . . . how valuable . . . if every woman should
> think how to nurse. (Nightingale, 1860/1969, p. 3)

Nightingale used the word *nurse* for "want of a better [word]" (Nightingale, 1860/1969, p. 8). She advocated for a new vision of nursing, one that looked beyond dependently following physicians' orders for patients' medications and treatments. A strikingly independent woman reformist,

Nightingale structured nursing care as an essential tool for the sanitary management of patients. She stressed that nursing "ought to signify the proper use of fresh air, light, warmth, cleanliness, quiet, and the proper selection and administration of diet" (Nightingale, 1860/1969, p. 8). Nurses, to Nightingale, were primarily sanitarians, with interventions emanating from the knowledge of sound sanitary practices extending from the individual to the general public. Nurses, physicians, sanitary engineers, and hospital designers and architects—all were necessary public health equipment. Nursing care complemented medical care, with all care dependent on good sanitary practices consistent with Nightingale's—and those of the Liberal wing of the Whig Party—social reform ideals. Nurses needed good, disciplined training to serve well as one component of the sanitary team improving the morbidity and mortality statistics of Britain—and of India.

With renewed interest, Nightingale turned again to the Nightingale Fund begun with much public fanfare, adoration, and acclaim in late 1855. At the time instituted, the Fund was nothing more than a mere distraction, a metaphoric gift from well-wishers unable—possibly unwilling?—to appreciate her true reform goals. In July 1860, the Nightingale School of Nursing opened its doors at St. Thomas Hospital in London. She handpicked her students—Nightingale nurses—who were trained in a 1-year program. Ultimately, graduates of the Nightingale School of Nursing, all unmarried and thus untethered to fulfilling the needs of husbands and children, became missionaries. Graduates were dispatched to serve in hospitals in England, Europe, and elsewhere in order to proselytize the knowledge of efficient sanitary principles of good nursing across much of the world. Nightingale was exceptionally clear that graduates of her school had not been trained merely to meet the workforce needs of St. Thomas Hospital. Eight years after the school was established, Queen Victoria presided over groundbreaking ceremonies for the construction of a new St. Thomas Hospital, in view of the Houses of Parliament (Dossey, 1999; Nelson & Rafferty, 2010)

For the fledgling school, 1872 was a pivotal year. Nightingale learned from probationers that classes were poorly delivered, if delivered at all. When a chief administrator at the school objected to her strong discipline and high ideals, Nightingale secured a new administrator, one willing to provide probationers' instruction according to her demands (Dossey, 1999).

Nightingale nurses were to be exemplary emissaries valuing discipline, moral character, and sanitary principles; to be less so meant dismissal from the school. In her May 1872 graduation address at the school of nursing, Nightingale appealed to the graduates to remain fresh, to avoid stagnation:

> What we can do depends so much upon what we are. To be
> a good nurse one must be a good woman; or one is nothing
> but a tinkling bell. To be a good woman at all, one must be an
> improving woman; for stagnant waters sooner or later, and

stagnant air as we know ourselves, always grow corrupt and unfit for use. Is any one of us a stagnant woman? Let it not have to be said by any one of us: I left this Home a worse woman than I came into it. (Nightingale, 1914, p. 5)

Nightingale School of Nursing, founded on her goal to improve morbidity and mortality through sanitary reform interventions, was a purposeful, self-conscious initiative to forcibly create standardized nursing training to diffuse sanitary health reform both nationally and internationally. In creating a school of nursing grounded in her guiding principles and values, Nightingale modeled the way for the profession of nursing for decades into the future. The sheer strength of her values influenced women to become pupil nurses—probationers—who shared Nightingale's vision of sanitation and social reform. Her sustained drive for excellence in sanitary, gentle nursing care provided in safe and clean environments captivated both the minds and the hearts of enrollees, empowering them to bravely nurse their patients. Her demand for self-discipline and accountability among nurses provided the foundation for strong, capable women to transform the public image of the Sairey Gamp midwife to that of a modern-era professional. Whether reviewing Nightingale's sanitary reforms, nursing school establishment, or hospital redesign, one common theme emerges—her strength of leadership.

Nightingale's somewhat strident confidence in her belief that the hospital environment was simply a mirror image of the society sponsoring it, coupled with her indefatigable energy and sustained attention placed on poor outcomes associated with hospitals, stimulated hospital reform. Nightingale again turned her attention to writing to promote her views on both hospital design and nursing care.

In 1863, Nightingale's *Notes on Hospitals* was published, deeply influencing hospital design and construction for decades into the 20th century (Rosenberg, 1989). Her *Notes* were basic instructions to hospital architects to improve sanitary conditions in hospitals by conforming to the various principles of construction she outlined in her book. Statistics served as her primary tool of persuasion. Turning to the mortality rates of three groups of hospitals—24 London hospitals, 12 provincial town hospitals, and 25 county hospitals—in the year 1861, Nightingale noted that the death rate was highest in London hospitals and lowest in county hospitals. "Here we have at once," Nightingale wrote, "a hospital problem demanding a solution" (Rosenberg, 1989, p. 4). Based on her experience, Nightingale stated, "a great deal of the suffering, and some at least of the mortality, in these establishments is avoidable" (McDonald, 2012, p. 50). Nightingale identified several ideals for construction essential to the health of hospitals. These ideals were elementary, including fresh air, light, ample space, and subdivision of the sick into separate buildings or pavilions. Subsumed in these principles are the additional realities of assuring effective sewage drainage and water flow, washable floors for disinfection, efficient kitchens and laundries, acceptable furniture for both patients and nurses, and appropriate accommodations for nurses residing at hospitals (Rosenberg, 1989). If hospitals were to be constructed to also support medical schools, then Nightingale advocated quite adamantly for her design—a design that would allow medical students to monitor patients recovering from sickness.

Several core concepts are intermeshed in Nightingale's *Notes on Nursing* (Nightingale, 1860/1969) and *Notes on Hospitals* (1863/1989), all operating under the umbrella theme of reform—social, public health, and management reform. Sanitation, central in Nightingale's efforts, underscored much of the nursing care services described in *Notes on Nursing* (Nightingale, 1860/1969), the first such effort to outline the essentials of nursing. In her construction of a nursing school program, organizational lines of authority and delegation were as central to predicting a quality school as the teaching materials. Viewing all people as equals in God's eyes, Nightingale advocated for improved conditions in workhouse infirmaries. Nightingale led efforts in nursing education and social reform that laid the groundwork for both public welfare reform and national health care reform in Great Britain. As Virginia Dunbar wrote in her foreword to the 1969 edition of *Notes on Nursing*, Nightingale lamented in 1860 that "bad sanitary, bad architectural, and the bad administrative arrangements [in hospitals] often make it impossible to nurse" (Nightingale, 1969, p. xiii).

Nightingale's prescient insistence on placing a trained woman nursing superintendent—called matron—in charge of nursing pupils and the training program itself revolutionized nursing services by centralizing the control of nursing to nurses (McDonald, 2013). The nursing superintendent position was thus upgraded, with defined authority and accountability. Power was diffused among men—physicians and hospital administrators—and women—nursing superintendents. Instead of serving as domestic servants, nurses now assumed status as operators of a separate field. Although battles between the genders ensued, nurses now were empowered to battle. Nightingale was firmly of the opinion that nursing was a service that opened doors of opportunity for women rather than serving as a vocation, as noted in her 1866 correspondence to her statistician-physician colleague, William Farr:

> I would rather than *establish a religious order open a career highly paid*. My principle has always been that we should give the best training we could to any women of any class, of any sect, paid or unpaid who had the requisite qualifications moral, intellectual and physical for the vocation of Nurse. Unquestionably the educated will be more likely to rise to the post of Superintendent, but *not* because they are ladies but because they are educated. (Baly, 1991, p. 75)

The nursing school program was one of "every day sanitary knowledge," as Nightingale wrote in her preface to *Notes on Nursing* (Nightingale, 1860/1969). Her *Notes on Hospitals* (1863/1989) and *Notes on Nursing* followed a common theme—sanitary reform, one from the perspective of hospital design and the second from that of direct patient care. These two volumes had different target audiences with themes remaining consistent. Her nursing care descriptions focused on ventilation and warming, health of houses, noise, diet, bed and bedding, light, cleanliness of houses and hospitals, personal cleanliness, observation of the sick, and documentation of the patient's status and care. Discipline, predictable care routines, and pride in one's work were prerequisites of being a Nightingale pupil nurse.

As these values began to permeate training schools of nursing in Great Britain, Nightingale turned her attention to the status of workhouse infirmaries, facilities established as a social welfare effort through the Poor Law Amendment of 1834. (Englander, 1998). Workhouse infirmaries had troubled Nightingale for many years. Therefore, when sought for advice on how to improve conditions in the Liverpool Workhouse Infirmary, Nightingale leaped at the opportunity. Twelve of Nightingale's graduates—"Nightingale nurses"—began working in the Liverpool Workhouse Infirmary in May 1865, shifting the workforce from Dickensonian Sairey Gamps to disciplined nurses well versed in the Nightingale curriculum (Dossey, 1999). The Liverpool Infirmary stands as a symbol of Nightingale's activism in public welfare reform. More interested in large-scale policy change than simply local, facility-based change, the success of reforms in the Liverpool Infirmary energized Nightingale to more aggressive activism, culminating in her "ABCs" for legislative amendments to the Poor Law. Nightingale's 1866 "ABCs" called for reforms in the infirmary system to include separation of the sick from the well pauper population, establishment of a single central administration, and placement of the entire system under responsible administration reporting to Parliament (McDonald, 2004). The "ABCs," although not fully implemented because of shifting political agendas, succeeded in informing subsequent legislation, particularly the Metropolitan Poor Act of 1867. Nightingale's efforts in social reform were part of an unrelenting, remorseless agenda that steamrolled through Britain, positioning the United Kingdom to embrace a national health care system years later.

As industrialization and subsequent urbanization accelerated in the latter half of the 19th century, the burgeoning hospital enterprise fundamentally changed Britain's basic ontology of health. With the hospitalization of the country, the locus of care now shifted from home to hospital while the focus gradually morphed from prevention and return to wellness to management of illness. Likewise, friendly visiting also changed, as might be predicted in cities where ladies' committees, often eager to participate in social reform movements and to demonstrate their talents at organization, sought tangible projects for engagement. Some ladies' groups supported programs for home nursing for the poor by providing basic care by untrained women (McDonald, 2009b). As this program of home care enterprise took hold, spreading in multiple neighborhoods in England, Nightingale noticed and was unnerved. Untrained individuals providing care in the homes of fragile, at-risk poor was a daunting development for Nightingale. Even as she orchestrated the training of nurses in hospitals consistent with the tenets of sanitary knowledge, Nightingale's basic assumption was that such trained nurses would deliver care to ill people in their homes. For her, hospitals existed for acute care management only.

Nightingale, once again, took action in the 1870s. With her mantra—only *trained* nurses can safely provide effective sanitary care—driving her actions, Nightingale turned her attention to district nursing. Collecting data on district nursing, Nightingale revealed that the majority of district nursing programs did not employ trained nurses. Outraged, she approached the Metropolitan and National Association for Providing Trained Nurses for the Sick and Poor, an organization established by her male colleagues William Rathbone, Henry Carter, and others, in 1875 to ensure at least basic care for poor residents (Baly, 1986; Dossey, 1999). Employing her oft-used strategy of influencing those in official power with undeniable data, Nightingale's report of existing district nursing programs stimulated the establishment of a central home for district nurses by the Metropolitan and National Association. Pupil nurses lived in the nurses' quarters of hospital training schools, which provided them structure and discipline under the authority of the nursing superintendent. Nightingale demanded similar arrangements for district nurses. Passionate that training was needed to meet the requirements of patients' needs, Nightingale bundled aspects of training specifically relevant to home care for nurse probationers in district training programs. District nursing programs in Britain, similar to private duty registries in the United States, evolved for the delivery of parceled nursing services through organized visiting nursing associations. Here was an emphasis on home, care, and wellness. As medicine advanced and hospitals flourished, this emphasis waned in Britain, as nurses assumed increasingly dependent roles to physicians and as hospitals began to be symbolic of health care. Nightingale's ontology of sanitation and public health conflicted with the public's idolization of technical advances, physicians, and specialization in health care. Regardless, nurses' training programs became standardized and accepted as a salaried career path for women, despite Nightingale's disdain for the unexpected twist in the road—the unpalatable shift in focus from caring for patients to caring for physicians.

As Nightingale turned 73, British and American nurse leaders planned to participate in the International Congress of Charities, Correction, and Philanthropy held in Chicago in June 1893, during the Chicago World's Fair. Nightingale served as advisor to those who orchestrated the first Nurses' Congress. During this historic World's Fair, American nurse leaders formed the American Society of Superintendents of Training Schools for Nurses, endorsing standard nurse training programs in hospitals (Ward, 2009). As hospital training schools flourished, unpaid pupil nurses became an indispensable intact workforce, a phenomenon contrary to Nightingale's personal ethos. She advocated for meaningful, paid work for women, not for work under conditions akin to slavery. In June 1867, Nightingale had written a friend "The ultimate destination of all nursing is the nursing of the sick in their own homes. I look to the abolition of all hospitals and workhouse infirmaries. But it is no use to talk about the year 2000" (Dossey, 1999, p. 298).

DEMYSTIFICATION

In 1907, 3 years before her death at age 90, Florence Nightingale was awarded the Order of Merit from King Edward VII, son of Queen Victoria. Nightingale was the first woman to receive this accolade, one that acknowledges those who have demonstrated exemplary service in the armed forces, distinguished themselves in science, or who promote art. At age 35, Nightingale's image as leader beloved to the British people was solidified through her work in the Crimea; at 90, she was a national icon. A complex confluence of factors shaped Nightingale's ability to lead. These factors are worthy of explication and demystification.

Although Jeffry A. Frieden (2006) is correct in noting that mercantilism was in decline by the time of the Napoleonic Wars, it is also true that the influence of the colonial mentality of command and control continued to exist as Victoria took the throne in 1838 and Nightingale arrived in Scutari. The managerial frame of reference that accompanied forced foreign trade was intractable, and advocates of reform would continue to face substantial opposition until the manufacturers of the early 19th century won the day by eliminating barriers to trade. A predecessor to our own global environment, the new manufacturing economy required another type of leader. Nightingale was part of that new brand of leaders.

To see the significance of her leadership in our own time, it is useful to reflect on the principles of leadership identified by Kouzes and Posner in 2011. Nightingale's behavior, as described in this chapter, emulates the principles of modeling the way, inspiring a shared vision, challenging the process, enabling others to act, and encouraging the heart as explicated by Kouzes and Posner. In 2013, Paul J. H. Schoemaker, Steve Krupp, and Samantha Howland identified abilities similar to those outlined by Kouzes and Posner that are needed in unpredictable environments such as the one in which Nightingale lived. Because uncertainty builds leaders, skills are needed in anticipation of opportunity, interpretation of complexity, extended inquiry, alignment toward common ground, acceptance of challenge, and commitment to decisive action. Even across a great distance, it is not too difficult to see Nightingale as our contemporary.

The simple fact of Nightingale's birth within an affluent British family was critically important to her development of leadership characteristics. Expected to become a pampered, tinkling bell of a wife to a well-chosen suitor, Nightingale prickled. Given that work was not demanded of her during her early life, and that she was exposed to influential figures conducting business with her father in their drawing room, Nightingale had time to study and be mentored by politicians, statisticians, policy experts, and others concerned with issues of social justice. Whirling within this salon of influential people, wealth, and education, Nightingale concretized the five attributes essential to leading as identified by Kouzes and Posner. She did not want a life of boredom. Provided an annuity by her indulgent father as a young woman, she was freed from the common financial constraints of daily life, allowing her absorption in topics that interested her: hospitals, nursing, theology, and literature. Disdainful of the paths that Victorian women chose, Nightingale emulated behaviors of men that she thought worthy and productive in the social reform political culture within which she was embedded. Had she been born a man, she may have groomed herself to serve as Britain's prime minister in the late 19th century. As she increasingly gained perspective on her intense desire to have a useful purpose in life, Nightingale became confident of herself, achieving the hubris that was reserved for men. In essence, she learned to anticipate threats to her progressive vision and strategically target opportunities to promote reform.

To synthesize the information she gathered, she learned to interpret complex streams of information. An elegant writer, she realized that style, tone, and content must vary for both the audience and the goals to be achieved. With a clear understanding of the religious values framing her actions, Nightingale honed her skills in writing—particularly writing for persuasion—as well as in interpersonal communication, artful manipulation of men in positions of influence, and goal-directed focus. To conduct extended inquiry, Nightingale wrote. She shared her opinions in belletristic language, inciting the British populace to outrage at crimes against soldiers, the poor, the sick, workhouse inhabitants, and anyone powerless in need of assistance. Faithful to her vow to do good for its own sake without the benefit of advancing her own reputation, she often allowed attribution to male colleagues in order to advance reform. A master at aligning her vision with the common ground of reformers in power and the British people, she knew how to target her reports and she was fearless in launching them. Nightingale exemplifies the practices of leadership as described by Kouzes and Posner. She always did her homework, identifying political support as trump cards to institute the changes she petitioned. In 21st-century terms, Nightingale conducted internal and external environmental scans prior to pushing her political agenda to colleagues in Parliament. Passionate on the page, she was never cited for lack of information to support her causes. Analyzing her visual rhetoric in the rose diagrams, Lee Brasseur (2005) praised Nightingale's understanding of making complex data clear to potentially resistant audiences. Along with Charles Joseph Minnard, who designed a visual of mortality in the Napoleonic Russian Campaign, Nightingale is cited as a leader in what is often termed the "Golden Age of Data Graphics" (Friendly, 2008, p. 509).

Born during the age of empire, Nightingale welcomed challenges on a grand scale. Given her predilection for sanitation, public health, and social reform, Nightingale framed all actions within that empirical mantra. Highly focused and very disciplined, when she realized that a problem existed, she employed her skills in statistics to determine the root cause. Subjective stories and emotional responses were rejected as useless; objective data derived scientifically was embraced. She deliberately moved as far away as possible from the stereotypical feminine attributes and behaviors of her time. Given that she functioned as a highly acclaimed social reform activist within the constraints existent in Victorian culture, Nightingale led remarkable change through her skills at exerting influence among those in power and through her prolific writing. She was economical in her friendships—all friends must have utility to further her causes. Ultimately, Nightingale became neutral toward her father, seeing him as lacking in tenacity as he refused to continue in politics once he lost an election. For Florence, commitment trumped empathy.

Nightingale never lost focus on sanitation, public health, and social reform. A decisive leader committed to action, her thoughts never scattered. From friendly visiting of ill friends and family members to the design of military hospitals, Nightingale walked a narrow path, becoming highly versed in all nuances of sanitary problems and associated morbidity and mortality. She was an expert in her field of sanitary knowledge, which she equated with nursing knowledge. Nurses, physicians, engineers, and others were all tools for sanitary improvement. She drove change in this field by meticulously collecting relevant data, analyzing data to identify patterns and trends, and subsequently disseminating her findings to individuals with the authority and power to make policy and to amend law. Her very passion also framed a certain intolerance of mediocre or poor performance. Far more decisive than the benign lady with the lamp, Nightingale was more likely to dismiss inept individuals than attempt to remediate them. Impatient and solitary, she sought guidance from divinity and her male colleagues. She kept one or two popular female press reporters in her inner circle, but only for specific purposes. Securing and retaining influential connections was critical to Nightingale. She believed in herself, in her own plans. She possessed confidence in her cause and her knowledge, never going off track to follow the causes of others. In fact, although she believed that women should have the right to vote, she believed more in advocating for women's utility and productivity. If a feminist at all, then she can best be labeled a reluctant one.

With keenly anticipatory vision for opportunity, superior interpretative communication ability, passionate inquiry through empirical methods, alignment toward common ground, unabashed willingness to accept grand challenges, and remorselessly decisive action, Nightingale led. The dark angel of nursing, she proclaimed in 1856 that she would eat straight through England to achieve her goals. She did just that.

TIMELINE

- May 12, 1820—Florence Nightingale is born Grand Duchy of Tuscany at Villa La Columbaia in Florence, Italy, to a wealthy British family; the family moves to Lea Hurst estate in Derbyshire, England; Florence has one older sister, Parthenope.
- February 7, 1837—First experiences a "Christian calling" to become a nurse while living at Embley Park in Wellow, Hampshire, England.
- 1844—Begins to visit hospitals.
- December 1844—Becomes the leading advocate for improved medical care in the infirmaries through the reform of the "Poor Laws."
- 1845—Declares her intention to become a nurse; she visits the convent of the Saint Vincent de Paul sisters, where she learns nursing theory.
- 1850–1855—Keeps a pet owl, Athena, as her constant companion, now mounted and on display in the Nightingale Museum.
- 1850—Makes her first visit to Protestant Deaconess at Kaiserwerth, where care was provided for the poor and which later became a training school for nurses and teachers.
- 1851—Spends 3 months training as a sick nurse at Kaiserwerth.
- August 22, 1853—Accepts the post of superintendent at the Institute for the Care of Sick Gentlewomen in Upper Harley Street, London.
- October 21, 1854—Sent to the Ottoman Empire.
- November 4, 1854—Arrives in Turkey with 38 nurses and is stationed at Selimiye Barracks in Scutari (Istanbul) to nurse British soldiers fighting the Crimean War.
- 1855—Nurses British soldiers through outbreaks of cholera and typhus.
- November 25 or 29, 1855—A public meeting to give recognition for her work during the war leads to the establishment of the Nightingale Fund for training nurses.
- August 7, 1856—After every patient has returned to Britain, she follows, meets with Queen Victoria at Balmoral and tells her about the defects in military hospitals and the need for nursing reforms; Nightingale plays a central role in the establishment of the Royal Commission on the Health of the Army.
- August 1857—After collapsing, Nightingale is sent to Malvern, a health care resort, where she is put on bed rest for exhaustion.
- 1858—In her report, *Notes on Matters Affecting the Health of the British Army*, Nightingale creates statistical charts to show the number of men who died from the conditions in the hospitals compared to those who died from battle wounds.

- 1859—Publishes her 136-page introduction to nursing, titled *Notes on Nursing: What It Is and What It Is Not.*
- 1860—Nightingale's attention turns to the morbidity and mortality rates of the British troops and citizens in India; she gathers statistics and recommends sanitation reforms; is elected the first female member of the Royal Statistical Society and becomes an honorary member of the American Statistical Association.
- August 7, 1860—Nightingale Fund is used to establish the Nightingale Training School at St. Thomas Hospital, London.
- May 16, 1865—The first Nightingale nurses begin working in the Liverpool Workhouse Infirmary.
- 1869—Dr. Elizabeth Blackwell and Nightingale open the Women's Medical College.
- 1883—Awarded the Royal Red Cross by Queen Victoria.
- 1892—With the assistance of the County Council Technical Instruction Committee, Nightingale organizes a health crusade in Buckinghamshire.
- 1896—Nightingale becomes bedridden but continues working on hospital plans.
- 1907—First woman to be awarded the Order of Merit from King Edward VII.
- August 13, 1910—Nightingale dies peacefully in her sleep (aged 90), 10 South Street, Mayfair, London; she is buried in the graveyard at St. Margaret Church in East Wellow, Hampshire, England.
- 1975–1992—Apart from Queen Elizabeth II, Nightingale becomes the only woman to be featured on a Bank of England note (at the beginning of this chapter); her portrait appears on the back of £10 Series D notes accompanied by a scene showing her tending wounded soldiers in Scutari; first issued in 1975, it ceased to be legal tender in 1994.
- 1989—Nightingale Museum is established on the site of the first Nightingale Training School at St. Thomas Hospital, London; remodeled and reopened in 2010.

QUESTIONS FOR DISCUSSION

1. Florence Nightingale, a wealthy and educated woman frustrated by the cultural ethos that constrained women's contributions to society in Victorian England, was awarded the Order of Merit from King Edward VII in 1907, 3 years before her death. She was the first woman to receive this prestigious award, generally reserved for distinguished service in the armed forces, science, or art. A reluctant feminist, if one at all, Nightingale led in an era marked by the oppression of women. What were Nightingale's attributes and behaviors that propelled her to successful leadership in *modeling the way* within this Victorian context?
2. Florence Nightingale promoted improved sanitation, public health, and social reform in Victorian England using statistics as the major driving

tool for change. Nightingale was elected to the Royal Statistical Society in 1858, the first woman ever elected to membership in this prestigious academy. An early evidence-based researcher, Nightingale's work led to reform within Britain's medical military services, the establishment of an army medical school and an army statistical department, and redesign of hospitals. Can you comment on Nightingale's statistical strategies, her data-collection and data-dissemination techniques, and her political acumen to ensure sustained incorporation of sanitary reform in her nation's health care system?

3. Leaders galvanize resources to effect change; Florence Nightingale did so in Victorian England, an era marked by the rejection of women in leadership roles. Nightingale deeply appreciated that power was the sine quo non for initiating change and social reform—she also knew that men held power. What resources did Nightingale employ in *modeling the way* to lead change? Consider Nightingale's use of family influence, family wealth, use of public press—particularly popular newspapers—and male politicians sympathetic to her social causes as you explore her use of resources to create change in this era of the British Empire.

4. Florence Nightingale has been referred to as the "mother of modern nursing," having established a school of nursing at St. Thomas Hospital in London in 1860 that incorporated principles of sanitary reform. For Nightingale, nurses were essential "public health equipment," members of a disciplined sanitary team improving the morbidity and mortality statistics of Great Britain and India. Explore the contrasting themes of Nightingale's career—the Lady with the Lamp during the Crimean War versus the Dark Angel of England who said she would "eat straight through England" to achieve her goal of reforming the British army. For Nightingale, the grand challenge was remorseless public reform. Was sanitary nursing care a tool for, or a stimulus for, such reform?

REFERENCES

Baly, M. (1986). *Florence Nightingale and the nursing legacy.* London: Croom Helm.

Baly, M. (1991). *As Miss Nightingale said . . .: Florence Nightingale through her sayings—A Victorian perspective.* London: Scutari Press.

Boyd, N. (1982). *Three Victorian women who changed their world: Josephine Butler, Octavia Hill, Florence Nightingale.* Oxford, UK: Oxford University Press.

Brasseur, L. (2005). Florence Nightingale's visual rhetoric in the rose diagrams. *Technical Communication Quarterly, 14*(2), 161–182.

Calabria, M. D. (1997). *Florence Nightingale in Egypt and Greece: Her diary and "visions."* Albany, NY: State University of New York Press.

Cook, S. E. (1914). *The life of Florence Nightingale: 1820–1861* (Vol. 1). London, UK: Macmillan.

Diamond, M., & Stone, M. (1981). Nightingale on Quetelet. *Journal of the Royal Statistical Society. Series A (General), 144*(1), 66–79.

Dickens, C. (1844/1899). *Martin Chuzzlewit.* New York, NY: Charles Scribner's Sons.

Dossey, B. M. (1999). *Florence Nightingale mystic, visionary, healer.* Springhouse, PA: Springhouse Corporation.

Englander, D. (1998). *Poverty and poor law reform in nineteenth century Britain, 1834–1914 from chadwick to booth.* London, UK: Longman.

Frieden, J. A. (2006). *Global capitalism: Its fall and rise in the twentieth century.* New York, NY: W. W. Norton.

Friendly, M. (2008). The golden age of statistical graphics. *Statistical Science, 23*(40), 502–535.

Gill, G. (2004). *Nightingales: The extraordinary upbringing and curious life of Miss Florence Nightingale.* New York, NY: Ballantine Books.

Goldie, S. M. (1987). *"I have done my duty" Florence Nightingale in the Crimean War 1854–56.* Manchester, UK: Manchester University Press.

Gourlay, J. (2003). *Florence Nightingale and the health of the raj.* Burlington, VT: Ashgate Publishing Company.

Hempel, S. (2007). *The strange case of the Broad Street pump: John Snow and the Mystery of Cholera.* Los Angeles, CA: University of California Press.

House of Commons. (1854–1855). *House of Commons Papers Volume 33.* London, UK: Parliament House of Commons.

Kouzes, J. M., & Posner, B. Z. (2011). *The five practices of exemplary leadership.* Hoboken, NJ: John Wiley & Sons.

Longfellow, H. W. (1857, November). Santa Filomena. *Atlantic Monthly, 1*(1), 22–23.

McDonald, L. (1998). Florence Nightingale: Passionate statistician. *Journal of Holistic Nursing, 16*(2), 267–277.

McDonald, L. (Ed.). (2001). *Florence Nightingale: An introduction to her life and family.* Waterloo, Canada: Wilfrid Laurier University Press.

McDonald, L. (Ed.). (2004). *Florence Nightingale on public health care.* Waterloo, Canada: Wilfrid Laurier University Press.

McDonald, L. (Ed.). (2009a). *Florence Nightingale: The Nightingale School.* Waterloo, Canada: Wilfrid Laurier University Press.

McDonald, L. (Ed.). (2009b). *Florence Nightingale: Extending nursing.* Waterloo, Canada: Wilfrid Laurier University Press.

McDonald, L. (Ed.). (2010). *Florence Nightingale: The Crimean War.* Waterloo, Canada: Wilfrid Laurier University Press.

McDonald, L. (Ed.). (2011). *Florence Nightingale on wars and the war office.* Waterloo, Canada: Wilfrid Laurier University Press.

McDonald, L. (Ed.). (2012). *Florence Nightingale and hospital reform.* Waterloo, Canada: Wilfrid Laurier University Press.

McDonald, L. (2013). What would Florence Nightingale say? *British Journal of Nursing, 22*(9), 542.

Neff, W. F. (1929/2006). *Victorian working women: An historical and literary study of women in British industries and professions 1832–1850.* Oxon, UK: Routledge.

Nelson, S., & Rafferty, A. M. (Eds.). (2010). *Notes on Nightingale: The influence and legacy of a nursing icon.* Ithaca, NY: Cornell University Press.

Nightingale, F. (1987). *Letters from Egypt: A journey on the Nile.* New York, NY: Grove Press. (Original work published 1849–1850)

Nightingale, F. (anonymously). (1851). *The Institution of Kaiserswerth on the Rhine: For the practical training of deaconesses under the direction of Rev. Pastor Fliedner, embracing the support and care of a hospital, infant and industrial schools, and a female penitentiary.* London, UK: London Ragged Colonial Training School.

Nightingale, F. (1969). *Notes on nursing: What it is and what it is not.* New York, NY: Dover Publications. (Original work published 1860)

Nightingale, F. (1914). *Florence Nightingale to her nurses: A selection from Miss Nightingale's addresses to probationers and nurses of the Nightingale School at St. Thomas's Hospital.* London, UK: Macmillan.

O'Brien, M. E. (2010). *Spirituality in nursing.* Burlington, MA: Jones & Bartlett.

O'Malley, I. B. (1934). *Florence Nightingale 1820–1856.* London, UK: Thornton Butterworth.

Poovey, M. (Ed.). (1993). *Florence Nightingale: "Cassandra" and other selections from "Suggestions for thought."* New York, NY: New York University Press.

Richardson, R. G. (Ed.). (1977). *Nurse Sarah Anne with Florence Nightingale at Scutari.* Chatham, UK: W & J Mackay Limited.

Rosenberg, C. E. (Ed.). (1989). *Florence Nightingale on hospital reform.* New York, NY: Garland.

Royle, T. (1999). *Crimea: The great Crimean War 1854–1856.* London, UK: Little, Brown.

Schoemaker, P. J. H., Krupp, S., & Howland, S. (2013, January–February). Strategic leadership: The essential skills. *Harvard Business Review*, pp. 131–134.

Vicinus, M., & Nergaard, B. (Eds.). (1990). *Ever yours, Florence Nightingale selected letters.* Cambridge, MA: Harvard University Press.

Ward, F. (2009). *On duty: Power, politics, and the history of nursing in New Jersey.* New Brunswick, NJ: Rutgers University Press.

Whelan, R. (2001). *Helping the poor: Friendly visiting, dole charities, and dole queues.* London, UK: Institute for the Study of Civil Society.

Widerquist, J. G. (1992). The spirituality of Florence Nightingale. *Nursing Research, 41*(1), 49–55.

Woodham-Smith, C. (1983). *Florence Nightingale 1820–1910.* New York, NY: Atheneum Books.

Williamson, L. (Ed.). (1911 and 1914/1999). *Letters from Miss Florence Nightingale on health visiting in rural districts and Florence Nightingale to her nurses.* London, UK: King.

FURTHER READING

Bullough, V., Bullough, B., & Stanton, M. P. (Eds.). (1990). *Florence Nightingale and her era: A collection of new scholarship.* New York, NY: Garland.

Clark, D. H. (1942/1960). *Source book of medical history.* Toronto, ON, Canada: General Publishing Company, LTD.

Coburn, C. K., & Smith, M. (1999). *How nuns shaped Catholic culture and spirited lives: American life, 1836–1920.* Chapel Hill, NC: North Carolina University Press.

Cromwell, J. L. (2013). *Florence Nightingale, feminist.* Jefferson, NC: McFarland and Company.

Fee, E., & Garofalo, M. E. (2010). Florence Nightingale and the Crimean War. *American Journal of Public Health, 100*(9), 1591.

Hebert, R. G. (1981). *Florence Nightingale: Saint, reformer, or rebel?* Malabar, FL: Robert E. Krieger Publishing Company.

Nelson, S. (2001). *Say little, do much: Nursing, nuns, and hospitals in the nineteenth century.* Philadelphia, PA: University of Pennsylvania Press.

Smith, F. B. (1982). *Florence Nightingale reputation and power.* Sydney, Australia: Croom Helm Ltd, Provident House, Burrell Row.

PART III

Inspiring a Shared Vision

Mother Mary Aikenhead:
A Life of Vision

Deborah Cleeter

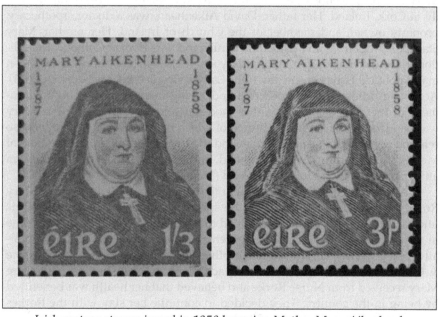

Irish postage stamps issued in 1958 honoring Mother Mary Aikenhead.

"The girl's mind was busy with a problem which she knew baffled the Philanthropists and Statesmen—but happily not the Saints" (Member of the Congregation, 2001, p. 11). Such was the worldview of Mother Mary Aikenhead (1787–1858). With confidence and humility, from the time she was a little girl, she took notice of those around her living in poverty and poor health, then began dreaming of how these individuals could have a better life. Regardless of how others saw a problem, even those in very powerful positions and with great authority, Mary felt led by the Lord to create opportunities to make the world a better place. Never satisfied just wishing that things could be better, Mary knew that action was necessary to change what she felt were appalling situations.

CHILDHOOD

Mary Frances Aikenhead was born in 1787 to a wealthy and prominent family in Cork, Ireland. Her father, David Aikenhead, was a doctor, apothecary, property owner, and member of the Church of Ireland. Her mother, Mary Stackpole, was from an aristocratic family and was Roman Catholic. In addition to the differences in religion, Mary's parents also had opposing views on many political issues of the day (Our Lady's Hospice & Care Services, 2014). Accepting differences in a peaceful and loving manner created an environment in the Aikenhead home that modeled tolerance and kindness. Mary was baptized in the Anglican Church of which her father was a member, also referred to as the Protestant Church and the Church of Ireland. At the time of Mary's birth and through her childhood, the family lived in Daunt's Square, an affluent neighborhood in Cork, Ireland (Member of the Congregation, 2001).

As a young child, Mary was sent to live with an Irish nurse, Mrs. Mary Rorke, and her family. Although the specific diagnosis of her ill health is unclear, Mary's father was determined to have her placed in the foster home in the countryside. Typically, her parents visited each week, and, occasionally, Mary went home to see her brother and sisters (Our Lady's Hospice & Care Services, 2014). The Aikenheads were very satisfied with the care Mary received from Nurse Rorke and believed that her health was benefitted by being in the country. They decided to continue her stay with the Rorkes (Member of the Congregation, 2001).

Calling her foster parents "Mammy Rorke" and "Daddy John," Mary regularly attended mass with the Rorke family. Their Catholic faith had a profound impact on Mary during the 6 years that she lived in their home and would provide an enduring foundation of service as she matured. While a little girl living in the Rorke foster home, Mary played with the poor children of the area, made many friends among them, and developed a lifelong empathy for those in need.

When Mary was returned home to Cork at age 6, the Rorkes also came to live with the family as staff in the Aikenhead household (Cathedral of St. Mary and St. Anne, 2014). Mrs. Rorke was engaged as a "nurse" to continue her care for Mary and also to care for her brother and sisters in the nursery. Mr. Rorke was given a post on the household staff as well (Member of the Congregation, 2001). Once settled again in her family home, Mary was then educated "befitting a young lady of her social class" (CatholicIreland.Net, 1999, p. 1). She attended a private school and learned to speak French fluently (Member of the Congregation, 2001). Mary joined the Protestant church, of which her father was a member, when she returned to Cork, but often accompanied her aunt to mass in the South Chapel of Cork (CatholicIreland.Net, 1999). Even as a young child, Mary recognized the differences between religions and was mindful that one day she would have to choose between them.

The Aikenhead home was often visited by prominent citizens, politicians, and religious leaders. Mary listened to the conversations of the social elite and was impressed by their importance (Member of the Congregation, 2001). Her introduction to influential people did not change her feelings toward her former playmates and friends made during her 6 years in the Rorkes's working-class neighborhood. During her early teen years, Mary's life is reported to have been quite difficult as she contemplated making decisions for her future. She was afforded the opportunity to take her place with the ascendancy class of her parents; however, she felt drawn to the poor and those cast out of society's favor (Member of the Congregation, 2001).

Mary's father, Dr. Aikenhead, was sympathetic toward the Irish Catholics and demonstrated compassion toward the poor. He was generous and, at times, outspoken about the discrimination of those living in poverty. Mary often accompanied her father on his patient rounds throughout Cork and saw firsthand his benevolence (Member of the Congregation, 2001). Her visits with her father to see his sick and poor patients created a continual unrest within Mary. These experiences were important in her personal, career, and leadership development.

While she was just a teen, Mary lost her father—her mentor. Following Dr. Aikenhead's deathbed conversion to Catholicism, Mary, at age 15, was baptized in the Roman Catholic Church. Finally, after moving between the Protestant and Catholic churches for all of her childhood, Mary, through confirmation, had become a Catholic of her own free will (Kerr, 1993). Her sisters followed her lead and also joined the Catholic Church (Our Lady's Hospice & Care Services, 2014).

As the eldest child and with her mother taken quite ill, Mary began to supervise the family business and finances as well as the family's social obligations (Our Lady's Hospice & Care Services, 2014). As a teenager, Mary had to assume adult responsibilities: running the household, attending dances and soirees, and managing family decision making.

People considered Mary to be serious, thoughtful, and an intelligent listener. She was able to spend time with learned men who often visited her grandmother's home and engaged in discussions about literature, culture, and religion (Member of the Congregation, 2001). Through these conversations, Mary learned of the work of St. Francis of Assisi in Italy and that of St. Vincent DePaul in France and, thus, came to believe that great change could be made through service to others. Concerned that Ireland did not have a leader such as these, Mary felt disheartened and did what she could in the poor areas of the city (Member of the Congregation, 2001). Her deep desire to help others motivated Mary to search for the best opportunities for her continued service.

THE NOVITIATE

At 17, Mary decided to follow God's call and offer her service as a nun. Not able to join a convent at the time of her decision, Mary spent the next several years developing a deep love of the church as she fulfilled her responsibilities in caring for her family (Member of the Congregation, 2001). At the age of 21, Mary went to Dublin to visit and stay for a short time with her friend Anne O'Brien. During this time, Mary traveled through the city with Mrs. O'Brien, visiting the poor and sick in their homes. She felt deep concern for the poor throughout this visit in Dublin. It was during this period that Mary met Father Daniel Murray who was working with Mrs. O'Brien in reaching out to the poor of Dublin (Our Lady's Hospice & Care Services, 2014). He became Mary's lifelong mentor and counselor.

In her early 20s, Mary was called home again to care for her ill mother. During this time, while still unable enter a convent, Mary began an intentional period of communication and planning with Father Murray. He was the Bishop Coadjutor of Dublin and was very supportive of her desire to create a new religious order to serve the poor and sick at home.

Finally entering the convent at age 25, Mary Aikenhead spent the next 3 years as a novitiate at the Bar Convent in York. Taking the religious name of Sr. Mary Augustine, Mary and her friend Alicia Walsh, Sr. Mary Catherine, embarked on their religious life of service together in the York convent (Our Lady's Hospice & Care Services, 2014).

While a novitiate at the Convent of the Institute of the Blessed Virgin at Micklegate Bar, York, Sr. Mary Augustine developed her prayer and life of service following the Ignatian spirituality: contemplation in action (Mary Aikenhead Ministries, 2013). Knowing that if she followed her calling to serve the poor, she could not join an enclosed order of nuns, Mary made a very important decision and embarked on a journey that would forever change her life and the lives of multitudes of others.

INSPIRING A SHARED VISION

"Exemplary leaders are forward looking. They are able to envision the future, to gaze across the horizon of time and imagine the greater opportunities to come" (Kouzes & Posner, 2007, p. 105). Two hundred years before

Jim Kouzes and Barry Posner began conducting their leadership research, Mary Aikenhead was exhibiting effective leadership behaviors and engaging people from multiple backgrounds and professions to join her in achieving her dreams. She was thoughtfully committed to her future and that of others from a young age. Mary's vision soon became the vision of many others, including Bishop Murray and other leaders within the Catholic Church administration, physicians within Cork and Dublin, and business leaders who held resources that would substantially help move her plans forward.

Kouzes and Posner (2007) believe that two essential concepts drive an individual's ability to effectively envision the future. Being able to "imagine a positive future" (p. 105) and "finding a common purpose" (p. 116) with others provides leaders with the foundation to turn possibilities into reality. Mary was exceptional at seeing the future through God's will for her and articulating a common purpose with those with whom she engaged in her leadership endeavors.

Visionaries dream of accomplishments that have a future impact that is greater than what they could ever achieve individually. It is through others that their dreams are fulfilled. A humble leader, Mary Aikenhead was steadfast in her acknowledgment and praise of those who shared her vision and acted on their unified purpose.

Mary's dreams were extraordinary for the time in which she lived and for the limited seemingly resources available, but she did not give in to common barriers. "They (leaders) imagine extraordinary feats are possible and that the ordinary could be transformed into something noble. They are able to develop an ideal and unique image of the future for the common good" (Kouzes & Posner, 2007, p. 105).

Appealing to common ideals through the description of aspirations is one way in which Mary Aikenhead engaged others in her vision. Kouzes and Posner state that "enlisting others" through "connecting to what's meaningful to them" aligns purpose and investment in the future (Kouzes & Posner, 2007, p. 134). The vision that Mary Aikenhead had from the time she was a little girl grew out of her passion for helping others and her love of God. The intentionality of her decisions, choice of supporters, and pathway for engaging others led to a shared vision that is still in place two centuries later.

"The poor are always the ones to suffer and no one seems to mind what happened to them. It's shameful! It's unfair!" (Kerr, 1993, p. 14). Often stating her indignation and compassion, Mary Aikenhead provided exemplary leadership even at a remarkably young age. She was able to clearly *envision the future* and *enlist others* as she stood strong within her local community and stated her concerns about the unjust treatment of the poor. One of Mary's fervent hopes was that "we shall each and all exceed in generosity" (Religious Sisters of Charity, 2007, p. 143). In 1816, a small group of the sisters began visiting the poor in their homes. This was the first formal movement of nuns actively helping the sick and suffering within Ireland (Kerr, 1993).

Many believe that it could be said that Mary Aikenhead and her sisters were the first "visiting nurses."

Her deep faith provided Mary with constancy in her personal mission to serve God in all things. A realist, she knew her personal limitations in seeking large-scale change. Not everyone saw possibilities as she did. Her reminder to "bear your own temper with patience" (Religious Sisters of Charity, 2007, p. 58) was stated as much for herself as for those working with her in service to others.

FOUNDRESS, CONGREGATION OF IRISH SISTERS OF CHARITY

High unemployment, cholera outbreaks, and the great famine had created enormous suffering throughout Ireland (Religious Sisters of Charity Ireland, 2013). Mary Aikenhead was filled with assurance that God wanted her to serve the unserved. Her life of commitment to social welfare emerged from life experiences, education, and her 3 years as a novitiate.

Following her training at the Bar Convent in York and prolonged planning with Bishop Murray, Mary Aikenhead founded the Religious Sisters of Charity in 1815 (Religious Sisters of Charity, 2013). Archbishop Murray was Mary's most formidable advocate. He believed in her vision and her ability to achieve it; his support and visibility were very important in helping to establish Mary's leadership credibility.

The first convent was opened in North William Street in Dublin at the same time that Mary was appointed Superior General for the congregation. Mary was determined to lead the newly created order in a manner different from any other religious congregations in existence at the time. The Sisters of Charity were devoted from the outset to actively serving the poor by visiting the sick poor in their homes (CatholicIreland.Net, 1999).

Building the religious congregation and its charitable service were enormous undertakings. Not always did Mary find it easy to fulfill her expectations and plans for a better life for the poor. "We must try to be truly humble—not in words but in the very core of the heart" she stated during times of trial (Religious Sisters of Charity, 2007, p. 189). Even some of those who initially supported her efforts became cynical and less than supportive. Administration of the congregation was difficult and, on many occasions, there occurred internal struggles and disagreements that threatened the future of the order (Member of the Congregation, 2001).

The Rev. Mother's confidence in the Lord and his path for her was demonstrated in her strong and powerful presence. Often seeming harsh and critical, Mary was direct and honest in her praise and reproach of her congregation. She was also known to have a lively sense of humor and was often heard laughing (Kerr, 1993). Loved by all and feared by many, Rev. Mother Mary Aikenhead was a steadfast leader who not only created a vison of a better future but also clearly had a plan of action to achieve her dream.

The growth of the Religious Sisters of Charity outside of Ireland came from a recognition of need. In 1838, the Superior General sent five sisters to Australia who eventually established the first convent in Parramatta. Shortly thereafter, the Jesuits in Preston, Lancashire, England, requested that Mother Mary open a convent there. This first English convent of the congregation was opened in 1840. Eight additional convents were established under the Superior General's leadership. The Religious Sisters of Charity were recognized for their commitment to helping the poor through the expansion of the congregation (O'Riordan, 2015).

MINISTRIES FOR PRISONS, SCHOOLS, AND ORPHANAGES

Mother Mary's vision to help the poor crossed many settings. Her journey started as a child noticing the living conditions of the poor and their resulting ill health, but she grew to embrace change for all aspects of the lives of those living in poverty. An advocate for large-scale change, she led the religious community to reach the poor wherever they were.

In 1821, the Religious Sisters were requested by the prison head to visit two young women who had been convicted of murder and sentenced to death. Following what he felt was a positive influence on these incarcerated women, the governor of Kilmainham Gaol asked whether the sisters would continue their visitation within the prison (Mary Aikenhead Heritage Center, 2014). Thus, the congregation started another valuable ministry for the Religious Sisters of Charity.

A proponent of education for all, Mary believed that education was a way to impact those born in poverty (Cathedral of St. Mary and St. Anne, 2014). In 1830, at the request of the Archbishop, Mother Mary led the Sisters of Charity in opening their first free school in Gardiner Street, Dublin. Another school was opened in Sandymount shortly thereafter. The Sisters of Charity partnered with Carmelite nuns, Society of Friends, and the Christian Brothers, and the congregations worked together to establish a number of schools within the metropolitan area. Many of these schools were orphanages as well (Member of the Congregation, 2001; Our Lady's Hospice & Care Services, 2014).

Through Mary's leadership, the Sisters of Charity became valued within the country as people who could achieve what they set out to do. Government and business leaders would approach the order with their needs and plead with the sisters to build new institutions and administer others. The sisters were seen as a powerful group of women who achieved their purpose in serving God through others.

HOSPITALS, NURSING, AND HOSPICE

Working within the slums and deplorable conditions within the poor areas of Dublin, Mary wanted to found a hospital that provided care to all regardless of their station in society or their ability to pay. The public hospitals were not staffed with trained personnel and were overcrowded. Mary wanted to establish a hospital that provided a higher level of care by trained nurses.

In a time of turmoil in Ireland, Mary led the ministry of caring for the poor during the devastating cholera epidemic. Her long-held dream of a hospital for the poor became more urgent as many people died from lack of care and terrible conditions. Her sister Anne, known as Sister M. Ignatius Aikenhead, died during the epidemic (Mary Aikenhead Ministries, 2013).

Although not a formally trained nurse herself, Mary secured nursing training for sisters within the congregation. In addition, she procured the honorary services of surgeons and physicians in preparation for opening St. Vincent's Hospital Dublin in 1834. This first hospital was dedicated to caring for the poor regardless of religious faith. St. Vincent's became the model on which many other of the congregation's hospitals were built and operated (Mary Aikenhead Ministries, 2013). At its opening, St. Vincent's was the first hospital in Ireland to be managed and staffed by women (CatholicIreland.Net, 1999).

Many troubles befell St. Vincent's Hospital during its first years. Financial problems, difficulties with unhappy staff, and expectations that could not be met caused great stress for Mother Mary. Through perseverance and unwavering dedication to Mary's vision, St. Vincent's did become a highly regarded teaching hospital. Even Florence Nightingale visited the hospital before opening her own nursing school (Kerr, 1993).

A strong advocate of trained hospital personnel, Mother Mary believed that nurses with formal skills were better able to provide care to the ill than the traditional untrained staff in the public hospitals. Not able to release any of her trained nuns because they were few in number and their purpose was to care for the poor in Ireland, Mary did not send her sisters to assist Florence Nightingale during the Crimean War when asked. She did offer prayers during the Crimean War for "the relief of the precious souls (of those) who die in this carnage and have none to pray for them" (Kerr, 1993, p. 17).

Mary's leadership of hospitals and the subsequent administration of the Sisters of Charity were highly regarded. Eighteen years after Mary's death, the congregation was asked by the governor to take over the administration of the children's hospital in Dublin. Only a few years in existence, the hospital had grown so quickly that new leadership was required to manage the facility (O'Riordan, 2015).

As the scope of service of the Sisters of Charity expanded, attention became focused on the dying. Hospice care originally served the sick, travelers, and others in need. History tells that these early hospices were founded by Christians in the eastern biblical lands for weary pilgrims. Mary Aikenhead's passion and vision inspired her followers and led them to focus on terminal care as a specialty. "Her spirit of love for the poor, of understanding their hardships, of dedication to their welfare was her legacy. . . . It was this spirit which conceived of the idea of a 'Hospice' for the dying" (Kerr, 1993, p. 13).

Not until 1879, when the Irish Sisters of Charity founded Our Ladies Hospice for the Dying, did the hospice become focused solely on the dying. This pioneering work was a continuation of Mother Mary's vision of service to the terminally ill (Kerr, 1993).

Ten other hospice facilities were established around the world and attributed to the movement of the Irish Sisters of Charity. Two of these were notable: the Sacred Heart Hospice for the Dying in Sydney, Australia, which opened in 1890 and St. Joseph's Hospice for the Dying in London, which followed in 1905 (Kerr, 1993).

LEADING IN THE FACE OF PERSONAL STRUGGLE

As a result of numerous health problems, Mary was confined to her wheelchair or bed for the last 27 years of her life. "Her vision and energy were not weakened by this confinement, but distilled into a deeper definition of service" (Religious Sisters of Charity, 2013, p. 1). While suffering from spinal problems, failing eyesight, rheumatism, and pulmonary deficiencies, Mother Mary found consolation in prayer (Kerr, 1993). Through courageous leadership, Mary continued to guide the community in its work developing new institutions, sending members on missions to France and Australia, and establishing outreach installations of the Religious Sisters of Charity.

On hearing the news of Mother Mary's death, a poor farmer stated, "That matchless woman! In her, Ireland's poor have lost their best friend" (Religious Sisters of Charity, 2013, p. 1). True to her deepest convictions and relationships with the common people of Ireland, the Rev. Mother Mary Aikenhead's coffin was borne by Irish laborers (Kerr, 1993). As Superior General of the religious order, she never strayed from her vision of helping those in need. The love that she had for others was returned by those she served.

GLOBAL LEGACY

Following her death in 1858, Mother Mary Aikenhead's work continued throughout the world. Legacies are difficult to define for many; however, for Mother Mary Aikenhead, this is an easy task. Her ministries and her influence on society throughout the world have provided the substance of her legacy as a global visionary leader. Instilling honor in service to the poor has created generations of followers who continue her dream and help millions of people around the globe.

One of many examples of this expansion occurred when five Irish nuns journeyed from Dublin in 1900 to bring comfort and care to the sick of London's East End. These Sisters of Charity were inspired by Mary Aikenhead's vision of 85 years before and were committed to their work in the overcrowded and disease-ridden inner city. The work of this early visiting group of nuns became St. Joseph's Hospice in Hackney. Still vibrant today, this hospice remains dedicated to its mission to help people of all faiths.

Mother Mary Aikenhead's dream of service to the poor continues in Nigeria, Zambia, Malawi, Australia, England, Scotland, Ireland, the United States, and Venezuela (Religious Sisters of Charity, 2013). Rev. Mother Mary has had a profound influence on religious organizations, health care, education, and social justice. Beyond the education and health care initiatives, the religious congregation led the establishment of the Foxford Woollen Mills in 1892 to improve social and economic conditions in County Mayo (Member of the Congregation, 2001).

The Mary Aikenhead Heritage Center is located on the grounds of Our Lady's Hospice in Harold's Cross, Dublin, Ireland. An extensive renovation of the center was completed in 2015, which now houses the official collection of historical documents and Mother Mary's living accommodations from 1845 to 1858 (Religious Sisters of Charity Ireland, 2013).

JOURNEY TOWARD CANONIZATION

Preliminary steps for Mother Mary Aikenhead's application for canonization were initiated in 1908 by Mother Mary Gertrude Davis, the Superior General of the Australian Sisters of Charity. Termed a "Cause," the journey for an individual to be pronounced a saint is often long and arduous; such has been the story for the process of the Vatican approval of sainthood for Mary Aikenhead (Religious Sisters of Charity, 2013).

Following many interruptions in the process, Pope Benedict XV signed the decree for the introduction of the Cause of Mary Aikenhead in March 1921. This decree officially opened the journey toward canonization; however, more church delays in Dublin, the two world wars, and political strife in Ireland slowed the progression significantly. The persistence of the promoters of Mary Aikenhead's Cause in Ireland and Australia has been formidable. At each setback, someone has taken the initiative to begin again (Religious Sisters of Charity, 2013).

Decades passed with minimal progress; however, the Cause continued. In March 2012, the Vatican provided notification that they were proceeding with the process for Mary Aikenhead to be declared Venerable (Religious Sisters of Charity, 2013). One hundred and seven years after the first letter was written to initiate the canonization process for Mary, the congregation and the world continues to await final proclamation from Rome.

EXEMPLARY LEADERSHIP

Rev. Mother Mary's commitment to her vision, which continues through her religious order, schools, hospitals, hospices, social service organizations, and numerous other institutions, has flourished since her death.

Mary was intelligent, diplomatic, purpose driven, and formidable. She was a businesswoman and a feminist, and had international influence. All of her gifts and talents were used in the service of God and the poor (Our Lady's Hospice & Care Services, 2014). A remarkable leader in social services, education, and health care, Mary Aikenhead demonstrated all five exemplary leadership practices described by Kouzes and Posner as the requisite characteristics of successful leaders.

In accordance with her vision of ministering to the poor, Mary inspired others to journey with her as they pioneered a new religious order, created new institutions in service to the poor, and subsequently changed the lives of millions of people throughout the world. Rev. Mother Mary Aikenhead was masterful at engaging others in her vision. She had worked among the poor in the worst possible conditions in the slums of Dublin and moved to the role of Superior General of the religious community that she created. Never losing sight of her calling, her spirituality permeated her being, her writings, and her legacy.

TIMELINE

- January 19, 1787—Mary Frances Aikenhead is born in Cork, Ireland, to a wealthy family and, shortly thereafter, is sent to live with Mary and John Rorke.
- June 6, 1802—Baptized as Roman Catholic.
- 1808—Moves to Dublin to live with friend Anne O'Brien.
- 1812–1815—Becomes a novitiate in the Convent of the Institute of the Blessed Virgin at Micklegate Bar, York.
- September 1, 1815—Appointed Superior General of the new congregation of Sisters of Charity in Ireland; first convent opens in Dublin.
- 1821—Prison ministry begins at Kilmainham Gaol.
- 1830—Sisters of Charity open their first school in Gardiner Street, Dublin, at the request of the Archbishop.
- 1831—As a result of multiple illnesses and over exertion, Mary becomes confined to her wheelchair and bed.
- 1832—Directs sisters during the plague (Asiatic Cholera) from her confinement.
- 1835—St. Vincent's Hospital is opened on St. Stephen's Green as the first hospital staffed by nuns in the English-speaking world.
- 1838—Mother Mary sends first five sisters to Australia; these are the first religious women ever to set foot in Australia; the first convent is opened in Parramatta.
- 1840—Jesuits in Preston, Lancashire, England, request assistance from Mother Mary; this leads to the opening of the first convent of the Religious Sisters of Charity in England.

- July 22, 1858—Mother Mary Aikenhead dies at the age of 71 in Dublin, Ireland, and is interred in the cemetery at St. Mary Magdelen's, Donnybrook, Ireland.
- 1872—The children's hospital is founded in Dublin; because of rapid expansion and need, the governor asks the Religious Sisters of Charity to accept responsibility of administering the hospital in 1876.
- 1879—Our Lady's Hospice is opened, the first such charity in Europe.
- 1892—The Sisters establish the Foxford Woollen Mills to improve social and economic conditions in County Mayo, Ireland.
- 1908—Application for canonization of Mother Mary Aikenhead is initiated.
- March 20, 1921—The decree for the Introduction of the Cause of Mary Aikenhead is signed by Pope Benedict XV in Rome.
- 1948—Three Religious Sisters of Charity arrive in Zambia to establish the first convent in Chikuni; the first congregation is established in Scotland at Clydebank.
- 1953—Five sisters are sent to Los Angeles, California, to work in the schools; their service expands to include care of the elderly and sick, the field of education, and social and pastoral ministries.
- 1958—Ireland issues two postage stamps honoring Mother Mary Aikenhead (see the beginning of this chapter).
- 1961—Sisters are sent to Lagos to serve in the Pacelli School for the Visually Impaired to care for children; this work expands to include running hospitals, schools, and pastoral service.
- 1995—The Historical Commission for the Congregation for the Causes of Saints unanimously passed the Positio on Mary Aikenhead.
- 2011—The Sisters of Charity Congregation sends sisters to Konzalendo to establish a community to work with the local people.
- 2014—The process for Mary Aikenhead to be declared Venerable proceeds; the Cause needs to be passed to the Cardinals, then to the Holy Father, and then to the Archbishop of Dublin to promulgate it.

QUESTIONS FOR DISCUSSION

1. As a child, Mary Aikenhead developed a keen sense of her future. What situations, key individuals, and motivators formed this vision for her future?
2. How did Mary Aikenhead *inspire a shared vision* among leaders from various fields and disciplines to support and advocate for her vision?
3. In times of disappointment, scarcity of resources, and often lack of supporters, what where the key elements of Mary Aikenhead's resilience, persistence, and commitment to her vision?
4. In what ways has Mary Aikenhead *inspired a shared vision* in others to sustain and expand her work?

REFERENCES

Cathedral of St. Mary and St. Anne. (2014). *Mary Aikenhead; Foundress of the Sisters of Charity*. Retrieved August 15, 2014, from http://www.catholicireland.net/mary-aikenhead-in-the-service-of-the-poor/

CatholicIreland.Net. (1999, November 30). *Mary Aikenhead: In the service of the poor.* Retrieved from http://catholicireland.net/mary-aikenhead-in-the-service-of-the-poor/

Kerr, D. (1993). Mother Mary Aikenhead, the Irish Sisters of Charity and Our Lady's Hospice for the dying. *American Journal of Hospice and Palliative Care, 10*(3), 13–20.

Kouzes, J. M., & Posner, B. Z. (2007). *The leadership challenge* (4th ed.). Hoboken, NJ: John Wiley & Sons.

Mary Aikenhead Heritage Center. (2014). *History.* Retrieved November 26, 2014, from http://www.rscmaheritage.com/

Mary Aikenhead Ministries. (2013). *Mary Aikenhead.* Retrieved August 15, 2014, from http://maryaikenheadministries.com.au/about-us/our-history-and-traditions/education-ministries/

Member of the Congregation. (2001). *The life and work of Mary Aikenhead: Foundress of the congregation of Irish Sisters of Charity 1787–1858.* Honolulu, HI: University Press of the Pacific.

O'Riordan, T. (2015). *Multitext project in Irish history. Emancipation, famine, and religion: Ireland under the Union 1815–1870—Mary Aikenhead.* Retrieved January 22, 2015, from http://multitext.ucc.ie/d/Mary_Aikenhead

Our Ladies Hospice & Care Services. (2014). *Heritage Centre.* Retrieved August 19, 2014, from https://olh.ie/about-us/our-heritage/

Religious Sisters of Charity. (2007). *The everyday wisdom of Mary Aikenhead.* Dublin, Ireland: Betaprint, Ltd.

Religious Sisters of Charity. (2013). *The history of the cause of Mary Aikenhead.* Retrieved August 15, 2014, from http://rsccaritas.ie/rscnews/487-history-of-the-cause

Religious Sisters of Charity Ireland. (2013). *Our foundress.* Retrieved August 15, 2014, from http://religioussistersofcharity.ie/mary-aikenhead/

FURTHER READING

University College Cork. (2015). *Multitext project in Irish history: Emancipation, famine & religion: Ireland under the union, 1815–1870—Mary Aikenhead.* Retrieved January 22, 2015, from http://multitext.ucc.ie/d/Mary_Aikenhead

Clara Barton: Angel of the Battlefield

Karen Egenes and Frances Vlasses

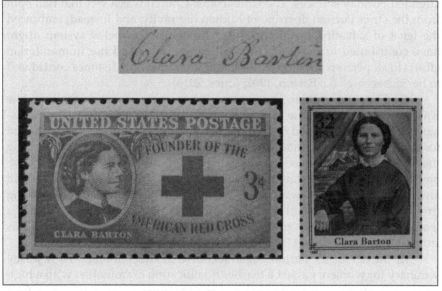

U.S. postage stamp issued in 1948 (left) and 1995 (right) honoring Clara Barton.

You must never so much as think whether you like it or not, whether it is bearable or not; you must never think of anything except the need, and how to meet it.

—*Clara Barton*

• • • • •

Clara Barton (1821–1912) was born in North Oxford, Massachusetts, on Christmas Day in 1821. She was the youngest of the five children born to Stephen and Sarah Barton. The family had deep roots in New England. Her father was descended from Samuel Barton, who came to the Massachusetts colony in 1640. Her grandfather fought in the American Revolution, while her father fought under General Anthony Wayne during the War of 1812.

Clara's siblings were responsible for much of her early education. By the age of 5, her brother David had taught her to ride a horse, and in a short time, her equestrian skills surpassed those of many men. When Clara was 11, David suffered a serious accident that left him an invalid for the next 2 years. During this time, Clara was responsible for providing the majority of his care, which included both basic comfort measures and the application of leeches. This experience may have helped to prepare Clara for the roles she would play later in her life.

The Barton family belonged to the Universalist Church and faithfully attended Sunday services. The Universalist Church was a sect that had split from the strict Puritan doctrine of human depravity, and instead, embraced the tenet of salvation for all, not just Christians. This belief system might have contributed to Barton's later willingness to extend her humanitarian efforts to all persons afflicted by disaster rather than only to those considered to be "deserving" (C. Barton, 1907; Jones, 2013).

As Clara grew older, she became increasingly shy and sensitive. She was short in stature, prone to obesity, and plagued by insomnia. The persistence of these traits caused her parents anxiety about a future course of action for their "difficult" daughter. They consulted L. N. Fowler, a lecturer visiting their town who specialized in phrenology, a forerunner of modern psychology. Following his assessment, Fowler predicted, "The sensitive nature will always remain. She will never assert herself for herself. She will suffer wrong first, but for others she will be perfectly fearless. She has all the qualities of a teacher" (C. Barton, 1907, pp. 112–115). Years later, Clara often repeated this story, stating she believed Fowler's words were prophetic.

At the age of 15, Barton began a course in education at a New Jersey seminary for women, passed a teacher qualification examination with a high score, and began a career in teaching that continued for the next 15 years. Barton taught in a variety of private schools in Massachusetts and New Jersey, and then settled in Bordentown, New Jersey. There she founded a free public school, one of the first in New Jersey. In 1 year, the school grew in size from 6 to 600 students. This growth required the town's citizens to secure a new school building at the cost of $4,000. Unfortunately, when the school was enlarged, Barton was replaced as principal by someone less qualified, a male teacher who had been born and educated abroad. Although Barton was well liked by her students, she was firm and held high standards for them. She corresponded with some of her former students for many years (Bacon-Foster, 1918).

In search of employment, Barton traveled to Washington, DC, to ask her Congressman and distant cousin, Alexander DeWitt, for help in her pursuit of a position as a governess. Instead, he recommended her to the commissioner of patents for a position as a government patent clerk (Pryor, 1987, pp. 60–61). In her appointment as one of the first female patent clerks, Clara Barton reputedly suffered much harassment from her male colleagues in the form of negative remarks, showers of spittle, and attempts to trip her as she approached her work space. At times, her managers required her to work at home in a small and dimly lit room in a boarding house to avoid the disruptions her presence in the workplace engendered. Barton's's perfect handwriting and hours spent copying legal documents by hand, however, led to a promotion and increase in salary after only 1 year (Jones, 2013). According to a close friend and daughter of Clara Barton's immediate superior, the chief clerk of the patent office praised Barton as "the best clerk we have ever had in this office" (Bacon-Foster, 1918, p. 284).

In 1856, when James Buchanan, who was sympathetic toward the continuance of slavery, was elected president, Clara Barton, who had been vocal in her opposition to slavery, lost her patronage position. She returned to Massachusetts and resumed her study of French and art with the hope of securing another teaching position. While in her home state, she resumed correspondence with some of her former students, writing to one that she hoped to secure a teaching position in the South, preferably in Mobile, Alabama (Bacon-Foster, 1918). In view of her strong abolitionist views and later work, this seems to be an unusual choice; however, it is indicative of her quest for new and challenging experiences. In 1860, when the newly formed Republican party came to power, Clara Barton was recalled to Washington and reappointed to her prior position, forsaking a suitor of many years who had recently proposed marriage. Enthralled by the promise of change that followed the election of President Lincoln, Barton gave her full support to the antislavery movement. The years that she worked in Washington seemed to give Clara the strength she would need for her future endeavors. During those years, she developed skills in organizational management, became confident in her abilities, and developed a sense of political activism.

Clara Barton was in Washington, DC, in April 1861, and witnessed the beginning of the Civil War, and foresaw the suffering the war would entail. Later that month, the Massachusetts Sixth Regiment, while en route to Washington, was attacked by rebels while marching through Baltimore. As the wounded volunteers streamed into Washington, Barton left her desk and rushed to their aid. Among the wounded, she recognized many as her former neighbors, classmates, and students. This early experience led her to bond with the ill and wounded soldiers she cared for throughout the war, often referring to them as "my boys" (Oates, 1994, p. 17).

At the beginning of the war, little thought had been given to the casualties of the war, the ill and wounded soldiers who would require medical and nursing care, as well as food, hospitals, and medical supplies to aid in their recovery. Dorothea Dix (see Chapter 8), who before the war had gained renown for her efforts to reform asylums and improve the care of persons with mental illness, was appointed superintendent of nurses for the Union Army. In this capacity, she was responsible for the recruitment of suitable women to serve as nurses for the Union Army and the coordination of the activities of these "nurses." At the time of the Civil War, no schools for the education of nurses had yet been established in the United States. Volunteers recruited by Dix had only a rudimentary knowledge of nursing care, gleaned primarily from personal experiences caring for sick family members. In addition, the U.S. Sanitary Commission, established by the government but supported by donations from citizens of the Northern states, raised money, gathered food and supplies, and mobilized resources to aid the sick and wounded soldiers. It took some time, however, before these efforts were sufficiently organized and functional to yield any demonstrable outcomes.

EARLY EFFORTS TO INSPIRE A SHARED VISION

Some women volunteers for the war effort eschewed the efforts of Dix and the U.S. Sanitary Commission, preferring instead to mount their own efforts. Included in this group of volunteers was Clara Barton. As sick and injured soldiers continued to stream into Washington, Clara Barton, acting independently, solicited clothing, food, and medical supplies from friends and relatives and distributed them to regiments in need. Her goal was to provide care to soldiers within days, or even hours, of their affliction. During the first years of the war, Clara Barton distinguished herself among fellow relief workers by her willingness to travel to battlefields and provide care on the front lines of the fray. She began to provide care on fields of battle in August 1862 during the Second Battle of Bull Run. But this was possible only after she had gathered personal warehouses of supplies, secured an army wagon and teamster for transportation, and persuaded reluctant army officers to issue her the passes necessary to travel to the front lines of battle.

A decade later, in a series of lecture tours, Clara Barton delighted in describing her Civil War service. It is believed, however, that many of her heroic exploits benefitted from a certain amount of personal embellishment. For example, in a tale often related, during the Battle of Antietam, as Clara Barton reached to the ground to offer a drink of water to a weary soldier, a bullet tore a hole in the sleeve of her dress, mortally wounding her patient. As the battle continued, she made repeated trips to the front to care for the wounded and comfort the dying soldiers. At a makeshift hospital, she assisted surgeons with sedation and restraint of patients, as well as with provision of lanterns so that care of the wounded could continue through the night (Oates, 1994).

Clara Barton launched similar initiatives later in 1862 during the battles of Cedar Mountain, Chantilly, Harpers Ferry, and Fredericksburg. Her work in these battles is considered to be the most significant of her service in the Civil War. Through her independent efforts, she was able to gather supplies, distribute them to sick and wounded soldiers, and provide nursing care to those in need. Her ability to provide aid quickly during these emergency situations helped thousands of soldiers whose needs could not be met by the poorly organized, government-sponsored mechanisms. These efforts also formed the framework for Barton's lifelong work.

By 1863, the efforts off the U.S. Sanitary Commission and army medical services had matured and become better systematized. As a result, Clara Barton found that the services she offered were increasingly marginalized. This proved to be a time, however, when Barton developed personal relationships that would influence her later life and work. In April of that year, Clara Barton joined her brother David in Hilton Head, South Carolina, where he had been appointed quartermaster. From this post, she witnessed the 8-month-long siege of Charleston, as well as the siege of Fort Wagner by the Massachusetts 54th Regiment, a unit composed entirely of African American troops. It was also at this time that Clara Barton had a brief romantic affair with Lieutenant Colonel John Elwell of Cleveland, Ohio, a married man who was an officer in the Quartermaster Corps. Before the war, Elwell had practiced both medicine and law and had served a term in the Ohio legislature. When they first met, he was a patient who had sustained a broken leg in a fall from a horse. He later wrote about his injury, "Two boys of the 62nd Ohio found me and carried me to our . . . hospital. . . . Clara Barton was there, an angel of mercy doing all in her mortal power to assuage the miseries of the unfortunate soldiers" (W. E. Barton, 1922, Vol. 1, pp. 251–252). During his recovery from the injury, Elwell also contracted yellow fever. But through his difficulties, Clara remained his nurse and constant companion. The couple found they shared many interests, including horseback riding and lively conversations, and spent increasing amounts of time together. Although Barton ended the relationship when she learned that Elwell's wife planned to visit South Carolina, there is evidence that, following the war, she continued to correspond with Elwell by mail, sharing fond memories of their time together and seeking his advice about matters of importance in her life (Oates, 1994; Pryor, 1987).

During the 4 years of the war, Clara Barton was present on 16 battlefields, in addition to the 8 months she spent in South Carolina during the siege of Charleston. A contemporary described her as "always calm, cheerful and well poised, and philosophical, but strict, firm, and unflinching in maintaining authority" (Harper, 1912, p. 703).

Jones (2013) asserts that Clara Barton's work on the battlefields of the Civil War developed in her the sense of humanitarianism that would be a force that drove her efforts for the rest of her life. She transferred the traditional Victorian virtue of "women as care givers" from the home to the battlefields and in the process demonstrated remarkable courage, a virtue not usually attributed to women of the era. Her work was based on her firm belief that the pain of wounded soldiers must be relieved as soon as possible. Thus, she expressed human sentiment, or concern for the welfare of others, blended with a rational call to action.

During the last months of the war, Barton became involved in a new venture, called by historians as "the search for the missing men," which would impact her later work. Of the Union soldiers known to be dead or imprisoned in the South, more than half were unidentified. More than 80,000 were listed on the government rolls only as "missing." Letters from distressed relatives flooded the office of the War Department, but because no information was available, the letters remained unanswered. Clara Barton, feeling a deep sense of injustice at the lack of response to these inquiries, personally asked President Abraham Lincoln if this correspondence might be routed to her and if she might officially respond to these letters. The President responded with the notice to the public, "To the friends of missing persons; Miss Clara Barton has kindly offered to search for the missing prisoners of war. Please address her at Annapolis, Maryland, giving name, regiment, and company of any missing prisoner" (Bacon-Foster, 1918, p. 296).

Because of the high mortality rates from disease and injury, many soldiers who died were quickly buried in unmarked graves. Although at the end of the war there were 315,555 known graves of Union soldiers, 143,155 of these were unmarked. In addition, 44,000 had been recorded, with no site of burial given. Over the next 4 years, Clara Barton answered more than 63,000 letters and identified more than 22,000 missing soldiers (Somervill, 2007, p. 59).

Clara Barton also established a Bureau of Correspondence for Friends of Paroled Prisoners, which carefully compiled lists of soldiers' names from hospital and prison rolls. Of particular concern was the Confederate prison in Andersonville, Georgia, where 13,000 Union soldiers were reported to have died in 1 year. During the summer of 1865, Barton supervised the disinterment, identification, and reburial of the bodies in graves with individual name markers. In addition, the graves of 4,000 Confederate dead were carefully marked. This work led to the establishment of Andersonville as one of the first national cemeteries in the United States.

Initially, Clara Barton financed this project using her own funds and spent over $8,000 to pay for maintenance of an office staff of 12. When her private funds were nearly exhausted, she appealed to Congress for funding to continue the work. In 1866, Congress appropriated $15,000 to reimburse Barton for the money that she, as a private citizen, had spent for a public cause. Although these funds enabled her to pay many of the bills she had accrued, they provided no salary for her work on this project.

DEVELOPING THE TOOLS TO INSPIRE A SHARED VISION

In 1866, Clara Barton, now almost insolvent after her search for missing soldiers, sought a means to support herself. During the Civil War, her fame had become so widespread that admirers across the country were eager to hear about her work during the war years. During this era, lectures by noteworthy persons were a popular form of entertainment. When she was first invited to give public lectures about her wartime experiences, Clara was overwhelmed at the thought and focused on what she perceived to be her deficiencies. In her childhood, she was thought to be painfully shy and sensitive. But motivated by her need for personal income, she signed a contract with a lecture bureau that charged from $75 to $100 per lecture. She traveled around the country, speaking to thousands of people. Clara Barton emerged as a gifted speaker with a soft and mellow voice, who captivated audiences with her descriptions of her wartime exploits. Newspaper accounts described her presentations as "animated, instructive, and enjoyable" (Oates, 1994). Barton distinguished herself from other persons on the lecture circuit through her use of stories to remind her listeners about the human costs of war (Jones, 2013). She proved to be one of the most highly paid lecturers of that time and was able to save $25,000 to use for her later work (Harper, 1912). Through her experiences on the lecture circuit, Barton was able to overcome the shyness that had haunted her during her earlier life. Further, she was able to develop persuasive skills that would benefit her in her later activities.

Clara Barton found the lecture circuit to be tiring. In 1869, she was scheduled to give a lecture but found herself before an audience, unable to speak. Throughout her life, Clara had experienced recurrent episodes of depression. It seems that the exhaustion of the travel involved in her work, coupled with the depressing effects of the constant repetition of her war memories, contributed to her physical and mental exhaustion. She consulted several physicians who advised her to spend some time in Switzerland to recover her strength. Her sojourn to Europe lasted until 1873 and introduced her to new ways of channeling her energies for her humanitarian efforts.

ROLE MODELS FOR INSPIRING A SHARED VISION—CLARA BARTON IN EUROPE

During her visit to Switzerland, Clara Barton was able to stay with friends. Charles Upton and his wife, whom she had known in both Massachusetts and Washington, were now engaged in diplomatic service for the United States in the Swiss city of Geneva. Clara was also invited to spend part of her visit with the family of Jules Golay, a Swiss citizen who had served in the Union Army and for whom Barton had provided care.

Soon after her arrival in Geneva, an event occurred that would influence the remainder of her life's work. Because news of Clara Barton's record of charitable activities had spread abroad, she was visited by members of the International Convention of Geneva, more commonly known as the Red Cross, a group with whom she was only vaguely familiar. The group, led by Dr. Louis Appia, inquired why the government of the United States had refused to give its consent to the Geneva Convention, also called the Treaty of Geneva, an international agreement of which she had no prior knowledge. These questions left Barton so surprised and perplexed that she asked her visitors for more information (Pryor, 1987). She was fascinated with the story that unfolded.

In 1859, Red Cross founder Henri Dunant was a Swiss businessman en route from his home in Geneva to the town of Soferino, who came upon a ferocious battle involving troops from France, Sardinia, and Austria. The battle, which would prove to be significant in the Wars of Italian Independence, had left 40,000 wounded soldiers to languish unattended on the field of battle. Dunant mobilized local residents to provide food, water, and bandages to aid the casualties of the battle and assembled makeshift hospitals in nearby villages. Over the succeeding years, Dunant was haunted by the memory of the men in agony, dying because they lacked the most basic care. He became convinced that similar tragedies should not be allowed to occur in the future. In 1862, he published, *Un Souvenir de Solferino* (A Memory of Solferino), which offered vivid accounts of the battle and its human costs. The book was so well received across the European continent that it garnered the attention of leading physicians and generals who agreed that some action must be taken. In 1863, the Convention of Geneva, a conference attended by representatives from 16 nations, was called to discuss the treatment of those wounded in battle. The following year, the Treaty of Geneva was written and signed by 11 countries. By the time Clara Barton first learned about the treaty, 32 countries had agreed to its terms. The Treaty of Geneva contained several key points: (a) In time of battle, ambulances and field hospitals, as well as the personnel staffing them, both volunteers and professionals, should be treated as neutral parties; (b) authorized workers should be able to enter the field of battle to distribute supplies and provide care; (c) casualties are entitled to care whether they were wounded in their own or in hostile territory; (d) seriously wounded soldiers should not be taken as prisoners of war but instead should be sent back to their own army for care; and (e) neutral workers caring for the wounded would be distinguished by a badge of a red cross on a white background (Pryor, 1987).

Clara Barton was both surprised and disheartened to learn that the U.S. government had been requested three times to sign the treaty but had refused on each occasion. In truth, there are a number of possible reasons for the government's refusal. At the time the Geneva Convention was called, the United States was embroiled in the Civil War and had little interest in international events. During the years that immediately followed, the United States was concerned with the process of reconstruction and recovery from the lasting effects of the war. Finally, the proceedings of the Geneva Convention were sent to the United States in French, and, thus without translation, could not be published in local newspapers. In 1866, Dr. Henry Bellows, the head of the Sanitary Commission during the Civil War, tried to interest government officials in the Treaty of Geneva but received the response that there probably would never be another war, and, if one occurred, a society such as the Sanitary Commission could be established to coordinate relief efforts (Harper, 1912).

Clara Barton was in Berne in 1870 when France declared war on Prussia (presently a part of Germany), launching the Franco–Prussian War. Although she was ostensibly in Switzerland for rest, Barton nevertheless convinced leaders of the Swiss Red Cross to travel to the battlefields of France to aid in the relief efforts. Antoinette Margot, a young Swiss woman who was fluent in English and French and who also aspired to be a battlefield nurse, was assigned to accompany her. At this time Princess Louise, Grand Duchess of Baden, only daughter of Kaiser Wilhelm of Prussia, visited Clara. She had read about Clara Barton's work during the Civil War and now came to ask for her guidance and assistance in the relief efforts. They eventually became lifelong friends. The city of Strasbourg in France had been defeated by troops led by Louise's husband, the Grand Duke, and the Duchess now asked Clara Barton to aid the citizens who had been harmed in the battle. Barton and her companion left for Strasbourg on August 6, 1870, stopping en route to observe field hospitals that had been set up to care for wounded soldiers who had been evacuated from the front lines. Clara longed to again provide nursing care on the battlefields as she had done during the Civil War. She repeatedly found, however, that her colleagues in the International Red Cross were unwilling to allow this.

When the women reached Strasbourg, they encountered members of the Swiss Red Cross who were providing aid to citizens of the city who had the greatest needs. The Swiss assigned Clara Barton to work with those persons who had been evacuated from the city during the battle and who had lost their homes and possessions. Barton developed a model of care that deviated markedly from the Red Cross members' traditional provision of care only to wounded combatants. She advocated for citizens who had been affected by the war to now be participants in the relief efforts aimed at helping in their recovery. Thus, she began a small business that involved the citizens of Strasbourg in sewing clothing. The garments produced aided those who had lost all of their possessions and also aided those without work. The relief efforts in Strasbourg were among the first attempts to involve citizens who had been affected by a disaster, a population whose needs had not been considered in the Treaty of Geneva (Jones, 2013). Barton continued to use this model when she organized relief efforts in the French cities of Metz, Montbéliard, Belfort, and later, in Paris. From that time forward, the main focus of her work would be provision of aid to citizens affected by war and other disasters (Bacon-Foster, 1918). Clara Barton also came to understand the effectiveness of Red Cross workers in their care of combatants and resolved to secure U.S. support for the Treaty of Geneva. She observed that the Red Cross workers were more efficient and better prepared than had been the Sanitary Commission workers during the American Civil War. After her 2 years of work with the French, Swiss, Prussian, and British Red Cross Societies, Barton promised her colleagues that she would devote the rest of her life, if necessary, to the introduction of the Red Cross movement in the United States (W. E. Barton, 1922). In turn, Clara Barton was praised by European dignitaries for the aid she had provided during the Franco–Prussian War. Kaiser Wilhelm presented her with the Iron Cross, the German government's highest honor, which had never before and has never since been awarded to a woman (Jones, 2013).

Unfortunately, Clara Barton's early attempts to *inspire a shared vision*, although effective, ultimately came at a cost to her credibility. Although her diary and accounts from her companion, Antoinette Margot, clearly indicate that both women never served on an actual field of battle in France, Barton nevertheless related that they had been personally involved in combat. It seems she embellished her accounts both to entertain her admirers and to enlist their financial support for her cause. She believed that necessary support could best be engendered through the use of strong words and the presentation of the events as both dreadful and in need of immediate attention (Pryor, 1987).

Unfortunately, Clara's work in Europe had taken a toll on her health. In 1873, she suffered another bout of exhaustion and depression, which caused her to return to the United States and to seek treatment in a sanatorium in Danville, New York. As she recovered her strength, she began to write newspaper articles about the work of the Red Cross in an attempt to gain public support. In 1887, when she had fully recovered her strength, she renewed her correspondence with Gustave Moynier, the president of the International Committee of the Red Cross (ICRC) and Dr. Louis Appia, a colleague of Moynier who had visited Barton when she first arrived in Switzerland. Both proved to be wise mentors to Clara Barton as she began her new endeavor. First, they cautioned her that under the rules of the ICRC, a country's national Red Cross would not be recognized until its government had signed the Treaty of Geneva. Barton's first action, therefore, should be to convince the U.S. government to agree to the terms of the Treaty of Geneva. Further, they warned that because the United States did not consider itself a military power and because the danger of war did not seem imminent, the government would be unlikely to see this action as a high priority. Historically, the United States had adhered to the warning of George Washington as he left office and avoided "entanglements" with foreign powers and had signed treaties with foreign governments only to bring an end to wars.

Dr. Appia sent Clara Barton a detailed plan for the establishment of a Red Cross Society in the United States: (a) seek publicity, (b) achieve government approval of the Treaty of Geneva, (c) found a national Red Cross Society, and (d) collect funds to support the national Red Cross. He further advised her to "surround yourself with a little body of persons full of goodwill and capacity, docile to your directions" (W. E. Barton, 1922, p. 128). Moynier appointed Clara Barton the agent of the ICRC and sent her a letter of introduction to present to Rutherford B. Hayes, the president of the United States, strongly encouraging him to accept the Articles of the Convention of Geneva. Unfortunately, during the years that Clara Barton was abroad, she had lost many of her prior contacts with persons of influence in the nation's capital. Those who remained had little power in the Hayes administration. Barton visited President Hayes at the White House and was warmly received. However, the letter of introduction was referred to the Assistant to the Secretary of State Frederick Seward, who had no interest in the proposal. During the 1860s, Henry Bellows and members of the Sanitary Commission had proposed the idea of a Red Cross Society to Seward, who remembered his refusal of their request, referred her to the record of this refusal, and regarded the matter as decided. Clara Barton later wrote,

> I saw that it was all made to depend on one man, and that man
> regarded it as settled. I had nothing to hope for then, but did
> not press the matter to a third refusal. It waited, and so did I.
> (C. Barton, 1922, Vol. 2, p. 146)

Clara Barton had learned much from her colleagues and mentors in Europe. She now needed to develop strategies that would appeal to the sentiments of the people of the United States, as well as to U.S. elected officials. To win acceptance, the idea of a Red Cross had to speak to the hearts of Americans.

INSPIRING A SHARED VISION—DEVELOPING NEW STRATEGIES

Because Clara Barton realized that she was unlikely to have any success in further appeals to members of the Hayes administration, she decided to wait until the election of a different president before making further attempts to secure approval of the treaty. As she waited, Barton embarked on a strategy to educate the American public about the value of a Red Cross Society. She gathered a group of friends, including the Swiss counsel-general, Switzerland's official representative to the United States, to form a "Society of the Red Cross." This committee aimed to bring public attention to the work of the Red Cross and to arouse public sentiment in favor of approval of the Treaty of Geneva. In 1878, the committee members published and circulated a pamphlet, *The Red Cross of the Geneva Convention: What It Is*, authored by Barton. In this publication, she presented the Red Cross as a national relief organization that would function during times of peace to "afford ready succor and assistance to sufferers in times of national widespread calamities, such as plague, yellow fever, and the like, devastating fires or floods, rail disasters, [or] mining catastrophes" (C. Barton, 1878, pp. 5–6).

Clara Barton expanded the idea of a Red Cross Society beyond that envisioned by Dunant. European Red Cross Societies had been formed to provide rapid relief to those injured in battle and actually had been cautioned by Moynier to limit resources expended in national relief efforts. But Clara Barton realized that in the United States, memory of the Civil War was fading and that the idea of provision of relief during "national calamities" would better speak to the concerns of the American public. She wrote,

> Our Southern coasts are periodically visited by the scourge of
> Yellow Fever; the valleys of the Mississippi are subjected to
> destructive inundations. . . . to gather and dispense the profuse
> liberality of our people, without waste of time or material,
> requires the wisdom that comes of experiences and permanent
> organization. (C. Barton, 1878, pp. 7–8)

Thus, Clara Barton and her committee members became the first in the international Red Cross movement to make disaster relief the central focus of its mission (Jones, 2013). Efforts to educate the American public and to win the support of persons of influence continued throughout the remainder of the Hayes administration.

Soon after the inauguration of President James Garfield in 1881, Barton renewed her efforts to secure government approval of the Treaty of Geneva. The new president was receptive to the idea. He urged its approval to Secretary of State James Blaine, who began correspondence with the ICRC and began arrangements to organize a branch of the Red Cross in the United States. In 1881, the original small committee was reorganized and incorporated as the Society of the Red Cross. President Garfield nominated Clara Barton to be its president, a position she held for the next 22 years. That summer, President Garfield was assassinated, a blow to the nation, but especially to the members of the newly formed Red Cross Society. However, his successor, Chester A. Arthur, proved to be equally supportive and recommended approval of the treaty in his inaugural address. The Treaty of Geneva was accepted by Congress and was signed by President Arthur on March 1, 1882.

President Moynier of the ICRC wrote to Clara Barton, "You must feel happy and proud at last to have attained your object, thanks to a perseverance and zeal which surmounted every obstacle" (Harper, 1912, p. 708). Bonfires were lit in Geneva in celebration of the acceptance of the treaty by the United States. In a proclamation of its mission, the stationery of the society read, "The American Society of the Red Cross organized under the Treaty of Geneva for the Relief of Sufferings of War, Pestilence, Famine, Fires, Floods, and other National Calamities" (Bacon-Foster, 1918, p. 307). The primary mission of the ICRC, however, was the provision of relief to casualties of battle, and the charter of the American Society required ratification by the nations of the ICRC. Using her well-honed skills in diplomacy, Clara Barton presented the case that because many disasters of various forms occur annually in the United States, for the American Society to be able to justify its existence, it should have the power to offer its aid in any national calamity. The nations of the ICRC accepted Barton's proposal, calling it the "American Amendment" (Harper, 1912).

For the first 10 years of its existence, the American Society of the Red Cross operated under the charter it had been granted by the District of Columbia. Barton and her colleagues realized, however, that for the Society to have the power and standing it required, a federal charter would be necessary. This could only be secured through congressional legislation. Although this would seem to have been a simple matter, Clara Barton spent several years lobbying members of Congress who were quite indifferent to her cause. During this time, Clara learned the important skill of political action, which is necessary for the inspiration of a shared vision.

In 1893, when Clara Barton's lobbying efforts were successful and a federal charter was granted, the Society was reincorporated as the American National Red Cross. Full recognition from Congress would not be attained until 1900. Congress failed, however, to allocate financial support for maintenance of the Red Cross, although the government of every other country in the Red Cross movement had established a mechanism to fund its national society. Thus, for 23 years, the cost of the Red Cross headquarters in Washington, DC, was borne entirely by Clara Barton. No salaries were paid to her staff except for a few temporary employees who provided fieldwork or secretarial services.

INSPIRING A SHARED VISION ON A LOCAL LEVEL

In August 1881, the first local branch of the American Red Cross, called a Red Cross Auxiliary Society, was established in Dansville, New York, Clara Barton's home during the years of her illness. In only a few weeks, other local branches were established in Syracuse and Rochester, New York. The value of the Society was soon proven in its rapid response to forest fires that swept across Michigan, leaving many families homeless and destitute. The local branches collected money and supplies, which were distributed by Dr. J. B. Hubbell, the chief field agent for the Red Cross and Clara Barton's personal assistant (Bacon-Foster, 1918).

Dr. Hubbell served as Clara Barton's assistant from 1881 until 1904. He took charge when she was away from headquarters and was sent to direct aid missions when she was unable to be away from the office. Barton met Hubbell when he served as a professor of science and principal of the Dansville Hygienic Seminary. He became interested in Barton's work and pledged to help her in the establishment of the American Red Cross. When he asked how he could best help the fledgling Society, Clara Barton asked him to attend medical school, in the belief that the presence of an educated medical doctor on her staff would add to the organization's credibility. Hubbell studied at the University of Michigan and received his medical degree in 1883. At many points in his education, however, he was called away to aid in various Red Cross relief efforts.

The first real test of the effectiveness of the Red Cross was its response to flooding in the Ohio and Mississippi river valleys in 1882, 1883, and 1884. The American Red Cross collected $175,000 in money and donations for the relief effort. Clara Barton rented a steamship, loaded it with supplies, and journeyed along the Ohio River, distributing supplies to those in need. When the flooding spread to the lower Mississippi River valley, the American Red Cross chartered another ship in St. Louis, stocked the ship with provisions, and traveled as far as the Mississippi Delta, bringing aid to many afflicted persons in areas too remote to have been reached through the government's relief efforts. The relief efforts of the American Red Cross were unique in that Barton collected and distributed clothing, seeds to replace lost crops, coal for heating homes, and feed for animals—all items needed for survival, which were not considered in government-sponsored relief efforts. Following the approach she had used during the Civil War, Barton traveled to the site of a disaster and personally comforted those in need.

Through her personal contact with disaster victims, Clara Barton strove to *inspire a shared vision* through collecting and sharing with the press personal stories of those who had been afflicted by the disaster. For example, a family of six children in Pennsylvania who had heard about the devastation caused by the flood staged a variety show to aid the victims and sent Clara Barton the $51.25 they collected. As Barton traveled along the flooded Ohio River, in Shawneetown, Illinois, she encountered a widow with six children who had been driven from their home by the flood. Clara used the funds from Pennsylvania to aid the family and notified the donors about the recipients of their generosity. The children in Pennsylvania responded, "Some time again when you want money to help you in your good work, call upon the 'Little Six'" (Jones, 2013, p. 41). Clara Barton sent the story to be published in the *Erie Dispatch*, the local newspaper of Erie, Pennsylvania. She then ordered 1,000 copies of the article, which she sent to other newspapers and included in the notes of thanks she sent to many of her donors. Thus, she was able to *inspire a shared vision* through astute use of the media, coupled with the establishment of a personal connection to her donors.

Later, in 1884, soon after Clara Barton returned from her flood relief efforts, the secretary of state appointed her to represent the United States at the International Conference of the Red Cross, which would be held in Geneva in September. At this conference, she was the only woman among the representatives from 32 nations. Her work was applauded through a resolution introduced by the representative from Italy, "This conference declares that in obtaining the accession of the United States of America to the Convention of Geneva Miss Clara Barton has well merited the gratitude of the world" (Bacon-Foster, 1918, p. 310).

In 1888, the American Red Cross aided victims of a yellow fever epidemic in Jacksonville, Florida. In addition to the Red Cross, many other agencies provided aid, including the U.S. Public Health Service and the U.S. Marine Hospital Service. When Clara Barton appealed to local Red Cross units around the country, the onetime leader of the New Orleans Red Cross responded by sending nurses to aid in the relief effort. Unfortunately, some of the nurses recruited for this effort proved to be less than professional and were accused of drinking to excess, theft, and general incompetence. In contrast, a group of educated nurses from Bellevue Hospital in New York City who joined the relief effort demonstrated the application of scientific principles such as attention to nutrition, hydration, environmental regulation, and treatment protocols in the care of the victims of yellow fever (D'Antonio & Whelan, 2004). Fortunately, a small group of the New Orleans Red Cross nurses performed valiantly through their establishment of a hospital and maintenance of quarantine in the severely afflicted town of McClenny, a short distance from Jacksonville. From this experience, Barton realized the importance of close supervision and guidance of local Red Cross chapters as well as the persons sent as nurses to disaster areas.

On the afternoon of May 31, 1889, a dam built by the exclusive South Fork Fishing and Hunting Club gave way, flooding the town of Johnstown, Pennsylvania, which lay in the valley below. In the wake of the disaster, 2,209 people were killed. Debris littered the town, thousands of residents were homeless, and parts of the city were covered with up to 30 feet of water. The club's members, who included industrialists such as Andrew Carnegie and Henry Clay Frick, had given little attention to either the maintenance of the dam or the threat it posed to the residents of Johnstown. The Philadelphia local Red Cross Auxiliary sent doctors and educated nurses who went door to door to locate sick and injured persons in need of medical attention. The medical and nursing staff further implemented sanitation mechanisms to prevent the outbreak and spread of waterborne diseases, such as typhoid fever. Clara Barton took charge of the distribution of food, clothing, and supplies to the flood victims. The Red Cross used donated lumber to construct temporary hotels that housed nearly one hundred families. Her goal was to provide care and comfort to those who were psychologically distraught as a result of the disaster. When the Red Cross's relief efforts ended in late October, Clara Barton was recognized in an editorial in the *Johnstown Daily Tribune* with the words, "The first to come and the last to go, she has indeed been an elder sister to us—nursing, soothing, and tending for the stricken ones" (C. Barton, 1898, p. 168).

In August 1893, a hurricane ravaged the South Carolina coast. Most affected were the Sea Islands along the coast, which were pounded by a 20-foot tidal wave. One of the greatest achievements of the American Red Cross was the aid it provided to the 30,000 residents who were affected by the storm and its aftermath. In 1890, 92% of the residents in the area most affected were African Americans. Many of these were descendants of former slaves who had labored in the rice plantations along the coast and retained many African traditions. Little media attention was given to this disaster, and because the nation was in the throes of an economic depression, little help was offered. Thus, the American Red Cross acted independently in its provision of relief and often was subjected to intense criticism. Complaints included that the African American victims of the storm were unworthy of aid and that any assistance provided would make them lazy and discouraged. Further, the argument was put forth that a disproportionate amount of aid was provided to the African American island residents, with little aid offered to the predominantly white residents along the coast. Thus, Clara Barton maintained the moral imperative of treating all victims of disaster equitably, regardless of race or ethnicity.

INSPIRING A SHARED VISION ABROAD—INTERNATIONAL RELIEF EFFORTS

During the 1890s, Clara Barton sought to expand the influence of the American Red Cross beyond the borders of the United States through involvement in crises abroad that demanded humanitarian aid. During the decade that followed its founding, the efforts of the American Red Cross had been confined to the United States. As the 19th century drew to a close, however, the spread of colonialism, improved communications and travel among nations, and an increase in missionary activities gave rise to the belief that more advanced nations had a responsibility to aid developing nations. Actually, international involvement seems to have been Clara Barton's vision as early as 1878, because in her pamphlet, *The Red Cross of the Geneva Convention*, she referred to "the misfortunes of other nations" (C. Barton, 1878, pp. 7–8).

Throughout this decade, opportunities for overseas involvement arose, the most significant of which were a famine in Russia from 1889 until 1892, a massacre of Christian Armenians in Ottoman Turkey, in 1895; and a Cuban struggle for independence from Spain from 1895 until 1898. Through these international relief efforts that were necessary to deliver aid to those in need, Clara Barton learned to balance her involvement with foreign governments with the need for the American Red Cross to maintain its neutrality.

Clara Barton was only partially successful in efforts to send corn, grain, and potatoes to Russia. Midwestern farmers quickly identified with the plight of starving peasants and willingly sent produce for shipment abroad. Barton had great difficulty, however, in raising the funds needed to ship the donations abroad. Further, she had difficulty coordinating the efforts of the American Red Cross with a rival, the Russian Famine Committee of the United States, which had been organized by American farmers who were weary of the delays Barton encountered in her attempts to ship contributions abroad. By the time the shipments reached the Russian peasants, they had endured the famine for nearly a year, and relief programs from their own government were beginning to show positive results. Americans, however, believed the relief effort mounted by Clara Barton had been a success. *The Christian Herald* proclaimed enthusiastically, "We have saved the lives of 125,000 Russians" (Jones, 2013, p. 68).

During the summer of 1895, reports were sent by missionaries and travelers abroad that Muslim Turks and Kurds had committed atrocities against the predominantly Christian Armenians. The ire of Americans was further raised by reports that schools and buildings that had been erected by American missionaries to bring "civilization" to the Armenians had been burned and razed. Because the nation of Turkey had ratified the Treaty of Geneva, Clara Barton, the president and representative of the American Red Cross, seemed the logical person to intervene in the crisis. Although she was 74 years old, Barton felt it was her responsibility to undertake this project, despite the knowledge that she would, once again, be venturing into potentially dangerous situations. When she was introduced to Tewfik Pasha, the prime minister of Turkey, by A. W. Terrell the U.S. ambassador to the country, both Clara Barton and Terrell presented their goals in strict humanitarian terms, stressing their concern for the welfare of both the survivors of the massacres and the missionaries attempting to provide aid. When asked to state her plans for the proposed relief effort, Barton later recalled saying,

> Our object would be to use [our] funds ourselves among those needing it, wherever they were found, in helping them to resume their former positions and avocations, thus relieving them from continued distress, the State from the burden of providing for them, and other nations and people from a torrent of sympathy. (C. Barton, 1898, p. 279)

The prime minister agreed to the relief effort and provided guards to escort Barton and her assistants on the four expeditions they made into the interior of the country. The group traveled hundreds of miles, bringing to the distraught Armenians medicine and supplies valued at $116,000. Both Clara Barton and Dr. Hubbell remained in Constantinople for 6 months, administering the distribution of aid.

In recognition of her work in Turkey, Prince Guy de Lusignan, Patriarch of Armenia, awarded Clara Barton the Brevet of Chevalier of the Royal Order of Melusine, which was conferred for her humanitarian services to the Armenian nation. Likewise, the Sultan of Turkey awarded Barton the decoration of Shefaket, also awarded for her humanitarian work. Despite the good that was accomplished by this mission, Barton was criticized by some Americans of Armenian descent for failure to prevent further massacres. Reportedly, 6,000 Armenians were slaughtered in the span of 2 days, only a few weeks after the American Red Cross team departed from Constantinople. Critics further claimed that Clara Barton had developed relationships with the Turkish prime minister and Sultan that were too cordial and that prevented her acknowledgment of the atrocities committed by Turkish officials.

In her work in Turkey, Clara Barton did much to extend the vision of Dunant, the founder of the International Red Cross. In this vision, the society aimed to provide immediate relief to the afflicted, rather than to prevent future crises. Further, in her mission to Turkey, Clara Barton demonstrated leadership through her maintenance of both religious and political neutrality. To successfully accomplish her aims, it was imperative that she refrain from actions that could be misperceived as sympathy to either the Muslim Turks or the Christian Armenians. Her success in this matter is evidenced by the awards she received from both sides in the conflict. When their steamship arrived in New York harbor, a member of her entourage told reporters, "It was not our work to investigate causes. We found the sufferers and did what we could for them" (Jones, 2013, p. 79).

INSPIRING A SHARED VISION—IN TIME OF WAR

During the summer of 1897, amid a growing number of reports of starvation among the peasant population of Cuba, concerned Americans repeatedly requested Clara Barton to send aid. Cuban revolutionary leaders were embroiled in a revolution against the government of Spain, which had ruled the island nation for over four hundred years. Early in 1896, the Spanish government removed peasants from their land and relocated them to detention camps. The peasants, called *reconcentrados*, now faced disease and death. Although President McKinley initially was opposed to U.S. involvement in the Cuban revolutionary efforts, he eventually agreed to a policy of provision of aid to the citizens of Cuba. In cooperation with Clara Barton and the secretary of state, President McKinley formed the Central Cuban Relief Committee to raise funds and collect supplies to aid the *reconcentrados*. Although Clara Barton was 76 years old, she agreed to the president's request that she lead the relief effort. She arrived in Cuba only 3 days after her meeting with the president, inspected the "dirt and filth" of the camps, and began to establish Red Cross distribution centers (Pryor, 1987).

In her efforts to aid the Cuban peasants, Clara Barton worked with General Ramon Blanco y Erenas, the commander of the Spanish armed forces in Cuba. Because Spain had been one of the first countries to sign the Treaty of Geneva and because he expressed compassion for the condition of the Cuban people, she sought to work with him as a colleague in the provision of aid. When she was later criticized for this alliance, Clara Barton defended her actions, stating she met with the Spaniards "as the head of the Red Cross of one country greeting Red Cross men of another." She continued that she did not "speak for America as an American, but from the Red Cross for humanity" (C. Barton, 1899, p. 546).

On February 15, 1898, the U.S. battleship *Maine* exploded and sank while it was moored in Havana Harbor, killing 250 persons. The ship had been sent to Cuba to protect U.S. citizens and their interests during the Cuban fight for independence from Spain. Although recent investigations have concluded that the explosion was caused by spontaneous combustion of the coal stored in the ship's hull, the American public accused the Spanish government of plotting the disaster (Maroldu, 2001). In April 1898, the Spanish government announced an armistice with the rebel forces and enacted a program to grant Cuba increased self-government. The U.S. Congress responded with resolutions that demanded full independence for Cuba and removal of Spanish forces from the island. Further, the U.S. Congress voted to allow President McKinley to send U.S. troops to ensure the removal of Spanish forces from Cuba. In response, on April 24, Spain declared war on the United States. This was followed by a U.S. declaration of war on Spain, which was made retroactive to April 21. With the outbreak of war, Barton bid farewell to General Blanco y Erenas and his staff and relocated the Red Cross headquarters to Tampa, Florida.

Only days before the start of hostilities, the *State of Texas*, a ship that had been commissioned by Clara Barton to deliver Red Cross supplies to the *reconcentrados* departed from New York, bound for Key West, Florida. Barton met the ship there and implored Admiral Sampson, the U.S. naval commander responsible for the enactment of a naval blockade that surrounded Cuba to allow the supplies to pass through the barrier. He responded that it was his responsibility to prevent aid from reaching Cuba despite Clara Barton's pleas that the responsibility of the Red Cross was to deliver immediate aid to combatants, regardless of their cause. But her resentment of the barriers to her mission that had been imposed by the U.S. military forces led to her choice to function independently, rather than in unison with the efforts of the army and navy.

Unable to begin the work she planned, Clara Barton remained in Tampa, the point of departure for U.S. troops leaving for Cuba. Her attention remained focused on the delivery of supplies and food to Cuban civilians, with little regard for the needs of the U.S. troops that were being assembled for the invasion of Cuba. Many of these troops languished in camps that lacked appropriate sanitation and soon fell victim to typhoid fever and malaria. To aid these troops, many relief groups, such as the American National Red Cross Relief Committee, were organized by concerned community leaders from all regions of the United States. These "auxiliary" Red Cross organizations were committed to raising funds to aid the army and navy in their efforts to provide medical and hospital care. These groups had been formed, however, without the knowledge or consent of Clara Barton—a fact she only later recognized as a threat to her leadership (Jones, 2013).

As hostilities on the island increased, Clara Barton, functioning in accord with the Red Cross mission to provide immediate relief, followed Theodore Roosevelt and his troops to Cuba. There, she once again encountered resistance from army medical personnel who opposed the presence of female nurses in military field hospitals. She noted in her diary, "All seemed interested in the Red Cross, but none thought a woman nurse would be in place in a soldier's hospital" (C. Barton, 1899, p. 557). On a battlefield in Siboney in Cuba, Clara Barton was dismayed to find wounded men with high fevers, lying on the coarse grass with no blankets under them. Her attempts to provide aid were rebuffed by U.S. Army surgeons who stated they were dealing adequately with the situation. The U.S. and Cuban field hospitals had been arranged in immediate proximity. Clara Barton and her staff then redirected their attention to the care of patients in the Cuban field hospital. When the American medics realized that the Cuban patients were clean, well nourished, and the recipients of excellent care, they changed their minds and requested the services of the Red Cross (Pryor, 1987).

In her memoir of the war, Clara Barton related an incident in which a young U.S. Army officer, who had been forbidden to ask for aid from the Red Cross in adherence with the U.S. Army's original policy, approached her with a request to purchase needed supplies for his men. Clara replied that she would not sell supplies to him, even if he offered her a million dollars. In desperation, he asked what he could do to obtain the supplies, to which she replied, "Just ask for them." With that, the officer gathered the supplies he needed and, with a bulging sack thrown over his shoulder, trudged back into the jungle to return to his troops. The young officer was Theodore Roosevelt who would soon be elected president of the United States (C. Barton, 1899).

During the Battle of El Caney, which was fought on July 1, 1889, victims were transported to Siboney for care. Nurses prepared gruel and a drink made from dried apples and prunes, which was nicknamed "Red Cross Cider." In her published memoir, Barton related that, dressed in a calico skirt and white apron, she worked from 16 to 18 hours each day, cooking and caring for sick and wounded soldiers. In addition, many soldiers and Red Cross staff members had contracted yellow fever, which required specialized treatment such as applications of ice.

Following the Battle of San Juan, Clara Barton heard that wounded men on the battlefield required care. In actions reminiscent of her work during the American Civil War, Barton loaded supplies into the only two wagons that were available and drove through tropical jungles to bring aid to the afflicted. Following the battle, military surgeons performed more than 400 operations in 2 days. Clara found the recovering patients, lying on the ground in pools of water, in conditions she assessed as much worse than any she had seen in her earlier work. She was welcomed by the more able patients with the cry, "There is Clara Barton. Now we'll get something to eat" (C. Barton, 1899, p. 649).

The work of Clara Barton and her associates was further recognized in Major Louis LeGarde's annual report to the U.S. War Department in 1898, for the "Base Hospital" at Siboney, Cuba. It states,

> As the wounded crowded upon us in numbers beyond anything we had any reason to anticipate, they came forward with cots, blankets, and other necessities. . . . For such help at a moment of supreme need, coming from people in no way connected with the military services, the deep sense of gratitude . . . cannot be conveyed by words. (Bacon-Foster, 1918, p. 341)

Ironically, for her work in Cuba, Clara Barton chose as her chief assistant, J. K. Elwell, the nephew of J. J. Elwell, the married officer with whom she had been romantically involved during the Civil War. In his memoir, J. K. Elwell wrote that he had met Clara Barton through his uncle, "who had been intimately acquainted with her during the Civil War" (Bacon-Foster, 1918, p. 330). He added that Clara Barton personally recommended him to President McKinley and that prior to the outbreak of hostilities, he had been appointed by the State Department to work with the U.S. consul general in Havana.

Hostilities ended on July 17, 1898, with the surrender of Spanish military forces to General William Shafter. In the Treaty of Paris, which was signed on December 10, 1898, Spain granted independence to Cuba, ceded Guam and Puerto Rico to the United States, and transferred its sovereignty over the Philippines to the United States for a payment of $20 million. At the conclusion of the war, the Spanish government presented Clara Barton with the "Diploma of Gratitude," a plaque engraved with a testimonial from the Red Cross of Spain for the aid she provided to Spanish soldiers (Harper, 1912). The people of Santiago, Cuba, erected a statue of Clara Barton on the town square (Frantz, 1998).

Clara Barton received criticism, however, for many of her actions in Cuba. Questions were raised about the aid she provided to Spanish troops during a time of war, her need to work independently with a concomitant inability to coordinate her efforts with other groups providing aid, and her decision to work on the battlefields rather than attend to administrative responsibilities in the Red Cross headquarters. This criticism would increase dramatically during the years that followed. Although her work during the Spanish–American War facilitated Clara Barton's efforts to *inspire a shared vision*, she neglected to consider a corollary of this leadership principle—the importance of coordinating efforts with others, sharing of intermediate goals, and delegation of work to others to make progress toward attainment of the vision.

ATTAINMENT OF THE VISION

On September 8, 1900, a devastating hurricane struck Galveston Island, off the coast of Texas, with winds of more than 125 miles per hour. Still ranked as the worst natural disaster in the history of the United States, the storm left 8,000 people dead and more than 25,000 homeless (D'Antonio & Whelan, 2004). Although Clara Barton was 78 years old and in poor health, she nevertheless traveled to Texas to aid in the relief effort. Although confined to a bed for over a week, she insisted on directing the clothing and food distribution efforts. She remained in Galveston for over 2 months, procuring lumber and planning the construction of houses on frail stilts, which were named Red Cross houses by locals. In her memoirs, she described fires that were kept burning for weeks to control the spread of disease from decaying corpses.

Following the disaster, her work was acclaimed in a resolution that was introduced in the Texas State Legislature on February 1, 1901, "especially does the Legislature thank Miss Clara Barton, President of the Society for her visit to the State and her personal supervision and direction of relief to those who were in need and distress" (Bacon-Foster, 1918, p. 347). This was to be Clara Barton's last relief effort.

Not everyone continued to be so enamored of Barton's work. The American National Red Cross Society had grown in both membership and in the scope of its activities. Many members believed that Clara Barton continued to work too independently without consulting with others, especially in regard to the collection of donations and the use of the Society funds.

In May 1900, the U.S. Congress approved an official federal charter for the Red Cross, to recognize the American Red Cross as the society responsible for fulfilling the obligations that the United States had agreed to through its acceptance of the terms of the Treaty of Geneva. Although the U.S. Congress had signed the treaty in 1882 and had approved a federal charter in 1893, it had never formally recognized the American Red Cross as its official agent. The charter specified that the American Red Cross would be responsible for the provision of aid to the sick wounded in times of war and would work with military officials to maintain communication between active service members and their families at home. Further, the Society was charged with maintenance of a system of national and international relief in times of peace to aid those afflicted by natural disasters. As an important addition, through this legislation, more power was given to the Society's executive committee, and a board of control was established.

Clara Barton had persistently sought to achieve this recognition for the American Red Cross, repeatedly lobbying members of Congress. Having achieved this goal, she decided to retire and submitted her resignation as president of the American Red Cross to the newly formed board of control at its meeting in July 1900. The board, however, refused to accept her resignation and praised her as "a greater heroine than Florence Nightingale" (Jones, 2013, p. 94).

Unlike the informal group of advisors that had loosely governed the American Red Cross since its founding in 1882, the new board of control was required to submit an annual report to Congress, which would need to include detailed information about contributions to the Society and funds expended in relief efforts. Throughout the years of her presidency, Clara Barton had developed her own unique method of fiscal management that was now exposed to the scrutiny of board members. Although many members of the board of control, including her nephew William Barton, were long-time supporters of Barton, some were detractors who believed the American Red Cross was in need of new leadership. These members, led by the socially prominent Mabel Boardman, called for a congressional investigation of the financial operations of the Society.

Unfortunately, through these new demands for fiscal transparency, serious flaws were detected in Clara Barton's methods of accounting. For example, Barton's approach was to wait for a new disaster to occur in order to secure the contributions needed to pay the debts the Red Cross had accrued from its involvement in a prior calamity. When Barton was asked to submit the American Red Cross account books for an audit by the U.S. Treasury Department, she brought an assortment of trunks, suitcases, hatboxes, and wooden boxes, which she had used to file these records. In addition, two of her most trusted employees were found to have embezzled funds from the Society; the Red Cross had issued no public financial statements until it was required to do so in 1900, and funds collected for the Society's relief efforts had been sent directly to Clara Barton, rather than being channeled through the Society's treasurer.

Clara Barton, who had always been sensitive to criticism, was distraught that she should be the subject of a congressional investigation. She wrote in February 1903, "All of this kind of life is so distasteful to me that I cannot carry it much longer . . . so humiliating that I can scarcely take it in or bear it" (Bacon-Foster, 1918, p. 352). Her only answer to the criticism she received was, "Let my life and work speak for themselves" (Harper, 1912, p. 711).

Although the congressional committee that conducted the investigation found that Clara Barton had done nothing wrong, it nevertheless questioned the accounting system for the Red Cross and the Society's distribution of funds. In 1904, at the age of 83, Barton resigned as president for the last time. In her letter of resignation, she wrote, "It is a pride as well as a pleasure to hand you an organization perfectly formed, thoroughly officered, with no debts and a sum of from $12,000 to $14,000, available to our treasury as a working fund" (Bacon-Foster, 1918, p. 354). This comment was undoubtedly a response to the board's expressed concerns about the financial status of the American Red Cross. Clara Barton had garnered these funds through sale of some of the Society's assets, including vacant lots in Washington, DC, that had recently increased in value.

For the final 15 years of her life, Clara Barton resided in her home in Glen Echo, Maryland. Originally built in 1891 as a warehouse for Red Cross relief supplies, Barton moved there in 1897, making it both her home and the headquarters for the American Red Cross. This may have indicated that she made little distinction between her personal life and her work. In her Christmas letter to friends that year, she outlined a plan for what she called "My Later Work." She wrote that now that the work of the Red Cross had, in her opinion, been totally taken over by the government, it was a "finished effort." She added, however, "You have never known me without work; while able you never will. It has always been a part of the best religion I have had." She now planned to initiate a program to provide "organized first aid to the injured" (Harper, 1912, p. 711).

In 1903, Clara Barton met with Edward Howe and recruited him to be superintendent for a new first aid department for the American Red Cross. Howe had been affiliated with a similar program, the St. John Ambulance Association, which had been initiated in Great Britain. He was now eager to bring the idea to the United States, and Barton was in full agreement. They envisioned an educational program that Red Cross auxiliaries could operate between relief missions. The program would provide training for school personnel, firefighters, police officers, and factory employees to enable them to provide rapid treatment for accidents they encountered in their work. Further, training would be provided to housewives to enable them to deal with family accidents and emergencies. The program could also provide a source of revenue for the auxiliaries through the sale of first aid kits and supplies and fees charged for classes. By the end of 1903, the governors of 24 states and territories, as well as the presidents of 19 state medical societies had voiced their support of the plan (Jones, 1913). This plan provides evidence that although Clara Barton was of an advanced age and showed frailty in many aspects of her life, she was nevertheless able to devise a creative plan for the expansion of the influence of the American Red Cross.

Although Clara Barton had planned to implement the first aid program in her retirement and the idea proved to be successful, the American Red Cross brought suit against her to own and direct the program. The Society argued that because Clara Barton had developed the idea for the program while she was president of the American Red Cross, it belonged to the Society. A weary Clara Barton decided not to engage in a battle for control of the program (Pryor, 1987).

During her final years of life, Clara Barton spent the majority of her time at her beloved Glen Echo, making frequent visits to a second home she purchased in Oxford, Massachusetts. In 1904, she wrote the book, *A Story of the Red Cross*, which although intended to be a history of the American Red Cross, was autobiographical in much of its content. In 1907, in response to a request from a young admirer, she wrote a book about her early life, *The Story of My Childhood*. Through her final years, Clara Barton continued to experience the episodes of depression that had haunted her through much of her life. She wrote, "The longer I live, the worse it gets, until now the menacing spirits hover about my poor beset pathway. . . . There have been no successes in my life, only attempts at success and no realization" (W. E. Barton, Vol. 2, 1922, p. 146).

In August 1911, Clara Barton made a final visit to her home in Oxford, Massachusetts, to visit family members. While there, she contracted pneumonia, which lingered for several months. Her health seemed to improve as she celebrated her 90th birthday on Christmas Day, 1911. As the winter wore on, however, her health continued to deteriorate. She died at Glen Echo on April 12, 1912. Friends held a memorial service for her there, and a burial followed in Oxford, Massachusetts, her birthplace and childhood home.

CLARA BARTON'S LEADERSHIP LEGACY

Kouzes and Posner (2012) describe *inspiring a shared vision* as a two-part process. A leader first envisions a future for the organization that is both exciting and desirable. The leader must have confidence the envisioned future is attainable and that he or she has, or can develop, the skills to bring the vision to reality.

Clara Barton envisioned a future for the provision of immediate care for those in need, for victims of both military actions and natural disasters. This vision was forged through her battlefield experiences nursing sick and wounded soldiers during the Civil War. Her ability to provide aid quickly during these emergency situations aided thousands of people whose needs could not be met by the existing, poorly organized, government-sponsored mechanisms. These efforts also formed the framework for Barton's lifelong work.

Jones (2013) asserts that Clara Barton's work on the battlefields of the Civil War developed in her the sense of humanitarianism that would be a driving force for her efforts for the rest of her life. Her work was based on her firm belief that suffering must be relieved as soon as possible. Thus, she expressed human sentiment, or concern for the welfare of others, blended with a rational call to action.

The possession of a vision is not enough. A leader must have the confidence to believe that he or she has the skills necessary to move the vision forward. Since her childhood, Clara Barton had been described as rather shy and lacking in social skills. Through her experiences on the lecture circuit, Barton was able to overcome the shyness that had haunted her during her earlier life. She was able to develop persuasive skills that would benefit her in her later activities. There is evidence, however, that her attempts to develop skills in persuasion sometimes worked to her detriment. At times, she embellished her accounts of her battlefield experiences, both to entertain her admirers and to enlist their financial support. She believed that support could best be engendered through the presentation of the events as both dreadful and in need of immediate attention, even if this involved a bit of exaggeration (Pryor, 1987).

In the second part of the process of *inspiring a shared vision*, the leader enlists others in the pursuit of the envisioned future. The process involves an ongoing dialogue with others in which the leader conveys an understanding of the hopes, aspirations, and values of others and presents the vision as one aimed at the common good.

Although Clara Barton had learned much from her colleagues and mentors on the International Red Cross Committee, upon her return to the United States she realized she would need to develop strategies that would appeal to the sentiments of her fellow citizens. To win acceptance, the idea of a Red Cross had to capture the imaginations of her fellow Americans. Because she realized that the memory of the U.S. Civil War was fading and that many Americans believed that the Unites States would never again be involved in a war, an idea of a Red Cross Society beyond that envisioned by Dunant would be necessary. Thus, the idea of provision of relief during "national calamities" would better speak to the concerns of the American public. Clara Barton wrote,

> Our Southern coasts are periodically visited by the scourge
> of yellow fever; the valleys of the Mississippi are subjected to
> destructive inundations. . . . to gather and dispense the profuse
> liberality of our people, without waste of time or material,
> requires the wisdom that comes of experiences and permanent
> organization. (C. Barton, 1878, pp. 7–8)

Her descriptions of the types of natural disasters that many Americans had actually experienced resonated with her audience and augmented her appeals for the support of a movement that would aid the "common good."

Efforts to educate the American public about the value of a Red Cross Society also formed an important strategy in Barton's attempts to enlist others in the pursuit of her envisioned future.

For example, Clara Barton authored a pamphlet, *The Red Cross of the Geneva Convention*, which presented the Red Cross as a national relief organization that would function during times of peace to "afford ready succor and assistance to sufferers in times of national widespread calamities, such as plague, yellow fever, and the like, devastating fires or floods, rail disasters, [or] mining catastrophes" (C. Barton, 1878, pp. 5–6).

Attempts to educate the public were most successful when they also appealed to the emotions of the audience. An example was Clara Barton's use of her personal contact with disaster victims to collect the stories of those who had been afflicted by the disaster. She then shared these experiences with the press. The example of the "Little Six" from Pennsylvania demonstrated her use of this strategy. Barton's use of local newspapers and the education of her donors through the use of newspaper articles further aided in her efforts to enlist others in the pursuit of her vision.

When Clara Barton's first attempts to secure congressional approval for the Treaty of Geneva were unsuccessful, she developed skills in lobbying members of Congress, the president of the United States, and members of his administration. These skills were also beneficial when Clara and her colleagues worked for congressional approval of a federal charter for the American Red Cross.

Perhaps Clara Barton's greatest aid in her efforts to enlist others in the pursuit of her vision was her adherence to the advice given to her by Dr. Appia. Barton took steps to surround herself "with a little body of persons full of good-will and capacity, docile to [her] directions" (W. E. Barton, 1922, Vol. 2, p. 128). To her advisory board and staff, she appointed people of unwavering loyalty, including William Barton, her devoted nephew; J. Elwell, the nephew of her former romantic interest; and Dr. Hubbell, who had pledged to help her in the establishment of the American Red Cross and, at her request, to aid the cause by earning a medical degree. Many of her supporters had been drawn to Clara because of the appeal of her humanitarian mission. They were impressed with her treatment of all victims of disaster equally, regardless of race or ethnicity. One of her contemporaries stated, "Clara Barton had one pronounced failing; she was never able to resist a plea for assistance" (Bacon-Foster, 1918, p. 350). In fact, during the congressional investigation Clara Barton endured, one of her detractors stated, "Nobody would testify against her—not even all our friends and relations in New England" (Jones, 2013, p. 111).

In her attempts to *inspire a shared vision,* Clara Barton was often the recipient of criticism; some of it perhaps well deserved. Leaders in the developing profession of nursing were sometimes harsh in their comments. Educated professional nurses did not emerge until the 1870s, when the first hospital-based schools of nursing, based on the Nightingale model, were established in New York, Boston, New Haven, and Philadelphia. While Clara Barton was single-handedly delivering care to soldiers in the jungles of Cuba, in the manner that she had during the American Civil War, a new movement was under way. In response to the horrendous conditions military personnel encountered in Cuba, the army set criteria for the selection of nurses who would serve there. All nurses were required to be graduates of a school of nursing and were required to furnish recommendations that addressed their health and character.

Leaders in the emerging profession of nursing had observed that Clara Barton was unwilling to work with government agencies that were organized to provide relief. For example, as late as 1864, when Barton was asked why she continued to work independently of the Sanitary Commission, she replied that she began her work before the Sanitary Commission was formed and had acquired so much skill in her work through practice that she might not be able to "work as efficiently" or "labor as happily" under the direction of those with less experience (W. E. Barton, Vol. 1, 1922). They had also experienced Barton's unwillingness to work with the educated nurses who had been sent by Red Cross auxiliary agencies to aid in relief efforts for victims of the Johnstown Flood, the Florida yellow fever epidemic, the conflict in Cuba, and other disasters' aid efforts in which she had participated.

Nurse leader Anna Maxwell, who in 1910 participated in the formation of the Army Nurse Corps, criticized Clara Barton stating,

> She resented having others take up and carry on . . . what she as one human being could not accomplish. . . . Professional nursing did not receive from her proper recognition. . . . Consequently, she was not willing that women prominent in the nursing profession who volunteered their service should be allowed their opportunity. (Maxwell, 1923, p. 619)

Nurse leader, Lavinia Dock, in her book, *A Short History of Nursing*, criticized Clara Barton for her failure to "identify herself with the growing movement to reform nursing," adding that Clara Barton was "rarely benevolent in spirit" (Dock, 1934, p. 150).

Psychiatrist and medical historian G. D. Evans (2003), in his analysis of Clara Barton's leadership, offers praise for her energy, creativity, and courage. As a psychiatrist retrospectively viewing behaviors that she consistently displayed over the course of her life as well as her family history, Evans asserts that she probably was afflicted by manic-depressive illness. This diagnosis is consistent with her episodes of disabling fatigue, interspersed with episodes of boundless energy and creativity. Evans uses this diagnosis as a partial explanation for the weaknesses Clara Barton displayed rather than as a denigration of her accomplishments and leadership abilities. Evans cites Clara Barton's greatest weakness as her "inability to manage a large number of people working toward a common goal" (Evans, 2003, p. 81). This opinion is similar to that held by other contemporaries.

Biographer Elizabeth Pryor (1987) also raised questions about mental health issues that may have plagued Clara Barton. She noted in particular the blind loyalty that Clara Barton demanded of her associates as well as her ruthless use of personal influence to achieve her goals. Historian Stephen Oates (1994) expressed concern about Clara Barton's paranoid tendencies in questioning the motives of those who criticized her work. A summary of these comments and criticisms indicates that Clara Barton had difficulty in the coordination of her efforts with those working toward a common goal. The key word in *inspiring a shared vision* seems to be "shared." A leader must be willing to share with others the tasks required for continued progress toward the attainment of the vision.

Robert Giffin (2000), a past president of the American Red Cross, pointed out that at the time Clara Barton founded the American Red Cross, it was a rather small operation. He quickly added that, in his opinion, Clara Barton lacked any sense of organization, stating, "There were numerous Red Cross movements, but they paid no attention to Clara Barton," (Giffin, 2000, p. 145). He further asserted that the Red Cross was able to grow only when Mabel Boardman, who succeeded Clara Barton in 1904, assumed control, stating that Boardman understood the importance of strong management and well-educated staff members. Anna Maxwell (1923) echoed these sentiments, stating that in Clara Barton's later years, the financial responsibilities in the management of a growing association proved to be too much for one who had always been accustomed to acting alone.

These weaknesses should not, however, diminish Clara Barton's leadership legacy. In fact, there is much to be learned by reflecting on her life and situation. Consider these:

- Clara Barton modeled a single-mindedness of purpose that is rare, yet required of leadership. She worked tirelessly, choosing to "go it alone" rather than being "side tracked" by the issues of other organizations/ agendas. Clearly, while she may have been affected by the criticisms of others, she stayed the course. This demonstrates, again, her passionate commitment to humanitarian efforts. For example, was her refusal to commit energy to the formation of professional nursing intentional in order to husband her strength for her own mission? She demonstrated excellence in political strategy but made choices along the way. Good leaders must be careful stewards of their actions and energies.
- Our society strives to respect individual differences related to disability. This was certainly not the case in Ms. Barton's lifetime. Yet, despite her struggles with mental disability, she formulated a leadership style and work ethic to achieve her goals. She leveraged her strengths to her advantage and produced successful outcomes of her interventions that could not be disputed. She would have benefited from our current emphasis on teamwork and team building, perhaps bringing together teams of individuals who could complement her weaknesses, thus avoiding her struggles with organization and finance in her later years.
- Consider the political expertise necessary for an individual to achieve an international sphere of influence such as Barton's. Politics do not come naturally to nurses. This aspect of leadership is often overlooked. It is often ignored in leadership development programs and formal nursing

educational programs. Most often, it is an "acquired taste" achieved through mentorship. Political action requires insight, excellent interpersonal skills, the ability to read and interpret behavior, group dynamics, and risk taking. Clara Barton certainly possessed this skill set. She serves as an inspiration to those who aspire to this level of change and sustainability. What would it be like to sit at the knee of a master, such as Barton, and be regaled with her analysis on navigating bureaucracy to meet the needs of individuals? Her story gives us just an inkling of this great talent.

Clara Barton was a true humanitarian. She showed great courage and worked tirelessly for the cause to which she had devoted her life: to bring humanitarian aid to those in need. She was repeatedly described as a person who was patient, diplomatic, calm, persistent, independent, proud, and determined to accomplish her goals. In spite of her weaknesses, her life exemplifies a triumph of the human spirit—the ability to overcome obstacles in the achievement of one's goals.

TIMELINE

- December 25, 1821—Clara Barton is born in North Oxford, Massachusetts, the youngest of the five children born to Stephen and Sarah Barton.
- May 1838—Secures first teaching position.
- 1850—Begins studies in the Clinton Liberal Institute in New York to further her education by studying writing and language.
- 1852—Founds a public school in Bordentown, New Jersey, which begins with six students, but enrollment soon grows to 600 students.
- 1854—Moves to Washington, DC, and secures a position as a clerk, one of the first women to hold a position with the U.S. government; she receives the same salary as the male clerks.
- 1856—Loses her position in the U.S. Patent Office because of a change in administration; returns to Massachusetts and resumes study of French and art with the hope of securing another teaching position.
- 1861—Returns to prior position in the U.S. Patent Office.
- April 1861—U.S. Civil War begins; the Massachusetts Sixth Regiment, while en route to Washington, is attacked by rebels while marching through Baltimore; among the wounded she recognizes many as her former neighbors, classmates, and students.
- August 1862–March 1865—Aids ill and wounded soldiers in the battles of Second Bull Run, Harpers Ferry, Antietam, Petersburg, Fredericksburg, and the Wilderness; earns the name "Angel of the Battlefield."
- March 1865—Abraham Lincoln appoints her general correspondent for inquiries about soldiers listed as "missing"; establishes a Bureau of Correspondence for Friends of Paroled Prisoners.

- Summer 1865—Attempts to identify the remains of those Union soldiers who perished while held at the Confederate prison at Andersonville, Georgia; this leads to the establishment of one of the first national cemeteries in the United States.
- 1869—Upon the recommendation of physicians, travels to Geneva, Switzerland, for recovery from fatigue.
- 1870—Works with members of the International Red Cross during the Franco–Prussian War.
- 1873–1877—Returns to the United States; suffers an episode of overwhelming fatigue for which she seeks treatment at a sanatorium in Dansville, New York.
- 1877–1882—Works tirelessly for U.S. ratification of the Treaty of Geneva.
- May 2, 1881—Founder and president of the American Association of the Red Cross; organizes the first branch of the American Red Cross.
- 1882—Treaty of Geneva is ratified by the Congress of the United States; the American Red Cross is chartered by President Chester A. Arthur and joins the International Red Cross.
- August 1888—Aids in relief efforts for victims of a yellow fever epidemic in Jacksonville, Florida.
- 1889—Aids in relief efforts for victims of a devastating flood in Johnstown, Pennsylvania.
- 1893—Aids in relief efforts for victims of a hurricane that brought widespread destruction to the Sea Islands, Georgia, North Carolina, and South Carolina; engendered criticism for assistance provided to African American residents of the Sea Islands.
- 1895—Travels to Turkey to provide aid to survivors of the Armenian Massacre.
- 1898—Works in Cuba during the Spanish–American War; publishes the book, *The Red Cross: A History of this Remarkable International Movement in the Interest of Humanity.*
- 1899—Publishes the book, *The Red Cross in Peace and War.*
- 1900—Aids victims of a hurricane that destroyed Galveston, Texas.
- 1904—Publishes the book, *A Story of the Red Cross: Glimpses of Field Work*; resigns as president of the American Red Cross in the wake of allegations of incompetence, inability to deal with expansion of the association, and fiscal mismanagement.
- 1906—Establishes the National First Aid Association of America.
- 1907—Publishes the book, *The Story of My Childhood.*
- April 12, 1912—Clara Barton dies at her home in Glen Echo, Maryland; she is buried in the family plot in Oxford, Massachusetts.
- 1921—The Women's National Missionary Association of the Universalist Church purchases Clara Barton's birthplace home with support from the Legion of Loyal Women, the Clara Barton Memorial Association, and members of the Barton extended family; they open the Clara Barton Birthplace Museum.

- 1948—The U.S. Post Office issues a commemorative postage stamp honoring Clara Barton (see the beginning of this chapter).
- 1974—Clara Barton's home, for the last 15 years of her life, in Glen Echo, Maryland, is established as the Clara Barton Historical Site by the National Park Service; it is the first National Park Service site dedicated to the accomplishments of a woman.
- 1995—The U.S. Post Office issues a second commemorative postage stamp honoring Clara Barton (see the beginning of this chapter).

QUESTIONS FOR DISCUSSION

1. Clara Barton's exemplary leadership led to a change in international policy and the eventual U.S. ratification of the Geneva Convention. Her leadership impact as an activist agent of change is still important today because the Treaty of Geneva still prescribes rules of humane treatment in times of war. Further, she and her colleagues became the first in the international Red Cross movement to make disaster relief the central focus of its mission; an action referred to as the "American Amendment" to the Treaty of Geneva. List current international challenges related to health promotion and health maintenance, as well to nursing and health care delivery. How can today's exemplary nurse leaders collaborate with others to inspire a shared vision and lead change in international policy in these areas of need?

2. In her youth, Clara Barton was often described as "shy," "sensitive," and even "difficult." What approaches did she use to move beyond these traits and establish herself as an innovator and leader of the American Red Cross? How can aspiring nurse leaders use similar methods to develop the ability to inspire others?

3. Clara Barton skillfully used the media (newspapers of the time) to share stories that demonstrated the value of the work of the Red Cross in relief efforts and inspired others to support her work. How can modern nurse leaders best make use of the media to engender support for nursing through sharing stories about nurses' work and its effects?

4. Although Clara Barton supposedly traveled to Switzerland for rest, she soon became involved in efforts to relieve the suffering of French citizens who had been devastated by the Franco–Prussian War. To be effective in this situation, it was necessary for her to develop sensitivity to the culture of the French people. What mechanisms did Clara Barton use to develop the cultural sensitivity required for her work? Through her life's work, what other groups did she encounter for whom culturally sensitive approaches were necessary? Describe situations in which a modern nurse leader is required to use culturally appropriate techniques.

5. Clara Barton had difficulty with delegation and might have benefitted from skills that team members could have provided. If Clara Barton had

been better able to work collaboratively with others, as she embarked on the formation and expansion of the work of the American Red Cross, what skills might she have sought in members she hoped to recruit to strengthen her "team"? What skill sets did Clara Barton lack that would have enabled the American Red Cross to function more effectively in its relief efforts?

6. An "accident of history," the American Civil War changed the life and vision of Clara Barton. For her entire adult life, she endeavored to *inspire a shared vision* of humane treatment of combatants in time of war. What are some of the national and international human rights challenges we face today and how can nurse leaders impact how they are addressed?

7. Clara Barton's international travels broadened her worldview and inspired her to collaborate with many others to address the health challenges of her day. Where have you traveled or where would you like to travel to see, firsthand, the health challenges confronting other people of the world? How might nurse leaders collaborate with others to meet these challenges? Who would be good partners to collaborate with in addressing these challenges and why?

8. Mentors were very important to Clara Barton in shaping and clarifying her vision. What mentors would you, or have you, identified who inspire and shape your vision of your preferred future of nursing, health care, and society? How have you, or will you, seek them out and pursue your vision of a preferred future?

9. As an exemplary nurse leader, Clara Barton *modeled the way* by tirelessly persevering in her pursuit of national and international change. How important are the characteristics of tenacity and perseverance in achieving a nurse leader's vision?

REFERENCES

Bacon-Foster, C. (1918). Clara Barton, humanitarian. *Records of the Columbia Historical Society, 21,* 278–356.

Barton, C. (1878). *The Red Cross of the Geneva convention: What it is.* Washington, DC: Rufus H. Darby.

Barton, C. (1898). The *Red Cross: A history of this remarkable international movement in the interest of humanity.* New York, NY: James B. Lyon.

Barton, C. (1899). *The Red Cross in peace and war.* New York, NY: American Historical Press.

Barton, C. (1907). *The story of my childhood.* New York, NY: Baker and Taylor.

Barton, W. E. (1922). *The life of Clara Barton, founder of the American Red Cross* (Vols. 1, 2). New York, NY: Houghton Mifflin.

D'Antonio, P., & Whelan, J. (2004). Moments when time stood still. *American Journal of Nursing, 104,* 66–72.

Dock, L., & Stewart, M. (1934). *A short history of nursing from the earliest times to the present day* (p. 150). New York, NY: Putnam.

Evans, G. D. (2003). Clara Barton: Teacher, nurse, civil war heroine, founder of the American Red Cross. *International History of Nursing Journal, 7*(3), 75–82.

Frantz, A. K. (1998). Nursing pride: Clara Barton in the Spanish–American War, *American Journal of Nursing, 98*(10), 41.

Giffin, R. (2000). American Red Cross national capital chapter marks 95th anniversary. *Washington History, 12*(1), 144–146.

Harper, I. H. (1912). The life and work of Clara Barton. *North American Review, 195*, 701–712.

Jones, M. M. (2013). *The American Red Cross from Clara Barton to the New Deal.* Baltimore, MD: Johns Hopkins University Press.

Kouzes, J. M., & Posner, B. Z. (2012). *The leadership challenge* (5th ed.). San Francisco, CA: Jossey-Bass.

Maroldu, E. J. (Ed.). (2001). Theodore Roosevelt: *The U.S. navy and the Spanish-American war.* New York, NY: Palgrave.

Maxwell, A. (1923). The life of Clara Barton. *American Journal of Nursing, 23*, 618–619.

Oates, S. B. (1994). *A woman of valor: Clara Barton and the civil war.* New York, NY: Free Press.

Pryor, E. B. (1987). *Clara Barton, professional angel.* Philadelphia, PA: University of Pennsylvania Press.

Sommervill, B. (2007). *Clara Barton: Founder of the American Red Cross.* Minneapolis, MN: Compass Point Books.

FURTHER READING

Barton, C. (1898). Our work and observations in Cuba. *North American Review, 166*(498), 552–559.

Bunker, E. (1957). The voluntary effort in disaster relief. *Annals of the American Academy of Political and Social Science, 309*, 107–117.

Burton, D. (1995). *Clara Barton: In the service of humanity.* Westport, CT: Greenwood Press.

Dock, L. (1922). *History of American Red Cross nursing.* New York, NY: McMillan.

Dulles, R. E. (1950). *The American Red Cross: A history.* New York, NY: Harper.

Epler, P. (1924). *The life of Clara Barton.* New York, NY: McMillan.

Gall, A. C. (1941). *In peace and war.* New York, NY: Crowell.

Kernoodle, P. (1949). *The Red Cross nurse in action.* New York, NY: Harper & Row.

Roberts, J. I., & Group, T. M. (1995). *Power, status, and political activism in the nursing profession.* Westport, CT: Praeger.

Schmidt, C. K. (2004a). American Red Cross nursing: Essential to disaster relief. *American Journal of Nursing, 104*(8), 35–38.

Schmidt, C. K. (2004b). One vision followed by thousands. *American Journal of Nursing, 104*(8), 36–37.

Williams, B. C. (1941). *Clara Barton, a daughter of destiny.* Philadelphia, PA: J. B. Lippincott Company.

PART IV

Challenging the Process

Margaret Higgins Sanger: The Law Shall Be Broken

Patricia K. Hindin

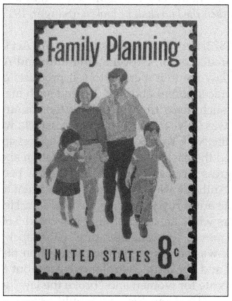

*U.S. postage stamp issued in 1972
honoring family planning.*

· · · · ·

THE LAW SHALL BE BROKEN

Woman has always been the chief sufferer under this merciless machinery of the statutory law. Humbly she has born the weight of man-made laws, surrendering to their tyranny even her right over her own body. For centuries she has been the helpless victim of excessive child-bearing. Meekly she has submitted to undesired motherhood. . . .

Against the State, against the Church, against the silent medical profession, against the whole machinery of dead institutions of the past, the woman of to-day arises. She no longer pleads. She no longer implores. She no longer petitions. She is here to assert herself, to take back those rights which were formerly hers and hers alone.

If she must break the law to establish her right to voluntary motherhood, *then the law shall be broken.* (Sanger, 1917, p. 4)

On March 3, 1873, the U.S. Congress passed "An Act for the Suppression of Trade in, and Circulation of, Obscene Literature and Articles of Immoral Use." This federal law made it a crime to sell products or distribute literature regarding contraception or abortion, to send such materials through the mail, or to import such items from outside of the country. One of the supporters of this bill was 29-year-old Anthony Comstock, who was an organizational leader for the New York Society for the Suppression of Vice. Wealthy New Yorkers formed the backbone of this organization and their money was used to lobby Congress for passage of the bill. The law became known as the Comstock Act and Anthony was appointed special agent to the United States Post Office, with the authority to enforce the new law. He held this position for the next 42 years while he successfully prosecuted 3,600 defendants and destroyed over 160 tons of "obscene literature" (Comstock Law of 1873, n.d.).

Mr. Comstock was successful in the prosecution of Margaret Higgins Sanger (1879–1966) and her birth control movement. But Ms. Sanger proved to be a tireless advocate for women and "broke the law" to defend women's reproductive freedom. The Comstock Act would restrict women's reproductive freedom for the next 101 years, that is, until the 1965 ruling of the U.S. Supreme Court, when *Griswold v. Connecticut* struck down the one remaining contraceptive Comstock law in Connecticut and Massachusetts. It was not until 1972 that the case of *Eisenstadt v. Baird* extended the 1965 rule to include unmarried persons as well, and the Comstock Act officially ended.

EARLY YEARS

On September 14, 1879, Margaret Sanger was born in Corning, New York, to Michael and Anne Purcell Higgins who were poor Irish immigrants. She was born sixth of 11 children. Her father was a stonecutter who worked in marble and sculpted statues for gravesites and churches. He was quite a radical and was taken with the writings of Henry George, who published *Progress and Poverty* in 1879, which was a discourse on the inequity of wealth in the United States and proposed a system of fair taxation as solution. The writings of Mr. George were not popular with the local Catholic Church, which owned a large portion of untaxed land in Corning. When Michael invited Mr. George to speak to the town workers, he angered the Church. As a result, the Church stopped providing marble commissions to Michael and it became more difficult to support an already poor family. He had to find work outside of town just to feed his large and growing family. He was an agnostic and had a different philosophy toward religion than his devoutly Catholic wife. The children were not brought up properly in the Church, and when Church members came to visit Anne with food baskets and invite her to attend services, Michael would not accept their assistance and sent them away.

The family could not afford the care of a doctor or midwife and Michael attended his wife during labor and managed the delivery of their infants. As Margaret became older, she was her father's assistant and helped in the births of her younger siblings. She remembered her mother as always either nursing a child or pregnant, while suffering from the debilitating symptoms of tuberculosis. Her mother experienced 18 pregnancies, 11 live births, and 7 spontaneous abortions during her marriage. Anne suffered from tuberculosis with miserable hacking, coughing, and the expectoration of bloody sputum. These symptoms were greatly exacerbated during each of Anne's pregnancies. Margaret cared for her mother in the last year of her life. She took charge of the household and managed four siblings under the age of 14 as well as her father. Anne passed away at the age of 42 from complications of her chronic illness, whereas her father, Margaret noted in her biographies, died at the age of 80. Her mother's multiple pregnancies and chronic health condition had a lasting effect on Margaret's view of women's role in marriage and society. Margaret associated her mother's early death with the toll that 18 pregnancies had taken on her body.

During this time, the major industry in Corning was the manufacture of glass light bulbs for the newly invented electric light developed by Thomas Edison. The owners of the glassworks company had moved from Brooklyn to Corning; they were attracted by the natural resources of water, coal, and sand necessary for glass production. In addition, there was an abundance of poor Irish immigrants and children as young as 12 who were willing to work long hours for low wages. To supplement the family income, Margaret's brothers attended school in the morning and then worked at the glassworks for the rest of the day.

The town was socially and economically divided between the small population of the wealthy, who lived on the hill in large beautiful homes, and the vast majority of the population, who worked in the glass factory and lived at the bottom of the hill in humble, overcrowded dwellings. When

Margaret reflected on her early years in Corning, she recalled that the families living in the poor areas of town had many children, with the women burdened with multiple pregnancies, miscarriages, and children they could ill afford to feed and clothe. In contrast, the wealthy women had few pregnancies, their children were healthy and well dressed, and they lived a social life of comfort and ease.

What did the wealthy and educated women know about reproductive health and methods to prevent pregnancies that the poor women did not? In these early years, unknown to Margaret, her life was to become a journey that would find the answers to this question and ignite the fire for her life-long passion of reproductive health care for women.

Margaret was to begin her education in class differences when she was allowed to attend a private school, Claverack College and Hudson River Institute, a coeducational boarding school, in Hudson, New York. She was a work–study student, and her two older sisters, who were working, provided some tuition assistance. The influence of the school on her developing philosophy was the first important step in educating her to become a future leader in the controversial area of reproductive health. Maggie Higgins, as she was known at the time, entered the world of the wealthy. Her school was housed in a Greek Revival mansion with running water and electricity. The furniture was beautifully made and she spent hours in the large school library where she studied a wide variety of subjects, from art to mathematics. Maggie appeared as the female lead in plays and she began public speaking, often debating women's rights issues of the time. She was learning to think critically about important social and political issues and developing her writing and public-speaking skills.

She absorbed the lifestyle of wealthy New Yorkers and learned how to dress and arrange her hair in a more sophisticated way. Maggie attended teas and dances. One of her classmates, a handsome young man from Long Island, became her first boyfriend. She was forming the foundational social skills and grace required for her future public life when she would influence wealthy donors and intellectual men and women in supporting her yet-unnamed cause. According to Baker (2011), Maggie "emerged as a fun-loving leader, organizing activities and, on more than one occasion, illegal escapades off campus" (p. 25). It was at this early point in her development that she stopped using the name "Maggie" and became Margaret Higgins, the unknown, future visionary of a new radical movement. Because money was scarce and she was needed at home to tend to her dying mother and the care of her siblings, Margaret never graduated from boarding school.

After her mother's death, Margaret rejected the role of surrogate mother to her brothers and father. Because she was an ambitious young woman, she did not want to take on the role of domestic servant, nor was she interested in work as a governess or teacher. Her dream of attending medical school at Cornell University was not possible without the proper undergraduate education, sufficient money for tuition, not to mention the unfortunate circumstance of being a female in a male-dominated profession. New opportunities, however, were opening up for young women in the newly expanding field of nursing.

Hospitals were starting nursing schools based on the principles developed by Florence Nightingale, and Margaret enthusiastically enrolled. In July 1900, she entered a 3-year nurses' training program at the White Plains Hospital in White Plains, New York. She worked on the women's ward and was proficient in gynecological care and the art of midwifery. She learned her nursing skills through apprenticeship on hospital wards and nursing theory from a textbook entitled *Text-Book of Nursing* by Clara Weeks-Shaw, and was lectured to by physicians. The topics of abortion and contraception were missing from her education. The Comstock Act, passed in 1873, was in effect and made the education involving birth control topics and the dissemination of birth control products illegal and subject to fine and imprisonment for anyone who broke the law. It was on the wards of White Plains Hospital that Margaret first heard the disturbing words of women after birth, asking her to tell them the secret of how to prevent more pregnancies. She was to hear these words over and over again throughout her nursing career while caring for obstetrical patients in New York City.

It is during her time as a nursing student that she became ill with weight loss, fevers, and night sweats—she was diagnosed with tuberculosis of the tonsils and lymph glands. She was treated by one of the physicians at the hospital but would bravely fight intermittent flare-ups of this disease for the next 20 years.

In the summer of 1901, she was sent to continue her education at the New York Eye and Ear Infirmary in New York City. It was at this time that she met a handsome young man at a dance, named William Sanger, who fell in love with Margaret. William was a student at Cooper Union, studying to become an architect, while earning a satisfactory salary working as a draftsman. He studied painting in the evenings and, unlike the men of Corning, he was Jewish and an educated, charming member of the Socialist Party. Margaret was intrigued and was very much attracted to this young man, so different from those she had known in her earlier years.

William began a courtship and soon asked Margaret to leave nursing school and become his wife. He made a good case for her to leave the hard work and stress of nursing for a life of intellectual rigor and pleasant living conditions with him. Margaret accepted this charming man's proposal, and in August of 1902, they eloped on one of her 2-hour breaks from her nursing duties. Margaret returned to the ward a married woman but the marriage was kept secret. Nursing students were not allowed to marry and were expected to live on hospital grounds with strict curfews and long hours spent working on the wards. Margaret wrote a letter of resignation to the school and left without completing her nursing education.

She and her new husband moved to the Bronx and began married life, living with his family. Margaret soon found herself pregnant with the unfortunate complication of her tuberculosis symptoms returning. Margaret was sent to the Adirondack Cottage Sanitarium under the direction of Dr. Edward Trudeau who was an expert in the treatment of this disease. She lived in an isolated cottage and followed the recommended dietary restrictions and fresh air regimens that were the state-of-the-art treatment of the time. Margaret returned to New York after about 6 months and her first son, Stuart, was born in what was described as a difficult delivery. Her health was again in jeopardy during the postpartum period and she agreed to return to the sanitarium with her infant and a wet nurse. Breastfeeding was contraindicated for women with tuberculosis as it was believed that the disease could be passed on in the mother's milk. This was a difficult time for Margaret, who spent over a year in treatment. She became depressed and weary of living the life of an invalid. The staff encouraged Margaret in her recovery and her tenacious spirit was revitalized to move forward and reject the invalid role.

She left the sanitarium in remission, and she and her husband built a large home in Hastings-on-Hudson, New York. This was a period of motherhood and middle-class living for Margaret. In her fearless way and against the advice of her physician, she had two more children while remaining healthy and free of disease. Margaret spent her days gardening, taking the children to the playground, and socializing with other mothers. She joined a women's literary group, and they read and discussed literature just as people do in today's book clubs. Margaret was rebellious and grew weary of living a life of middle-class privilege. She began searching for inspiring work and intellectual stimulation. Meanwhile, William changed his career path, resigned his job as an architect and draftsman, and devoted himself to full-time painting. Margaret wanted to move back into the city; the house was put up for sale, and the couple began a new direction in their lives.

THE MAKING OF MARGARET SANGER

In the winter of 1910, the couple and their three children moved to 135th Street on Manhattan's Upper West Side. William spent his time painting in a Greenwich Village studio, working to become an artist. Margaret embarked on two new pathways that would put her career in motion. She joined Branch 5 of the Socialist Party of New York and resumed her nursing work even though she had not completed her nursing diploma.

As a new member of the Socialist Party, she became active in the Committee on Propaganda. She spent time on the streets of New York handing out booklets and newspapers on Socialist ideology and speaking to people, explaining the principles of the movement. Branch 5 was composed of Greenwich Village bohemians who were some of the premier intellectual and radical thinkers of the time, such as Jack Reed, a Harvard graduate and journalist; Bill Haywood, the leader of the Industrial Workers of the World; Emma Goldman, a well-known and early supporter of contraception; Jessie Ashley, a wealthy lawyer who spent her money supporting radical publications and providing bail for her jailed comrades; and Anita and John Block, publishers of the daily Socialist paper, *The New York Call*. It was with these intellectuals that Margaret began to find her voice. The Blocks were impressed with her logical thinking and asked her to speak at meetings and write for a popular column in their paper called "The Women's Page." Always resourceful, Margaret's first lecture was on the social conditions of the day as seen from the perspective of a trained nurse. Gradually, she began to include in her lecture series the dangerous topic of sex education. She wasted no time in taking the opportunity to *challenge the process* by directly writing and publicly speaking on this forbidden topic.

She fearlessly moved on to write and publish in the *New York Call* "What Every Mother Should Know, or How Six Little Children Were Taught the Truth." Margaret urged mothers to teach their children age-appropriate sex information using nature (the birds and the bees) as a metaphor for human physiology. She attended evening gatherings at Mabel Dodge's home on Fifth Avenue. Ms. Dodge was a wealthy intellectual and Jack Reed's lover. At Mabel's evening salons, the group discussed the radical ideas of the day, including the dangers of capitalism and religion, the concern over the government's censorship of art and literature, and the importance of sexual liberation.

During these evening salons, Margaret passionately discussed her ideas on sex education, which was the emerging discipline known as "sexual hygiene." Margaret explained to the group the significance of educating women in methods to prevent pregnancies as well as infections of sexually transmitted diseases, in particular, syphilis and gonorrhea. She shared her views on sexuality as a pleasurable component of human love and not just for the purpose of procreation. She instructed her friends in methods to simulate and prolong sexual enjoyment for personal fulfillment and satisfaction. These Greenwich Village intellectuals of 1912 were engaged in the exploration of "free love" and experimented with alternative relationships, taking multiple sex partners and lovers, or partners and lovers of the same sex. They were the rule breakers who laid the foundation for the Beat Generation of the 1950s and the hippies of the 1960s, who moved into Greenwich Village and espoused the same principles of free love.

Margaret, always a shrewd propagandist, was searching for an alternative to the word *contraception* in order to give her lectures and writings a signature phrase. It was during one of these gatherings at Mabel's apartment that the term *birth control* was conceived (pun intended) and she now had a new name for her evolving work. She educated herself in the important human sexuality literature of the day. Margaret read the works of the English

Malthusians, especially the writings of Havelock Ellis, a renowned sexologist and the author of a group of works entitled *Studies in the Psychology of Sex* and Edward Carpenter's *Love's Coming of Age*. Malthusianism is a philosophy that is grounded in the work of Reverend Thomas Robert Malthus as described in his 1789 book, *An Essay on the Principle of Population*. Reverend Malthus was concerned with the continuous growth of populations and the notion that this growth would not keep pace with the supply of food. He believed that population growth should be restricted by moral restraints such as abstinence, delayed marriage, and limiting marriage among people living in poverty or with mental deficiencies. Population limitation would ensure a sufficient food supply and a strong genetic pool. As a man of religion, the Reverend was not a proponent of artificial means of contraception; he believed in the principle of self-control. English Malthusianism was an outgrowth of this movement. It was composed of people who believed in the importance of population control and the relationship between too many people and a decreasing food supply. As opposed to the Reverend Malthus, however, this group was very interested in the use and development of artificial means of contraception and not in favor of limiting sexual intercourse in an effort to prevent pregnancy.

Simultaneously, as Margaret was expanding her knowledge of sexuality and forming new ideas on reproductive health, she needed to supplement the family income, so she resumed her nursing career. She worked as a public health nurse for the Henry Street Settlement House founded by Lillian Wald (Chapter 9). The Lower East Side of Manhattan had a large and poor immigrant population and was an area targeted by public health nurses. In this dirty and overcrowded environment, the disease of tuberculosis was uncontrolled. Much of the public health nurses' work was dedicated to teaching hygienic practices to the population in an attempt to stop the spread of infection.

Margaret soon became impatient with this work, and, with her usual self-confidence, began her own nursing practice. She focused on obstetrical and gynecological care and delivered babies with the midwifery skills she learned as a nursing student. While attending home visits to these poor women, Margaret would be transported back to the wards of White Plains Hospital. She would hear the same questions again, the pleading voices of women, asking for advice on how to prevent more pregnancies.

It was not uncommon for her to attend gynecological cases in which women suffered from the consequences of abortion, including complications such as excessive bleeding or unresponsive uterine infections. In spite of abortion not being allowed by law, women had information on ways to abort pregnancies even with the knowledge that they risked disastrous outcomes. Women used folk remedies, such as applying hot mustard plaster compresses to the lower abdomen or using over-the-counter herbal preparations, sold in pharmacies or newspapers to "bring on the monthlies." Abortions cost

$5 and were performed by both knowledgeable practitioners, such as mid-wifes and physicians, and untrained local people found in the neighborhood. To save money, poor women used household items to induce self-abortion, such as wire coat hangers, knitting needles, crochet hooks, hairpins, scissors, and buttonhooks (Reagan, 1997).

In the summer of 1912, Margaret was called to care for Sadie Sachs, a young woman recovering from a uterine infection after an abortion. Sadie asked the same question that Margaret had been hearing since nursing school, "How can I prevent any more pregnancies?" The doctor, who attended her, offered the same unsatisfactory and routine answer, telling the young woman to have her husband "sleep on the roof" (Baker, 2011, p. 50). It was illegal for physicians and nurses to provide contraceptive and aborti-facient information to patients as a result of the Comstock Act. In addition, the Act made it illegal to use the U.S. Post Office to send contraceptive equip-ment, such as diaphragms, condoms, or educational materials describing contraceptive methods, through the mail. The special agent in the U.S. Post Office had the authority to not allow distribution of censored materials and to arrest and imprison anyone involved in sending this material.

A few months later, Margaret was called back to Sadie's apartment; she had had another abortion and this time she did not recover. Sadie Sachs, at the age of 28, was dead from complications of septicemia. The death of Sadie and Margaret's inability to prevent this tragic occurrence was a defin-ing moment for Margret. She walked throughout the city that night reflecting on the needs of poor women and the unnecessary death of Sadie. Returning to her apartment defiant, she decided to *challenge the process,* which did not allow reproductive decision making and family limitation to be a choice for women. She would defy and confront the Comstock Act and rebel against religious teaching. She was determined to prevent pregnancies and avoid the practice of illegal abortion. She would become the visionary who would stop women from dying by preventing unwanted pregnancies so no more abortions would be performed; she would be the risk-taker who would give women their reproductive freedom; and she would be the fearless one to dis-tribute birth control education in spite of the Comstock Act. She would use her passionate writing and speaking abilities to *inspire a shared vision* among her intellectual and wealthy friends. Armed with the monetary resources of her liberal Greenwich Village friends, together they would bring important birth control education to the women of New York City. But Margaret would not stop at the local level; she would travel throughout the United States and Europe and make her movement, her birth control movement, accessible to all women.

Contraceptive science had its limitations when Margaret entered the field of birth control education. A survey conducted by Dr. Clelia Mosher on the contraceptive practices of married women of the upper middle class between the years 1892 and 1920 provides insight into the state of the science of the time. Dr. Mosher's qualitative sample size was small ($N = 41$). She asked women to describe the methods of contraception they used during their marriage. Women reported the following in order of the most frequently used method to the least frequent: (a) douche, (b) safe period/rhythm method, (c) withdrawal or coitus interruptus, (d) condoms, (e) cervical caps/diaphragm, (f) suppository jelly or foam powder, (g) abstinence, and (h) no method of pregnancy prevention at all (David & Sanderson, 1986).

Products were advertised in newspapers and pharmacies and sold as health-promotion items to maintain female hygiene. The words "contraceptive" and "birth control" were never used or implied in the product endorsements. Cleanliness was advertised as a virtue, the advertised goal to keep women free of germs with the unsaid words and, it was to be hoped, free of sperm. These products included vaginal jellies, antiseptic douches, suppositories, foaming tablets, and sponges. The bases of the products were antiseptic chemicals, which had no effect on destroying sperm. Nonoxynol-9, an effective spermicide, had not yet been developed.

A common recommendation was for vaginal douching either before or after intercourse with homemade preparations of water with salt or vinegar to maintain feminine hygiene. We know today that neither of these preparations functions as a spermicide. Lysol antiseptic soap was a product actively marketed for women, as a must for female hygiene, with the unstated implications that it was an effective spermicide. The pre-1953 formula contained cresol, a phenol compound reported in some cases to cause inflammation and burning of vaginal tissues. Douching with Lysol was an inexpensive method of birth control that could be purchased over the counter as a hygiene product to assure "dainty feminine allure." Unfortunately, information from a 1920 to 1930 survey shows a very high failure rate for douching as a contraceptive (Pasulka, 2012).

It is interesting to note that the recommendation by health professionals and the Church was for couples to practice the safe period/rhythm method and it was the second most common method reported by the women in this study. Reproductive endocrinology was in its early days of building knowledge and information regarding hormone ebbing and flowing and the actual timing of ovulation was not known until the mid-1930s. This method did not perform well as a contraceptive in the early 1900s because the science of when ovulation occurs was not understood (David & Sanderson, 1986).

Condoms are the oldest method of barrier contraception with evidence of use in ancient Egypt. In 1564, an Italian anatomist, Gabriello Fallopio, made a linen sheath to fit the penis and this was used as protection against syphilis. History claims that he used this application on 1,100 men and all of this population stayed free of the disease (Youssef, 1993). In the memoirs of Casanova, it is noted that he used the condom as a contraceptive with much success. The early condoms were made from the intestines of sheep, calves, and goats. It was not until the development of rubber by Charles Goodyear in 1839 that condoms became more user-friendly; the introduction of latex in the 1930s allowed a stronger product with a longer shelf life. Condoms were marketed as a health promotion product to prevent sexually transmitted diseases (Youssef, 1993).

Cervical caps and diaphragms have a long history as contraceptives. In 1823, a German gynecologist, called Wilde, noticed that women in a particular farming area had only two or three children instead of the usual rates of one pregnancy every 2 years. A midwife in this region had found that putting an object in front of the cervix prevented pregnancy. Wilde took this practice idea and made a wax form of a woman's cervix. From this, he made a rubber cap to fit the cervix perfectly and developed an effective barrier method of contraception. Diaphragms, invented in 1880 by another German physician, were promoted by the Dutch family planning movement. Dr. Aletta Jacobs opened the world's first clinic in Amsterdam in 1882 and introduced the Mensinga diaphragm to the Dutch population. Diaphragms and cervical caps were available and legal in Europe and were effective means of preventing pregnancies; however, a physician was required to properly fit the device (Cervical Caps and Diaphragms, 2010).

Margaret was a strong advocate for the cervical cap and diaphragm as birth control methods but had to overcome a number of obstacles before she could bring this method to the United States. In the fall of 1913, Margaret, William, and their three children moved to Europe, arriving in Liverpool, England. Margaret would educate herself regarding the English and Dutch practices of reliable contraception. Margaret soon became a part of the group of intellectuals who gathered regularly in the Clarion Cafe. Her new friends in Liverpool introduced her to the London Neo-Malthusians, under the leadership of Dr. Charles Vickery Drysdale and his wife, Bessie. One of the activities of this group was to publish a monthly journal entitled *Malthusian*. The journal supported contraceptive practices during sexual intercourse in order to prevent pregnancy, not just the use of abstinence. The Drysdales introduced Margaret to the renowned sexologist Havelock Ellis, whose work she had read back in New York. Margaret found a mentor and like-minded spirit and teacher in her relationship with Mr. Ellis. They became companions and lovers and enjoyed an intense intellectual and sexual relationship. They agreed on the inappropriate role of government and religious censorship of contraception and the banning of literature and products related to the prevention of pregnancy.

Havelock, educated as an anthropologist and scientist, introduced her to the world of sexual literature. She read *Male Continence; or Self-Control in Sexual Intercourse* by John Humphrey Noyes, and *Karezza* by Alice Stockham, in which the male partner satisfies the female and then ejaculates outside of the vagina. Havelock encouraged Margaret to spend time in the reading room of the British Museum library, where she educated herself in statistics and the new field of demographics. She read widely on topics related to reproduction, sexuality, and contraception. Armed with more knowledge, a new project was taking form in Margaret's mind.

The complication to her relationship with Havelock was that they were both married to other people. The troubles of the Sanger marriage were now out in the open. The couple separated and eventually divorced. William moved to Paris to continue studying his painting while Margaret returned to New York with the children. Once settled back in New York, she was ready to start her campaign, which would include writing, speaking, education, and the opening of a birth control clinic for poor women. She was to publish a radical monthly magazine that presented information on ways to prevent pregnancy and educate women, especially poor and working-class women, on sexuality.

PUBLIC SERVICE AND PROGRESS IN BIRTH CONTROL

Margaret was a resourceful woman who was not concerned that she had no money to finance her birth control project. According to Baker (2011), "She made a list of possible subscribers, found sponsors, pleaded for loans from friends, and asked for grants from a special fund of the Free Speech League, set up by the University of Pennsylvania-trained physician, Dr. Edward Bliss Foote" (p. 75). She worked very hard and raised the funds to start her publication.

In March 1914, the first edition of *The Woman Rebel*, covered in brown wrapping paper, was available on the streets of New York for 10 cents per copy and sent via the mail. The U.S. Post Office was monitoring the publication and stopped its delivery. In August of 1914, Margaret was served a warrant by the Post Office inspector for violation of four counts of the Comstock Act. She was arrested and indicted for sending birth control information through the mail. Margaret posted bail, thus making the decision not to go to jail. She left the country through Canada, returned to Liverpool, and toured the Netherlands for the next year.

She traveled to the clinic of Dr. Johannes Rutgers at The Hague, who was a socialist and member of the Dutch Neo-Malthusian League. She was instructed in the anatomical variations in women's pelvic structures and learned to measure and fit cervical caps and diaphragms. She toured clinics throughout the country and was impressed by the attention and instruction given to women regarding contraceptive use and the successful practice of this model of contraceptive care. This was the model she would use for her new clinic. She decided it was time for her to go home and face the consequences of the Comstock Act violations. Being Margaret, however, she smuggled diaphragms and cervical caps on board the ship as she traveled back to the United States. Shortly after her return, her young daughter Peggy came down with a virulent form of pneumonia and died from the infection.

Public support was with the grieving mother and the prosecutor decided to drop the old Comstock Act charges against her. Margaret proceeded with her plan and opened the first birth control clinic in Brooklyn, New York, on October

16, 1916. She modeled the way with her premier hygienic and private clinic for women in New York. The purpose of this quiet space was for women to learn from trained nurses about their own reproductive physiology and safe methods of family limitation. She set high standards for this clinic based on her time visiting and learning from excellent clinics in the Netherlands. This singular clinic was the practice model for clinics that she would eventually open throughout the country. A report of the event appeared in the March 1917 edition of *The Birth Control Review*. The staff consisted of four women: Margaret; her sister, Ethel Bryne, a trained nurse; Miss Fania Mindell, the clinic interpreter, who spoke English, Yiddish, and Italian; and the receptionist, Miss Elizabeth Stuyvesant. Weeks before the clinic opened, the women had flyers made in three languages, including English, Yiddish, and Italian, and walked from building to building in the neighborhood, handing out invitations that read:

Mothers!
Can you afford to have a large family?
Do you want any more children?
If not, why do you have them?
Do not kill, do not take life, but prevent.
Safe, harmless information can be obtained of trained nurses
at 46 Amboy Street, Near Pitkis Ave., Brooklyn
Tell your friends and neighbors. All mothers welcome.
A registration fee of 10 cents entitles any mother to
this information. (Stuyvesant, 1917, pp. 6–7)

The first day the clinic opened with 45 mothers, along with their children, waiting in line to learn about pregnancy prevention. The clinic consisted of two rooms, the first for the collection of demographic information regarding the woman's name, religion, address, nationality, number of children, and husband's trade and salary. The second room was for instruction in douching and diaphragm fittings. Margaret reported that she and her sister Ethel fitted 488 women with diaphragms in the first 10 days of the clinic's operations (Cervical Caps and Diaphragms, 2010). The terms *diaphragm* and *pessary* seem to have been used interchangeably. The pessary was available at pharmacies and the indication for their use was for support of the pelvic floor and for reducing the discomfort caused by various stages of uterine prolapse. An advantage of the pessary was that it covered the cervical os, or opening to the uterus, thus preventing sperm from entering the uterus and fertilizing an egg. By using this barrier method of birth control, a pregnancy could be prevented (Cervical Caps and Diaphragms, 2010).

Within 10 days of its opening, the clinic was closed down by the police and the women arrested, charged with violating the New York Penal Code for opening a clinic and providing unlawful information in violation of the state's obscenity laws. Margaret was released on $500 bail, which was paid by her supporters. She used the occasion to keep her birth control movement in the press and in front of the public. She was an attractive and interesting woman to interview and always made time to speak with journalists or the public regarding the rights of women and reproductive freedom. She told the press that she would not be stopped and she would reopen her birth control clinic (Baker, 2011).

The Brownsville trial began on January 29, 1917, in the Kings County Courthouse. Margaret was found guilty, but the panel of judges offered a deal to her attorney. If she would stop all of her activities regarding birth control, her sentence would be suspended. She would not be fined $5,000 and she would not be sent to jail for 30 days. The court wanted the case to be resolved quietly and did not want any more publicity and public sympathy for Margaret and her birth control movement. It was not possible for Margaret Sanger to stop her passionate life's work. Margaret chose jail and was sent to the Queens County Penitentiary. Her time in jail only made her more renowned among her supporters and won her new public support. Now the hero who had sacrificed for the cause, she was in demand to speak at lunches and organizations, and her birth control movement received positive publicity.

MAJOR ACCOMPLISHMENTS

After her trial, Margaret was more determined than ever to continue her fight. She energetically planned a new publication to educate and change the opinions of Americans regarding contraception. Her publication was boldly entitled *The Birth Control Review* and it became available to the public in February 1917. Margaret was the editor, a role she held until 1928. Her strategy was to educate and make people aware of the use of safe and effective methods of birth control. She spent the next 40 years of her life working toward this achievement.

In 1921, Margaret organized the first American Birth Control Conference in New York City under the newly formed national organization, the American Birth Control League. Archbishop Hayes used his influence with the police to close the meeting. The public and press came to support her, expressing their concerns over the violation of her First Amendment rights and too much power being imposed by the Catholic Church. In 1922, the first birth control world tour was established, with Margaret attending conferences held in Japan, China, and Hawaii.

Margaret next opened birth control clinics across the country, using the Crane exception as her legal justification to do so. Judge Frederick E. Crane ruled that if the Comstock Act prevented a licensed physician from taking proper care of patients, then the law was unconstitutional. He further stated that the law did not allow physicians to provide immoral advice to their patients. The law did, however, allow a physician to provide contraceptive advice to a married patient for the medical purpose of preventing or curing disease. By 1937, there were 377 birth control clinics across the country with physicians at the head of the organization using the Crane exception ruling (Net Industries and its Licensors, 2014).

In 1923, Sanger founded the Clinical Research Bureau of the American Birth Control League and had the physicians in her clinics keep demographic records and conduct research on birth control methods. In 1925, she organized the International Birth Control Conference in New York City. A thousand delegates from 18 countries attended this conference and heard 150 experts in the field presenting scientific papers and research reports on new findings in the field of human reproduction.

In 1923, Margaret and her second husband, millionaire Noah Slee, illegally imported diaphragms from Germany, the Netherlands, and Japan. In 1932, Margaret had a Japanese manufacturer send a package of diaphragms to a supportive New York physician. The U.S. Customs authorities confiscated the package. Margaret filed a lawsuit and, in 1936, the court case, the *United States v. One Package of Japanese Pessaries*, was heard. A federal appellate court ruled that the package could be delivered and that the government could not interfere with a physician in the treatment of his patient (David & Sanderson, 1986). This ruling was another small step in the developing judicial debate stating that the law cannot interfere with the physician–patient relationship and a physician's recommendations for treatment or prevention of disease.

In 1950, Margaret renewed her friendship with Katherine McCormick, a wealthy woman and heir to the vast International Harvester fortune. Katherine was interested in birth control and wanted to know where the greatest financial need was and what the current state of birth control research was. Margaret knew that financial support was needed for research. Together, the women reviewed the major research projects that were being conducted and selected the work of an obscure researcher in Massachusetts, Dr. Gregory Pincus. His work focused on mammalian eggs and sperm and the effects of the hormone progesterone, in mediating the physiological process of conception. The women wanted him to develop a safe and easy-to-take pill that would interfere with conception and function as a highly effective contraceptive. After conversations with Pincus, the women endorsed his research and Katherine provided him with $10,000 in start-up funding, followed by $150,000 for the remainder of the first year. By 1967, Dr. Pincus had received $2 million from Katherine and additional money was left to him in her will. Another researcher, Dr. John Rock, started human trials using progesterone to strop ovulation. He was the first to demonstrate anovulatory cycles in his study sample. Katherine McCormick provided financial support for both men's research. She and Margaret wanted an oral contraceptive developed and they wanted it quickly. In 1955, Margaret convinced Dr. Pincus to present his paper demonstrating the anovulatory effects of progesterone at an international conference in Tokyo. In 1957, the pharmaceutical company Searle applied for a license based on Pincus's trial with 897 women. As a result, the first-generation oral contraceptive, Enovid, was ready for the market. Margaret saw her dream, held since the 1930s, become a reality.

For her entire career, Margaret Sanger provided exemplary leadership in the struggle for women's reproductive health. She made her last public appearance in New Delhi in 1959 at the International Planned Parenthood Federation Conference. She was tired and ill, having had two heart attacks and gallbladder surgery, and had been experiencing signs of dementia since the late 1950s. She returned to Tucson, where she had a home near her son and his wife. Leukemia was diagnosed in 1962, which further weakened an already battle-weary woman. Her family decided to place her in a nursing home in July of 1962, where she lived out the remainder of her life. Margaret Sanger passed away on September 16, 1966.

On October 16, 1916, Margaret Sanger *modeled the way* when she opened the first birth control clinic in the United States in Brooklyn, New York. She established this clinic based on the standards of care she observed while visiting clinics in the Netherlands and learning accurate methods of fitting diaphragms from physicians. The clinic was closed by police within 10 days, but it became the prototype for future clinics, which she would open once she was legally free to do so. Margaret's opportunity came with her stunning victory in 1936, of the case of the *United States v. One Package of Japanese Pessaries*. Judge Crane ruled that the law could no longer interfere with the patient–physician relationship and health promotion recommendations. Margaret used the patient–physician ruling as a rationale for reopening birth control clinics. She accomplished this by hiring physicians for her clinics who would provide reproductive health care and education to women. Her organization was named the American Birth Control League and, in 1942, was renamed Planned Parenthood. This name is still in use today.

Margaret Sanger left behind a vigorous legacy of reproductive health care. There are now more than 700 Planned Parenthood clinics, which provide services to 2.7 million people annually in the United States (Planned Parenthood, 2015). She began her life as a poor girl whose heart was unsettled seeing her mother's generation of women suffering endless pregnancies, miscarriages, and death from septic abortions while being encumbered with too many children. She lived a full and accomplished life, working tirelessly for reproductive freedom for women. She *encouraged the hearts* of the brave women who attended her first birth control clinic by showing them they could do this; they could practice birth control. For the next 40 years, Margaret continued to *encourage the hearts* of women across the country as she strived for safe, legal, and effective birth control.

TIMELINE

- September 14, 1879—Margaret Sanger is born, the sixth of 11 children, to Michael and Anne Higgins, a poor, Irish immigrant family in Corning, New York.
- September 1895–1898—Attends Claverack College and Hudson River Institute, a coeducational boarding school, Hudson, New York, as a work–study student.
- July 1, 1900—Starts a 3-year nurses' training program at the White Plains Hospital, White Plains, New York; Margaret works on the women's ward and is proficient in gynecological and midwifery care.
- 1901—Diagnosed with tuberculosis during her nurses' training program.
- August 1902—Marries William Sanger, architect and artist, during a 2-hour break from her nursing duties; nurses in training are not allowed to marry and she resigns from the program before completing her nursing diploma.
- 1903—Reactivation of tuberculosis causes her to spend 6 months at the Adirondack Cottage Sanitarium.
- 1903—First son, Stuart, is born.
- 1903–1904—Tuberculosis is reactivated after her son's birth; returns to the sanitarium with her infant and wet nurse and stays for over a year.
- July 1908—Second son, Grant, is born.
- May 1910—Third child, a daughter, Margaret, known as Peggy, is born.
- Winter 1910—The Sanger family moves from Hastings-on-Hudson to New York City.
- Spring 1911–1912—Joins Branch 5 of the Socialist Party of New York; begins writing for the New York Call, a Socialist newspaper; writes "What Every Mother Should Know, or How Six Little Children Were Taught the Truth" and "What Every Girl Should Know"; restarts her nursing career.
- 1912—Sadie Sachs dies from septicemia—a defining event for Margaret.
- 1912—The term birth control originates.
- September 1913—Sanger family moves to Europe; William paints and Margaret studies European methods of contraception; Margaret and William separate; he stays in Paris; she returns to Greenwich Village.
- March 1914—Margaret's first 8-page publication entitled The Woman Rebel is distributed, covered in brown wrapper and purchased on the streets of New York, where it is sold for 10 cents.
- August 1914—Is served a warrant by the Post Office inspector for violation of four counts of the Comstock Laws; she is arrested and indicted for sending birth control information through the U.S. mail.
- February 1915—Flees the country rather than stand trial; crosses the English Channel and goes to the Netherlands; learns to fit cervical caps from Dr. Johannes Rutgers, a Socialist and member of the Dutch Neo-Malthusian League; visits birth control clinics throughout the Netherlands and designs future clinics on this model.

- 1915—Returns to New York to face trial but has public support when her daughter, Peggy, dies and the charges are dropped.
- October 16, 1916—Opens the first birth control clinic in Brownsville, Brooklyn, and is arrested after 10 days of operation; spends 30 days in jail.
- March 1917—Publishes first edition of *The Birth Control Review*.
- 1921—Organizes first American Birth Control Conference in New York City; Archbishop Hayes uses influence with police to close the meeting; press and public come to her defense.
- 1922—First birth control world tour takes place with conferences in Japan, China, and Hawaii.
- 1923—Founds the Clinical Research Bureau of the American Birth Control League; marries millionaire J. Noah Slee.
- 1925—Organizes International Birth Control Conference in New York City.
- 1931—New York Academy of Medicine passes resolution to support birth control.
- 1932—Diaphragms are mailed from Japan to a supportive doctor in New York City; U.S. Customs confiscates the illegal contraceptives; Sanger files a lawsuit, *United States v. One Package of Japanese Pessaries*.
- 1935–1936—Travels to India, China, and Hawaii with Edith How-Martyn, honorary director of the Birth Control International Movement in London; together they establish 50 birth control teaching centers.
- 1936—*United States v. One Package of Japanese Pessaries* is settled; the U.S. Circuit Court of Appeals rules that it is legal to import contraceptives and that the government cannot interfere with a doctor providing contraceptives to patients.
- 1937—American Medical Association endorses birth control.
- 1948—Organized Cheltenham Congress on World Population and World Resources in Relation to Family.
- 1950–1951—Margaret, together with wealthy friend Katherine McCormick, reviews current research on hormones and the prevention of ovulation.
- 1952—International Planned Parenthood Federation is founded.
- 1953—Ms. McCormick, with input from Margaret, provides financial support to Drs. Gregory Pincus and John Rock for the development of the first oral contraceptive.
- 1959—American Public Health Association endorses birth control.
- 1959—Margaret moves to Tucson and retires from public life.
- 1965—The U.S. Supreme Court decides the case *Griswold v. Connecticut*, strikes down the remaining Comstock Laws in Connecticut and Massachusetts, but only for married relationships.
- September 6, 1966—Margaret dies at the age of 86, having battled mental confusion and dementia since the mid-1950s and a leukemia diagnosis, which occurred in 1962.

- 1972—*Eisenstadt v. Baird* extends the 1965 Comstock ruling to include nonmarried couples; after 101 years, the Comstock Act is ended; the United States issues a postage stamp honoring family planning (at the beginning of this chapter).

QUESTIONS FOR DISCUSSION

1. Margaret Higgins Sanger *challenged the process* by fighting for women's access to reproductive health care. In what ways has the leadership of Planned Parenthood continued this fight and enlarged the scope of women's health care?
2. On October 16, 1916, Margaret Sanger *challenged the process* by opening the first birth control clinic in Brooklyn, New York. What are some of the differences and similarities between the services offered at that first clinic and the current clinic services offered by Planned Parenthood?
3. Identify the major strengths of Margaret Sanger's leadership skills that enabled her to cultivate a national and international birth control movement. Think about the age-old question: Are leaders born or made, or perhaps a little of both?

REFERENCES

Baker, J. H. (2011). *Margaret Sanger: A life of passion*. New York, NY: Hill and Wang.

Cervical Caps and Diaphragms. (2010). *Highlights of the Percy Skuy history of contraceptive gallery*. Cleveland, OH: Case Western Reserve University. Retrieved from http://www.case.edu/affil/skuyhistcontraception/online-2012/Cervical-Caps-Diaphragms.html

Comstock Law of 1873. (n.d.). In *West's encyclopedia of American Law* (2nd ed.). St. Paul, MN: West Publishing Company. Retrieved from http://legal-dictionary.thefreedictionary.com/Comstock+Law+of+1873

David, P., & Sanderson, W. (1986). Rudimentary contraceptive methods and the American transition to marital fertility control, 1855–1915. In S. L. Engerman & R. E. Gallman (Eds.), *Long-term factors in American economic growth* (pp. 307–390). Chicago, IL: University of Chicago Press. Retrieved from http://www.nber.org/chapters/c9685

Malthus, R. T. (2014). In *Wikipedia. The free encyclopedia*. Retrieved from http://en.wikipedia.org/wiki/Thomas_Robert_Malthus

Net Industries and its Licensors. (2014). *New York Sanger: The door is opened: Civilly disobedient*. Retrieved from http://law.jrank.org/pages/24655/New-York-v-Sanger-Door-Opened.html

Pasulka, N. (2012). *When women used Lysol as birth control: A look back at shocking ads for the popular, dangerous, and ineffective antiseptic douche*. Retrieved from http://www.motherjones.com/slideshows/2012/02/when-women-used-lysol-birth-control/lysol-douche-cobweb

Planned Parenthood. (2015). *Planned Parenthood at a glance*. Retrieved from https://www.plannedparenthood.org/about-us/who-we-are/planned-parenthood-at-a-glance

Reagan, L. J. (1997). *When abortion was a crime: Women, medicine, and law in the United States, 1867–1973*. Berkeley, CA: University of California Press. Retrieved from http://ark.cdlib.org/ark:/13030/ft967nb5z5/

Sanger, M. (1917). Shall we break this law? *Birth Control Review, 1*(1), 4. Retrieved from http://babel.hathitrust.org/cgi/pt?id=hvd.hnp3k3;view=1up;seq=10

Stuyvesant, E. (1917). The Brownsville birth control clinic. *The birth control review: Dedicated to the principle of intelligent and voluntary motherhood* (Vol. 1, pp. 4, 6–7). New York, NY: Da Capo Press. Retrieved from http://babel.hathitrust.org/cgi/pt?id=hvd.hnp3k3;view=1up;seq=23

Youssef, H. (1993). The history of the condom. *Journal of the Royal Society of Medicine, 86*(4), 226–228. Retrieved from http://www.ncbi.nlm.nih.gov/pmc/articles/PMC1293956/

FURTHER READING

Coigney, V. (1969). *Margaret Sanger: Rebel with a cause*. Garden City, NY: Doubleday.

Eig, J. (2014). *The birth of the pill: How four pioneers reinvented sex and launched a revolution*. New York, NY: Macmillian/W. W. Norton.

Kouzes, J. M., & Posner, B. Z. (2011). *The five practices of exemplary leadership: Government*. Hoboken, NJ: John Wiley & Sons.

Murphree, V., & Gower, K. K. (2013). Making birth control respectable: The birth control review, 1917–1928. *American Journalism, 30*(2), 210–234. doi: 10.1080/08821127.2013.788464

Sanger, M. (2004). *The autobiography of Margaret Sanger*. Mineloa, NY: Dover Publications. (Original work published 1938)

Suitters, B. (1968). Contraception in ancient and modern society. *Royal Society of Health Journal, 88*(1), 9–11.

Sister Elizabeth Kenny: Conviction and Controversy

Mary Kamienski

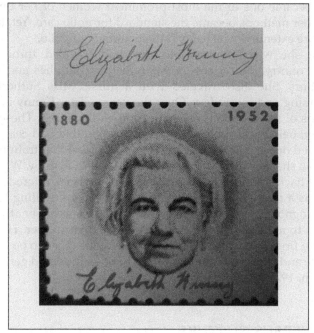

Sister Elizabeth Kenny 1952 "Fight Against Polio" seal, issued in 1952.

"I want them rags that wells my legs."
—E. Kenny and M. Ostenso

• • • • •

These words were uttered by a young child who was stricken with polio and treated using the Elizabeth Kenny method. Elizabeth Kenny (1880–1952) was a remarkable woman who challenged the entire medical community as well as the social customs of her time. She was an Australian bush nurse with a vision, or perhaps an obsession about the care and treatment of poliomyelitis victims. She became world famous for her innovative approach to the treatment of these patients. Although she was well loved and respected by patients and families, her approach to treating polio patients was contrary to the medical community's beliefs and she battled much resistance to advance her methods. In spite of this, she persevered throughout her entire career in teaching what would eventually become known as the "Kenny method." In doing so, she achieved great success in preventing deformity and paralysis in children, as well as adults, who were stricken with this devastating disease.

In spite of the fact that Sister Kenny was never a licensed nurse, she eventually became one of the most prominent women of her time. By the mid-1940s, her methods became the standard for polio care. Yet, her impact on health care extended well beyond the treatment of polio.

Before she was 30 years old, she had traveled throughout the Australian countryside for several years helping families and caring for sick neighbors. She also traveled with a nurse, Miss Sutherland, and learned nursing and midwifery. Over the years, Sister Kenny offered several versions of stories about her education and training. These included a story about being educated in a private hospital that had ceased to exist or had burned down. She admitted to one individual that training was too expensive, so she went into nursing with a friend in Sydney. Whatever her educational background and despite her apparent lack of credentials, her reputation as a nurse began to grow. She was always willing to try even when the prognosis for her patients was poor. She was never afraid to give her opinion to a physician, or anyone else for that matter. Her patients always came first. She was considered by her colleagues to be a good and caring nurse and she was remembered for her beautiful and gentle nursing hands (Cohn, 1975, p. 60).

NATURE VERSUS NURTURE

Nature versus nurture is not a question often used when discussing leadership. Are good leaders born or can they be taught and developed over time with experience? A look at Sister Elizabeth Kenny's early life suggests she was born with strong characteristics that would lead to success in her career. The circumstances of her early life, however, definitely played a role in creating this nurse leader who challenged the medical establishment in many areas, the most prominent being the treatment of polio.

Elizabeth Kenny was born of Irish immigrants who came to Australia as a last resort after losing their home owing to the fact that her great-grandfather guaranteed a loan for a friend who later defaulted (Cohn, 1975). Her great-grandfather Richard Pearson was from County Donegal and he headed for Australia in 1841 with his wife and children in tow. One of his daughters, Elizabeth, later became Sister Kenny's maternal grandmother (Yoder, 1942).

The Kenny family name is Gaelic for "sprung from fire" (Cohn, 1975, p. 14). Those who knew Elizabeth Kenny would attest to the fact that she seemed to have a fire burning inside that allowed her to accomplish great things. The Kenny family clan lived in County Kilkenny, where the Kilkenny men had a fierce reputation for being independent. They were described as being contentious and contrary (Cohn, 1975).

Bravery, courage, and a fiery spirit were integral parts of Sister Kenny's personality. Her father, Michael, was born in Ireland. He was a farmer until age 27, when he took advantage of an unexpected opportunity to immigrate to Australia. When Michael Kenny met Mary Moore, daughter of Jim Moore and Elizabeth Pearson Moore, they married and moved onto a new home-stead. Michael later moved his family many times and finally settled outside the town of Warialda where Elizabeth was born on September 20, 1880. She was the fifth child although an earlier sibling, the "first" Elizabeth had died of bronchial pneumonia prior to Eliza's birth (Cohn, 1975).

Over the years, the family moved many more times, and five more children were born to the Kennys. Elizabeth was rarely called by her given name. Her family called her Liza or Eliza (Cohn, 1975). She had traits of her father and became a wanderer at a very young age (Cohn, 1975). Her mother had to tie her to a stump at the early age of 9 months to keep her safe. When she was 4, she tried to fly. When she fell, she seemed to have learned a lesson for a time (Cohn, 1975). Eliza and her sister Julia wandered about and saw the Aboriginal corroboree, a festival of the Aborigines, who are also famous wanderers (at the time, the term "Abos" was frequently used and the term "Aborigine" was also used; Cohn, 1975). In spite of her fear of being captured by these "Abos," she continued to explore her world.

The Kennys were very poor and the girls' dolls were usually dressed-up bottles or rags. When one of the dolls developed pneumonia, Eliza decided the dolls needed a hospital. She organized her first hospital and put poultices on her doll "patients" (Cohn, 1975).

Eliza's interest in and knowledge of human anatomy was piqued when she was a child and fell and broke her arm. She stayed with Dr. Aenas McConnell, who treated the complex fracture in his home. He had a wonder-ful library that contained a skeleton. She played with the skeleton for hours and learned how to trace muscle from origin to insertion. Dr. McConnell became a lifelong mentor and friend to Eliza (Cohn, 1975).

Shortly after her long recovery, Eliza asked Dr. McConnell how to help her brother Willy improve his physique, which she considered skinny and frail. He prescribed a program of calisthenics, which Eliza supervised. Eventually, Willy was able to isolate his principal muscles through voluntary contraction and he developed biceps so well defined they looked like fruit (Cohn, 1975). So, in spite of her lack of a formal education, Eliza had become very knowledgeable about the actions of muscles.

THE VISION

Although Eliza was never formally trained as a nurse, in 1911 she decided to ride her horse into the outback and treat those in need. There is no mention anywhere regarding her desire to be a nurse. She was, however, always eager to reach out and help wherever there was a need. There were few physicians in the area. Sister Kenny was self-appointed and she did not bother to apply for a formal nursing job, as she did not have the required qualifications. The need for health care in the bush was so great that many were not concerned that she did not have a certificate to practice nursing and many did not even know what a "certificate" was (Cohn, 1975). They were simply grateful to have someone to care for them.

Elizabeth's decision to join the military in 1915 was instrumental in enhancing her reputation as a legitimate nurse. She did not have the credentials necessary to join the Australian Army Nursing Service. She did obtain references and testimonials from her long-time mentor, Dr. Aneas John McDonnell. He stated she was a capable nurse, but even this this did not get her into the military. As usual, Elizabeth was unstoppable. She simply boarded a ship and sailed to England where she found a bed in a nurses' club. She reported for duty to a general who ordered her to France for special duty (Cohn, 1975). After this, she was to help transport Australian casualties back home. There is controversy over exactly how this happened. There are no records indicating anything about her training or licensure as a nurse. At the time, there were ships full of severely wounded soldiers and sick civilians being returned home. Elizabeth was popularly known as "Eliza" and wore the drab gray nurse's uniform and a cape with a red lining. She watched; she learned. She became officially known as "staff nurse Kenny."

Her next assignment was on a "dark" ship carrying 600 wounded and sick Australians (Cohn, 1975; Fairley, 2008; Rogers, 2014). Dark ships sailed with no lights in order to avoid submarine attacks. It was during this 4-week journey that she performed another of her "muscle miracles" (McKinnon, 1935). A soldier had been shot through both shoulders and was completely paralyzed in his arms; yet he was able to walk off the ship in Melbourne carrying his own pack. He credited a nursing sister with working with him in "reeducating" his muscles. The nursing sister was Elizabeth Kenny. That soldier later returned and reenlisted.

In 1916, Elizabeth was promoted from staff nurse to sister, which was equivalent to first lieutenant (Cohn, 1975). She used this title for the rest of her life. She continued to serve in many areas both on board ships and in Australian hospitals. During these assignments, she remembered the first polio patients she encountered in 1911 when she started her career as a bush nurse (Cohn, 1974). She started to watch the meningitis patients who moved through the acute phase of the disease but continued to remain paralyzed and deformed. She had only a vague knowledge of meningitis, but she did know about muscle rehabilitation. It was reported that she made the men think about their muscles and got them up and walking. She worked hard to position and reposition her patients at regular intervals (Cohn, 1975; Rogers, 2014). She was convinced of the need to reeducate both the mind and the muscles.

Sister Kenny served more time in danger zones that any other nurse of her time. In 1918, the influenza epidemic was rampant. All measures to treat these patients were futile and the men on board ships died. At one point, she and another nurse were left to care for 500 ill and wounded patients. After this ordeal, she was given a furlough and the armistice was signed. But she remained in the military and became a head nurse in a hospital in Brisbane.

When she became ill in 1919, Kenny was discharged with a pension. She had been diagnosed with pericarditis and was told that she had a short time to live. When given this prognosis, she got up out of bed, dressed, and said, "If I only have a short time to live, I better get busy" (Cohn, 1975, p. 64).

This prognosis led her to seek advice about her condition from a specialist in Stuttgart. She traveled to Ireland first, where her Catholic relatives convinced her to travel to Lourdes, where she spent 6 weeks. Later she saw the specialist who had nothing to offer, so she returned home. She had now used 4 months of her "allotted" time. She still suffered from poor health but was determined to return to work.

Sister Elizabeth started working with a young girl who had cerebral palsy. Working with this child, using her muscle-training regimen, brought her serious criticism from physicians. The child progressed and was finally able to walk. Dr. McDonnell agreed the child had improved and encouraged Eliza to continue her treatments with warm water and massage. She worked with this child for 3 1/2 years until she could walk with a stick, ride horseback, and write letters. To some, her walking looked like painful hobbling, but to those who knew the child before the treatments, it was a miracle. Eliza continued her country nursing during these years. As a rule, she took no money because she had her war pension.

COMMITMENT TO THE VISION

Sister Kenny's passion was her work. She knew how to stir controversy and was expert at using the politics of medicine through the media to challenge the establishment. Elizabeth Kenny spent her entire life challenging the process. She battled mostly with men and appeared to enjoy these encounters. On more than one occasion, she stated, "I won't let any man boss me" (Cohn, 1975, p. 100). She embraced chances to question the status quo and to think creatively. She had the ability to learn quickly through observation and her experiences. Although nurses were expected to show deference to physicians, Eliza's style was in direct opposition to this practice. She was quick to question the expertise of any physician.

Elizabeth Kenny was never naïve about the need to use influence in order to change the care for polio victims in Australia and in the United States. She was determined to eradicate what she referred to as an attitude of medical laissez-faire.

Elizabeth Kenny became famous for her contentious nature. She simply did not back down. On one occasion, a physician wanted to operate on a child for appendicitis in the hospital where Elizabeth was working, an old, one-story wooden house. She advised the physician that she did not believe the diagnosis was accurate. When the doctor replied, "Who are you to say?" she responded by telling him, "I'm sorry. This is my hospital" (Cohn, 1975, p. 49). She refused to prepare for the surgery. She felt that if the child died, she would be responsible. Believing this physician incompetent, she had the child transferred for treatment by her mentor, Dr. McDonnell. The child did not have appendicitis (Cohn, 1975).

BEYOND POLIO

In 1926, Sister Kenny was called to care for a severely injured child named Sylvia and was to accompany Sylvia on the trip to the hospital. The Nobby motor ambulance had been engaged to make the 30-mile trip to the Toowoomba hospital. As a military nurse, Sister Kenny had witnessed the death of many soldiers while being transported over rough terrain. When the Nobby ambulance arrived and prepared to transport this child on a canvas stretcher, Elizabeth said she wanted to use her own stretcher. Eliza's creativity and imagination allowed her to adapt to the situation. She had a heavy door removed from a linen cupboard and placed the child on this door. She immobilized Sylvia with strips of sheeting and packed hot water bottles around her to reduce shock. The child fell asleep within a few miles and they continued on until they were about 7 miles from their destination where they were involved in a head-on collision with an oncoming vehicle. Although Sister Kenny injured her shoulder in this crash, the child was not hurt. When the child recovered completely after 6 weeks, Dr. McDonnell was impressed and stated, "I think you saved your patient's life" (Cohn, 1975, p. 78). He suggested that Sister Kenny get a patent for her stretcher.

She immediately drew up a design of this stretcher and had a friend's son build a full-size version. Her completed invention had a firm base to keep the spine straight, coil springs, a mattress, a canopy, hot water containers, and rubber-tired wheels. She called it the "Sylvia" stretcher. It was patented and manufactured, but total sales were only 30 after more than a year's efforts to market the invention. She firmly believed, however, that her stretcher was effective and offered the best care for transporting sick and injured patients. She refused to take it off the market. By 1930, the stretchers were in general use throughout Australia, although many ambulance companies found them to be large and cumbersome. Eliza continued to collect her self-negotiated guaranteed fee from the manufacturers. Between this fee and her military pension, she had gained some financial security and much experience in living, selling, arguing, and cajoling. This experience served her well as her career continued on its path, focusing more and more on the care and treatment of patients with polio.

Sister Kenny relied heavily on intuition, coupled with science, to develop her ideas about effective treatment for polio victims, as well as in her other endeavors. Her creation of the Sylvia stretcher, the first backboard for transport, stemmed from her understanding of the physiological stress placed on the body of a trauma victim and the need to immobilize the patient during transportation.

SOCIETAL VALUES

Eliza's inability to conform to public opinion was not restricted to her nursing career. She was proud of her physical size and strength. She disregarded the belief that it is vulgar for women to be robust and that they should be lady-like and delicate (Rogers, 2014). In the early 1900s, Australian women did not leave home unless they married. As a spinster, Elizabeth was expected to remain home and care for her mother. Not so Eliza! She believed nursing was her destiny (Cohn, 1975; Rogers, 2014).

In an effort to conform to societal values, she told several people that she had a relationship with a man named "Dan." She saw him often and told him she would marry him after she finished her preparations to become a nurse. He wanted her to give up this notion and pressured her to get married. On the last occasion of their courtship, they were preparing to go to a picnic and a dance. A young boy approached her frantically and said his father was away and his mother was about to have a baby. Dan objected, but Eliza was determined to help. He forced her to choose between marriage to him or her vocation. For Eliza, there was no option, no choice. She rode off with the young boy and never looked back (Cohn, 1975).

With Eliza so involved in other activities, her mother, Mary Kenny, became lonely. Eliza heard of an 8-year-old girl from a broken home. The child was named Mary Stewart and she was placed for adoption or a foster home. Eliza made the arrangements, and in 1925, formally adopted her. This was a rare event for a single woman. She now legally had a daughter. Perhaps it was a calculated move as the child remained with Eliza's mother, Mary, to keep her company while Eliza traveled around the countryside on Country Women's Association affairs and bush nursing. As little Mary Stewart grew, she later traveled with Sister Kenny and was an active part of Eliza's polio work.

NOT A NURSE

Registration for nursing became official in New South Wales in 1906 and in Queensland in 1912. There is no evidence that Sister Kenny ever applied to be "grandfathered" as a licensed nurse and she joined no nursing associations. So how did she become a recognized uniformed nurse? It appears she commissioned a tailor to make her a nurse's outfit. She had a red silk Nightingale cape worn beneath a longer cape of dark velvet. She wore a white uniform with a white belt and a dark velvet nurse's cap with a stiff crown. She put this on and just became "nurse" Kenny. She displayed confidence and determination. She looked like a nurse, she acted like a nurse—she literally became a nurse. Throughout her career, her education and qualifications were questioned, but she rarely responded to any questions about her early years.

Sister Kenny met her first polio patient in 1911. A 2-year-old named Amy was unable to move and her body was twisted. The child was whimpering in great pain. Eliza did not know what was wrong. She was unable to straighten Amy's legs. She prayed and waited for an answer from the doctor. During that night, two more children several miles away became ill and could not stand or walk. The physician finally answered with the message that the children had infantile paralysis. She was told there was no treatment and to do the best she could to treat the symptoms. Eliza was devastated. After much prayer and contemplation, she decided to treat the contracted muscles that appeared shortened and tightened with hot packs (Cohn, 1975).

Within a week, there was a polio epidemic afflicting six of the 20 children in the district. Eliza went from house to house putting hot poultices on the children's painful arms and legs. In each case, after a few days, the pain subsided and Eliza began to gently move the affected limbs. She encouraged the children to remember how to move them. Almost a year passed until she saw Dr. McDonald again. When he asked how the children had fared, he was astounded when Eliza stated that they were all well and without any paralysis or pain. They had all completely recovered. Elizabeth Kenny's crusade had begun.

Eliza lived in her parents' home during this part of her career, but many times she stayed in a shack in the bush. She rode many miles on horseback to visit outback areas. She delivered babies and cared for the sick and injured. She did not ask for a fee, but often received payment in the form of a rooster, a leg of lamb, or a cut of beef. Once she even received an armchair from the relative of a grateful patient.

THE REALITY OF POLIO

Polio was a frightening reality during these years. It is a potentially fatal infectious disease. It is a virus transmitted mainly from person to person either from contaminated feces to hand to mouth or from oral secretions. The disease is most common in the summer and fall. During these months, children congregate in groups at swimming pools and playgrounds and physically interact, which increases the threat. The primary nervous system targets are motor cells and the nerve cells that control all voluntary motion. In severe cases, the motor cells in the spinal cord's anterior horn, which is part of the cord's vital gray matter, are affected. The name *poliomyelitis* comes from the Greek *polios* (gray), *myelos* (marrow), and *itis* (inflammation; Cohn, 1975; Rogers, 2014).

The symptoms may progress to a high fever, unrelenting headache, and nausea. This may lead to nuchal rigidity (stiff neck) and back with painful arm and leg muscles. This, may in turn, progress to permanent paralysis and, eventually, muscle wasting (Centers for Disease Control and Prevention [CDC], 2014).

In Kenny's time, physicians believed the twisted necks, spines, hips, knees, legs, and feet and the flail joints of polio patients were caused by healthy muscles pulling on weak ones. They logically believed prevention of distortion could only be accomplished by splinting the affected parts so they could not become distorted. The common treatment was to strap the affected limbs to wooden or wire splints or place them in plaster casts. Sometimes the entire body would be fastened to a rigid frame with stiff arm and leg pieces. Knees were held in a slightly flexed position, with the legs in plaster. This immobilization would be continued for at least 10 to 14 days. In many cases, however, this was continued for 2 or 3 months, sometimes 6 months or even a year. In some cases, the splints might be removed for part of the day and some exercise might be started. This treatment was inconsistent and exercise regimens ranged from 1 hour to 12 hours. Practices varied widely (Cohn, 1975).

There was a small group of individuals who called for more physical therapy, which, at the time, was an unfamiliar term. Rehabilitation, in a modern sense, simply did not exist. The therapy that did occur was mainly directed at treating paralysis after it occurred and not at preventing it. Only those with ample financial resources were able to receive any long-term treatment.

Eliza had seen this immobilization treatment and considered it a desecration of the body. She said the children looked as if they were being crucified. They moaned in pain and agony and begged for the splints to be removed. Eliza began to work with many of these patients during the acute phase of the illness. This practice was contrary to all medical beliefs about the treatment of polio. She taught patients about their muscles. She told them to concentrate on the muscle. She persisted day after day with her treatment with hot packs and re-educating the muscles to move. One physician said, "She's a saleswoman. She talks the patient into thinking he's better when he really isn't" (Cohn, 1975, p. 83). But other physicians said that she knew that constant, graded exercise could obtain good results, if the paralysis was not irreversible.

Dr. McConnell, who had remained Eliza's mentor over the years, advised her that the medical community would not be kind to a reformer. He told her that, if she had courage, the time would come when her work would be recognized. He also advised her to never fight with the medical profession or she would make no progress. Sister Kenny did not learn this lesson. As the years passed, she became more and more confrontational and she continued to meet resistance, although her methods were proven over and over to be effective.

One physician said that her methods could never be more than of limited value with chronic paralytics but did agree her treatment should be applied to new patients. This signaled a major change. In her earlier days treating polio victims, she was never allowed by physicians to treat patients in the acute phase of the illness. This physician suggested that a more scientific comparison of old and new methods should be done. This was never done in Australia or anywhere else (Cohn, 1975). In a historical case analysis, however, the author claims Sister Kenny made "bold assertions, obtained scientific validation, learned from experience, used publicity and opposed resistance" (Oppewal, 1997, pp. 83–87).

In 1937, a widespread polio epidemic occurred in Australia. Eliza traveled, treated polio patients, and began to feel sure of her success. In 1938, a crucial report of the Queensland Royal Commission was released. It damned Sister Kenny's treatment methods. Of 47 cases studied, the majority showed no effective improvement, a few worsened, and a few improved. It proclaimed that her numerous treatments for paralysis were unnecessary. Her response to this report was to demand that the commission produce the deformed patients (Cohn, 1975). Even this did not stop her quest to open more treatment centers. Sister Kenny was relentless in her pursuit to gain acceptance of her treatment method from the medical community.

The governments of Queensland, New South Wales, and Victoria supported her. They stated the government was "satisfied." The existing clinics would stay open and the new ones would continue to be organized. In Melbourne, because it was polio season, the authorities compromised and said she could have a section of 22 beds in the Children's Hospital branch. She would be allowed to treat patients coming out of the acute phase of the illness, as long as the parents requested her treatment.

Still, this tenacious woman did not rest. She focused on her treatment and pushed for more and more centers and hospitals. Eight clinics were now operating in Australia. She left for London and waited for a report on the success of her treatment. This report said she claimed to cure poliomyelitis completely, which was not true and this caused her to become angry yet again. The rest of the report was mixed. They agreed that her refusal to splint had not caused the deformities and disaster that orthopedists had predicted. Her next reaction was depression. Finally she thought of her mother's advice that "he who angers you, conquers you" and "the greater the fight, the greater the victory." She focused on the fact that the British report admitted that removing splints caused no harm (Cohn, 1975). This was her victory.

The challenges continued. When she heard of a modified Kenny treatment being used in her Newcastle clinic, she rushed there only to realize that, although they were using her name, she had no control over the facilities. They were responsible to their state governments, not to her. Eliza became more depressed but she did not remain discouraged. She constantly sought ways to learn and grow from these experiences (Cohn, 1975).

Eliza decided to concentrate on Brisbane and asked to be assigned to a hospital ward with acute polio cases. She was refused. She defied state law and medical custom by turning one of her treatment rooms into a ward and placing two new polio patients in the room. She was officially told to dismiss the patients, but she ignored the order. The demands that she dismiss these patients continued, but Sister Kenny maintained that these patients could not be safely discharged from hospital supervision. She suggested that they be moved to Brisbane General Hospital where she could supervise their treatment. This request was approved, which was a triumph for Kenny. She had manipulated the system in order to gain what she wanted, the opportunity to care for polio patients in the acute phase of the disease (Cohn, 1975).

Because she was rehabilitating disabled people, Kenny believed the state government should help support her efforts. Several doctors eventually wrote a letter on her behalf to the health minister and asked the government to explore the training of therapists under her direction. When she arrived in Queensland to demonstrate her therapy, she was greeted by Dr. Crawford, president of a branch of the Australian Massage Association, the then physical therapy society. Sister Kenny had not enlisted any physiotherapists because she felt they had too much to unlearn. This angered Dr. Crawford who greeted her in what she considered an unwelcoming manner. She became haughty and suggested they cancel the demonstration (Cohn, 1975).

The demonstration was not canceled; however, an observer said her demonstration was crude and seemed to suggest that she had a charm or gift that traveled from her brain though her arm to the child's arm and on to the child's brain. She became incensed at this implication and the meeting ended. The next day, Kenny attempted to lecture to a medical audience and was greeted with stark silence. When she stated she did not believe in casts, splints, or immobilization, one doctor responded that this was criminal. The audience reacted with looks of disgust and jeering laughter and the session was adjourned. These reactions from the medical community continued throughout her life (Cohn, 1975).

Kenny did, however, have some supporters in the medical community. She was able to establish a government clinic on an experimental basis for the training of therapists. Although she had operated small bush hospitals in the past, this was the first government support she had received. The son of the proprietress of the Queen's Hotel, Dr. James Vivian Guinane, was doing his surgical training in England. When he returned, he brought Sister Kenny physiotherapy texts, taught her some physiology, and improved her knowledge of anatomy (Cohn, 1975) in an attempt to ameliorate criticism of her lack of knowledge and training.

But the fight continued, and although many applauded her success, there were many who were sure that there was trickery involved or misdiagnosis of patients. The commission's report was quoted for years. The medical community in Australia, as a whole, would not accept her. World War II finished her career in Australia. She was no longer criticized but was largely ignored. The Queensland government had spent substantial money on her clinics but William Smith, Queensland's premier, felt she was not a political asset and decided she should be dispatched to avoid controversy. The decision to send her to America was made, and she concluded this was perhaps the best solution (Cohn, 1975).

THE AMERICAN FRONTIER

In 1940, Sister Elizabeth Kenny left her home and country and went to America. She brought her daughter, Mary, with her. Mary had become expert in the Kenny method. Eliza's purpose was to demonstrate her methods to American doctors. She was determined to obtain the approval of the American medical society. During her stay in America, she opened many Kenny treatment centers. Many are still in existence, but with the eradication of polio resulting from the development of the Salk vaccine, these centers now have a different focus. There were centers in Minneapolis, New Jersey (which no longer exists), and her favorite, the Ruth Home in El Monte, California. The Sister Kenny Rehabilitation Associates in Minneapolis is perhaps the best known center and is still in operation. The new name, the Courage Kenny Rehabilitation Institute, is a reflection of the woman after whom it was named. Certainly, Elizabeth displayed remarkable courage throughout her long career. She provoked controversy wherever she traveled, but she was a determined and outspoken woman who believed in herself and had the confidence and courage to persevere.

Kenny may have had her greatest successes in her 11 years in America. She was able to open many clinics, and she lectured to physicians, obtained financial support, and treated many victims of polio. She became a celebrity in her own time. In fact, in 1946 her life story became a movie, *Sister Kenny*, starring Rosalind Russell. Kenny and Russell became close friends after she treated Russell's nephew who had contracted polio. Some other celebrities who were treated by Sister Kenny were Alan Alda, actor; Dinah Shore, singer; and Majorie Lawrence, Australian opera singer. Cartoonist Al Capp was an amputee and became involved in the Sister Kenny Foundation during the 1940s and 1950s. She has been referenced in *An American Christmas Carol* and an episode of *The Waltons*.

Sister Kenny recognized the high status granted to physicians in American society. She was driven to be accepted by them. She realized that challenging the male-dominated medical establishment meant using a different approach. She was 5'10" and had a typical Australian Irish sense of humor and she used this effectively most of the time. Although she found it uncomfortable, she developed a feminine persona and dressed in large, dramatic hats and flowers. She often referred to herself as a mixture of Florence Nightingale and Marie Curie (Cohn, 1975). She was never "antiscience," although her treatment ideas were considered unorthodox. She claimed her clinical work and observations led her to believe that polio was not a neurotropic disease but a systemic one. This theory was debated endlessly, and in 1950, virologists discovered the poliovirus was spread through the body by blood (Rogers, 2014). She was convinced that scientific theory must be based on clinical evidence. She did not trust clinical trials that relied on tissue pathology rather than the living body. This allowed her detractors to state that she lacked an understanding of science (Cohn, 1975).

While in America, Sister Kenny met with President Franklin D. Roosevelt, who was a victim of poliomyelitis as a young boy. He created his own polio treatment center but it was fairly primitive and did not reverse his paralysis. Although he did not actively oppose her, he did not support the Kenny treatment method. Little has been recorded about her encounter with him.

Sister Kenny remained focused on her clinical practice, although she also worked tirelessly to reeducate the medical community. The patients, therapists, and nurses she worked with were a central part of her mission. They often saw her practice as one of constant struggle and sacrifice. They were inspired by her commitment and used her experiences as a way to obtain autonomy and acceptance from physicians.

Sister Kenny was fierce in her determination to provide the care that she believed was optimal for polio patients. She observed patients treated with her method recovering at higher rates than those treated with the traditional methods of splints and braces. She believed that clinical trials were not necessary when the proof was right before her eyes. This is perhaps her greatest legacy. In an era of evidence-based medicine and large-scale clinical trials, a keen clinical observation still has its place. Kenny once wrote about her opponents, "They have eyes, but they see not" (Kenny & Ostenso, 1943, p. 202). She was not a scientist but a crusader.

Charisma is not a term that has been associated with Sister Kenny. She was often caustic and sarcastic but not cruel. She could be intimidating to some because of her height and demeanor. She responded or reacted to the situation at hand in many instances. She was a role model in clinical practice but she was not a good communicator. This, of course, put her at a disadvantage with the medical community. Her constant controversy with physicians became tiresome to many of her supporters. She did not inspire the creation of strong interdisciplinary teams. Some have said that she sometimes lied and often exaggerated. She was never content to let an idea settle but used to hammer at everyone with her beliefs. She often made claims she could not substantiate.

Elizabeth battled, was defeated multiple times, accepted that, and changed her ideas when she had to. When she became depressed over her defeats, she retreated, recovered, and then went onto a fresh start. In the end, she was successful in revolutionizing treatment for poliomyelitis, whereas her impact went far beyond the treatment of polio.

In 1942, *TIME* magazine reported that her amazing method had an 80% recovery rate, thus forcing doctors to recognize her nonconventional work (Fairley, 2008). A 1943 article in the *Journal of Bone and Joint Surgery* reported that patients who underwent the Kenny treatment were,

> more comfortable, have better general health and nutrition, are more receptive to muscle training, have a superior morale, require shorter periods of bed rest and hospital care, and seem to have less residual paralysis and deformity than patients treated by older conventional methods. (Fairley, 2008)

In 1943, the University of Rochester, which was a site for studies conducted by Dr. Schwartz on polio spasm and pain, awarded Kenny the honorary degree of doctor of science. This represented a major victory for Sister Kenny. The university president, Alan Valentine, said, "In the dark world of suffering you have lit a candle that will never be put out" (Cohn, 1975, p. 170). Shortly after this, she was awarded another honorary degree by New York University and she became a doctor of humane letters as well as of science. Sister Kenny did not, however, see these awards as an advantage in promoting her treatment.

In 1951, the Gallup poll named Kenny the woman whom Americans admired the most in the world. Eleanor Roosevelt had previously been the recipient of this honor. The National Foundation for Infantile Paralysis, which is now known as the March of Dimes, also supported her efforts financially and conceptually.

THE WAR RAGES ON

Orthopedists remained Kenny's fiercest opposition. They were struggling with achieving their own professional recognition as specialists. They had actually abandoned the practice of using rigid immobilization for polio patients, but they were reluctant to publically advertise this fact. In 1942, a committee of three orthopedists were charged to visit 16 clinics in six cities and examine 740 patients. They spent time with Sister Kenny, albeit much of the time was spent in argument. In 1944, Dr. Jonathan Ghormley presented the committee's conclusions at the annual American Medical Association meeting. He purported that muscle reeducation had been the basis for orthopedic treatment for many years. He reported that nerve cell destruction, not untreated spasm, was the most important cause of crippling and that 50% to 80% of polio cases recovered spontaneously. This committee condemned the "Kenny publicity" that they felt was misleading the public but did suggest that it had provoked the medical profession to reevaluate their traditional methods of treatment. As might have been predicted, Sister Kenny's response to this report was confrontational. She demanded to know where they had visited these patients and clinics; however, the committee refused to release any names or locations (Rogers, 2014).

During her time in America, Sister Kenny seemed to create miracles. In Jersey City, she examined an 8-year-old polio patient who had been treated for 8 months but was unable to lift his head or sit up. An orthopedic surgeon, Dr. Nicholas Ransohoff, planned to transplant a strip of muscle from the boy's hip across his abdominal wall in order to help him sit up. Sister Kenny asked to see the boy and to apply the Kenny treatment. According to her, in 30 minutes, the patient was walking (Cohn, 1975).

Yet, Elizabeth Kenny did not believe in miracles. She said that she was seeking to restore mental awareness. Her claim was that patients stopped using the muscle because of the pain in the acute phase of the disease. She said that in some cases, a long course of relaxing heat, stimulation, and reeducation would restore movement, whereas in others, restoration might happen quickly with her commands to "relax" and "think" as she moved the affected limb. This, she said, allowed the patient to be free from pain and use voluntary nerve pathways to move the crucial muscle (Cohn, 1975).

Elizabeth Kenny visited health centers in 14 countries. She advised the Soviet Union that she had no politics but did not like theirs. She had a private audience with Pope Pius XII (Cohn, 1975). When she returned to Australia in 1947, she made a formal report to her Australian medical sponsors and visited the Kenny clinics. Dr. Stubbs Brown, fellow of the Royal College of Surgeons of Edinburgh, past president of the Queensland Branch of the British Medical Association, and distinguished senior orthopedic surgeon at Brisbane General Hospital, asked Sister Kenny if she would trust him with her bag and its contents. She replied, "I would trust you with anything except a case of polio" (Rogers, 2014, p. 16).

Although she was gentle in her speech and was said to be polite, Sister Kenny never learned to communicate in a nonconfrontational manner. She was well known for her rapier wit and quick responses and was particularly caustic to physicians (Cohn, 1975).

Perhaps her most important contribution to nursing leadership was her determination and stamina to continue in the face of opposition. She believed in her vision and was willing to dedicate her life's work to achieving success. She was motivated, not by personal gain, but in the belief that her method was the right treatment for polio patients. Thousands of patients and families would attest to her success.

Some have called her the founder of modern physical therapy; however, the World Confederation for Physical Therapists does not agree and suggests that Kenny's contribution to patients with polio was unique but controversial. Her muscle reeducation techniques are still used today in some individuals who have lower motor neuron lesions (Fairley, 2008).

Long after her death, her concept of polio and its treatment were viewed as unique. Sister Kenny encouraged physicians and therapists to focus on the functioning of the neuromuscular system, which had an impact on physical medicine and rehabilitation. More important, her treatment provoked research on neuromuscular physiology; on kinesiology; and on the entire science of motion, walking, and balance. She helped reshape therapeutic approaches to virtually all disabilities. In 1930, she advocated restoring usefulness and self-care. It is believed that she actually saved physical therapy, which had become invisible when orthopedic physicians came on the scene.

Sister Kenny did not restrict her knowledge to polio victims, but utilized similar concepts in her approach to all areas of patient care. She applied her ideas to all illnesses and disabilities. Although the use of hot packs to relieve pain and muscle spasm was important, the paramount contribution was her therapeutic aggressiveness. She was vehement in her belief that rest for patients was an abuse. She strongly advocated for patient and family involvement in all aspects of treatment of illness and disability. She was always a crusader (Cohn, 1975).

The polio menace ended in 1955 with the development of the Salk vaccine, followed by an oral vaccine discovered by Albert Sabin. Although Elizabeth Kenny may be largely forgotten because polio has been all but eradicated, she left a legacy for thousands of patients (Cohn, 1975).

Sister Elizabeth returned to her home in Australia and died on November 30, 1952, at the age of 72, from complications of Parkinson's disease. There is a small museum in Nobby, Australia, which displays artifacts and documents regarding the history of her life. The Sister Kenny Memorial Fund awards scholarships to students with an interest in remote and rural nursing (Townsville City Council, 2014).

Sister Elizabeth Kenny was courageous and tenacious. She was combative and confrontational when she felt it was necessary. She had a vision that some might say was tunnel vision. She could only see her way and remained very focused on her treatment options. At times, this was not to her advantage. But she did save, literally, thousands of children and adults from crippling disabilities. One physician said that her opposition to rest as a treatment for polio helped to end a century of the "abuse of rest." This is widely accepted today, many years after Kenny's death.

Over the course of her career, this remarkable woman continuously challenged the processes of her time. Her efforts were tireless in obtaining interest in and funding to teach her method. Involving as many individuals as possible in her quest, she did achieve great success although she was never completely convinced of that fact. Although she gained notoriety for her method of treating polio victims, her legacy continues today. Kenny's belief that patients need to take personal responsibility for their own rehabilitation continues to be an essential tenet in health care. Patients and their families were always her focus; family-centered care is an important model in health care today.

TIMELINE

- September 20, 1880—Elizabeth Kenny is born in Warialda, New South Wales.
- 1909—Assumes the role of a qualified nurse.
- 1911—Opens a cottage hospital at Clifton.
- 1911—Begins her travels as a bush nurse.
- 1911—Treats first polio patient.
- 1915—Volunteers to serve in the Australian Army Nurse Corps.
- 1919—Supervises a temporary hospital to care for victims of the 1919 influenza epidemic.
- 1925—Adopts her daughter, Mary Stewart.
- 1926—Designs and manufactures the Sylvia stretcher.
- 1937—Opens and operates many treatment centers supported by the governments of New South Wales, Queensland, and Victoria.
- 1937—Widespread polio epidemic begins in Australia; travels to care for the victims.
- 1938—Report of the Queensland Royal Commission is released condemning the Kenny method for treating polio.
- 1940—Sister Kenny is dispatched to America by the Queensland premier.
- 1942—Sister Elizabeth Kenny Institute is established in Minneapolis, Minnesota.
- 1943—Receives the honorary degrees of doctor of science by the University of Rochester and doctor of humane letters from New York University.
- 1946—Rosalind Russell stars in the movie *Sister Kenny*, about Kenny's life.
- 1949—Sister Kenny Memorial and Children's Playground are unveiled.
- 1951—Named the woman whom Americans admired most in the world; returns home to Toowoomba, Australia.
- November 30, 1952—Kenny dies of Parkinson's disease at the age of 72; Sister Elizabeth Kenny "Fight Against Polio" seal is issued (see the beginning of this chapter).
- 1955—Sister Elizabeth Kenny Foundation is established.

- 1963—Sister Elizabeth Kenny Art Show for Artists with Disabilities.
- 1975—Sister Elizabeth Kenny Institute merges with Abbott Northwestern Hospital.
- 2014—Sister Elizabeth Kenny Memorial Fund provides scholarships to students attending the University of Southern Queensland; Sister Kenny Rehabilitation Associates in Minneapolis remains in operation.

QUESTIONS FOR DISCUSSION

1. Sister Elizabeth Kenny *modeled the way* for many nurses to overcome barriers in their practice. She was relentless in her determination to achieve her goals and was adamant that those working with her do the same. How can today's nurse leaders achieve the same success in the face of existing regulatory barriers?
2. There is no doubt that Sister Kenny was *challenging the process* when she challenged the medical model of her day. Are today's nurse leaders challenging the current model of health care delivery? How can we, as nurse leaders, challenge the status quo?
3. Sister Kenny was fearless and took many risks to achieve her goals. What are the risks nurse leaders of today must take in order to change nursing, the health care system, and improve the health of society?
4. Sister Kenny did not exemplify *encouraging the heart* by formally acknowledging her colleagues' accomplishments; yet they followed her into very nontraditional nursing practices of the time. How can nurse leaders of today encourage other nurses and interested others to pursue new, innovative, and unique ways of improving nursing, health care, and the health of society?

REFERENCES

Centers for Disease Control and Prevention (CDC). (2014). *What is polio?* Retrieved October 31, 2014, from http://www.cdc.gov/polio/about/index.htm

Cohn, V. (1975). *Sister Kenny: The woman who challenged the doctors.* Minneapolis, MN: The University of Minnesota Press.

Fairley, M. (2008). Sister Kenny: Confronting the conventional in polio treatment. *The O & P Edge,* 7(11). Retrieved October 15, 2014, from http://www.oandp.com/articles/2008-11_09.asp

Kenny, E., & Ostenso, M. (1943). *And they shall walk.* St. Paul, MN: Bruce Publishing Company.

McKinnon, E. (1935, February 8). A biographical sketch of Sister Kenny. *Sydney Morning Herald.* Retrieved from http://www.smh.com.au/

Oppewal, S. (1997). Sister Elizabeth Kenny, an Australian nurse and treatment of poliomyelitis victims. *Image: The Journal of Nursing Scholarship,* 29(1), 83–88.

Rogers, N. (2014). *The polio wars.* New York, NY: Oxford University Press.

Townsville City Council. (2014). *The strand*. Retrieved October 31, 2014, from http://www.townsville.qld.gov.au/townsville/heritage/townsville/Pages/chronology2.aspx

Yoder, R. (1942, January 17). Healer from the outback. *Saturday Evening Post*, pp. 18–19.

FURTHER READING

Kenny, E. (1955). *My battle and victory: History of the discovery of poliomyelitis as a systemic disease*. London, UK: Robert Hale.

Clara Louise Maass: Servant Leader Undaunted

Carol Emerson Winters

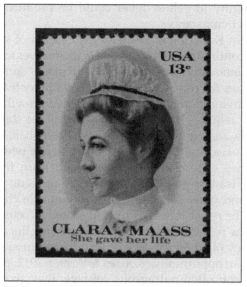

U.S. postage stamp issued in 1976 honoring Clara Louise Maass.

• • • • •

While it is not the objective of a true martyr to seek applause, the acknowledgements of Maass's sacrifice by both her professional colleagues and the world at large are rightly deserved. Through recognition, she can continue to be an inspiration for those who devote their lives to serving others, to those whose lives are based on principle, and to those who in a more modest sphere may just desire to help one other human being. (Herrmann, 1985, p. 56)

Clara Louise Maass (1876–1901) was passionate about nursing American soldiers during the Spanish–American War of 1898, especially those suffering from yellow fever. She qualifies as an *exemplary leader* as defined by Kouzes and Posner (2012). Even in her early 20s, Clara Maass was unaccepting of the current thought regarding the etiology of this mysterious, dreaded disease. She *challenged the process* by betting her life on the theory that immunity to yellow fever could be produced by inoculation under controlled circumstances.

Findings from Kouzes and Posner's exploration of successful leaders suggest that they continuously look outside of themselves to seek challenging opportunities for innovative initiatives that will make "something meaningful happen" (Kouzes & Posner, 2012, p. 157). Exemplary leaders *challenge the process* and are convinced and convince others that growth, transformation, and improvement require changing every aspect of the status quo—people, processes, systems, and strategies. These mover-and-shaker leaders, in spite of resistance, mistakes, and delays, persist to generate new ideas, methods, and solutions. They experiment, take risks, and learn from their experiences. Exemplary leaders guide others through ambiguity, adversity, transition, recovery, and other seemingly unsurmountable challenges. Kouzes and Posner describe *personal best* leadership as being focused on significant departures from the past and new approaches of doing things in places yet to be discovered. They often do not seek or wait for permission or instructions before leaping on an opportunity (Kouzes & Posner, 2012, p. 160). Exhibiting a *can do* attitude and often outrageous courage, they accept the challenge with high purpose and motivation, which results in stirring things up.

Clara Louise Maass, a New Jersey native, was "possessed by an overmastering inner drive; hers was to serve humanity through seeking to free the world from the ravages of disease" (Herrmann, 1985, p. 51). She sought out opportunities to serve and welcomed and persevered the hardships of travel to nurse in unfamiliar, distant, tropical military bases steeped in known dangers of war and disease, much as her idol, Florence Nightingale, had done in the Crimea. In spite of stern admonitions, Clara Maass chose to deny herself personal pleasure, comfort, and health in her determination to offer nursing care to U.S. soldiers hospitalized from wounds and, more prevalently, tropical illnesses in Savannah, Georgia; Jacksonville, Florida; Manila, Philippines; and Santiago and Havana, Cuba. Upon arrival in Havana, she interviewed Dr. Walter Reed and other members of Havana's Yellow Fever Commission about their experiments with yellow fever. Taking the ultimate risk, she sacrificed herself for the experimentation and advancement of yellow fever research by volunteering to be bitten by infected *Stegomyia* (*Aedes aegypti*) mosquitoes. Her death (a) gave credence to the theory that these infected mosquitoes were the vectors of yellow fever and (b) disproved the hypothesis that immunity to yellow fever could be produced by inoculation (immunization) in a controlled environment. Unfortunately, the results of the latter could not have been determined in any other manner.

SPENDING CHILDHOOD AS AN ADULT

Clara Louise Maass, though a "charming, animated and ambitious girl" (Guinther, 1932, p. 172), was no prima donna. She was born on June 28, 1876, in East Orange, New Jersey, into a poor family, which had immigrated to America with other Germans seeking religious freedom and better opportunities. While still a young child, as the eldest of nine children, Clara Maass was expected to assist her mother, Hedwig, with the housekeeping and childcare duties. The wages that her father, Robert, earned as a grocer, farmer, and seasonal worker in the East Orange hat mills, proved insufficient to support his rapidly expanding family.

At 10 years of age, Clara Maass, a student at Northfield Elementary School, sought employment as a mother's helper in a private home. Her compensation was room and board and time off to attend school. A year later, her family moved to a farm in Livingston where she is remembered by her classmates for her "honey-blond hair and her eternal optimism" (Cunningham, 1968, p. 35). Clara's family moved back to East Orange when she was 12 years old, where she attended East Orange High School and resumed her job as a mother's helper. Three years later, at age 15, she abandoned her secondary studies in order to obtain full-time employment and to continue to help support her family. At the Newark Orphan Asylum, she worked 7 days a week feeding, dressing, and sewing for the orphans. Here she earned $10 a month, sending half to her mother.

TRAINING SCHOOL FOR NURSES

At a time when there were limited career options for women, 17-year-old Clara Maass, inspired by Miss Nightingale's dedication in nursing soldiers during the Crimean War and her desire to help her economically struggling family, decided to pursue nursing. From early childhood, she was considered to have had "an unusual spirit of service which constantly grew and for which she sought expression in nursing" (Guinther, 1932, p. 173). In the fall of 1893, she applied to join the second class of the Christina Tref Training School for Nurses at Newark German Hospital. It had been publicized that applications would be accepted from women between 20 and 40 years of age with proof of physical ability, spoken English, and a minimum of a general school education. She was scrutinized by a young and stern head nurse, Anna Steebler, who approved of her small and wiry frame, coiffed and knotted hair, and her wire-rimmed glasses. Clara Maass also passed the other entrance requirements of being plain, unadorned, and accustomed to drudgery and hard work. It was expected that during the 2 grueling years of classes, offered predominantly in German and Latin (when the physicians taught), the female trainees (nursing students) would earn $5 per month. At the end of their first year, they could accept private nursing cases with their wages paid directly to the hospital. Upon graduation, they received a $100 bonus (Cunningham, 1968; Herrmann, 1985).

In 1894, Carrie Frank was the only nursing student out of six who graduated in the first class. A year later, at the age of 19, Clara Maass, along with her three classmates, Sophie Bruckner, Sarah Filer, and Madeline Gill, graduated in the class of 1895. After graduation, Clara remained at Newark German Hospital but supplemented her income with private nursing cases. Three years later, the hospital directors offered Clara Maass the head nurse position in recognition of her high-quality work (Cunningham, 1968).

THE SPANISH–AMERICAN WAR

On February 19, 1898, Spain blew up the U.S. battleship *Maine,* in the harbor in Havana, Cuba. On April 20, U.S. President McKinley demanded that Spain withdraw from Cuba and issued a declaration of war, which became known as the Spanish–American War or the War of 1898. During this war, American casualties were small, with 10 times more deaths occurring in the hastily constructed army camps resulting from the epidemics of typhoid fever, malaria, dysentery, and food poisoning. Nursing care of Cuban patients was provided by lower class servants whose work was considered so inadequate that the Spanish word for nurse, *enferma*, was considered a derogatory term (Herrmann, 1985).

Nurses were desperately needed and the Nurses' Associated Alumnae of the United States and Canada, renamed the American Nurses Association (ANA) in 1911, offered their nursing services but the U.S. Army refused. It is conjectured that Army officials were prejudiced against women serving with them in the field. The primary objection to the nursing services offered by the Nurses' Associated Alumnae was that this organization had only been in existence for a short time and it was not recognized as the representative body for nurses. Additionally, their proposal was received 1 day after the Daughters of the American Revolution (DAR) had volunteered. The DAR vice president and physician, Dr. Anita Newcomb McGee, had been appointed as director of the Army Nursing Service and acting assistant surgeon in the U.S. Army even though she had no administrative experience.

After the war, Dr. McGee, Associated Alumnae, and influential citizens proposed bills to establish a permanent, sanctioned nursing corps to no avail. In 1900, after numerous surgeons testified about the work of the contract nurses during the war, the Army Reorganization Bill proposed that the Nurse Corps be a part of the U.S. Army Medical Department. Members would consist of hospital nursing school graduates supervised by a hospital nursing school graduate. The bill was finally passed on February 2, 1901, with Dr. McGee, a physician, having to resign as director of the U.S. Army Nurse Corps because she was not a nurse (Donahue, 1996).

With the outbreak of the Spanish–American War, Congress authorized employment of women who were nurses on a contract basis, providing them with $30 per month, room, and board. Dr. McGee preferred that the contract nurses be graduate nurses endorsed by their own schools who had passed health examinations and received clearance by the DAR. Approximately 8,000 volunteer nurses became contract nurses, with 1,600 being graduate nurses. Large numbers of the Catholic orders served, especially the Daughters of Charity. The first contract nurses were appointed in May of 1898 and they were stationed in army hospitals located in the southern United States, Puerto Rico, Cuba, Hawaii, and the Philippine Islands. Heretofore, these army hospitals were staffed by corpsmen who were lacking in training and experience. The corpsmen engaged in unsanitary practices, such as using the same bucket for food and excrement, thus spreading diseases throughout the camps (Donahue, 1996).

Because she could not enlist in the military, Clara Maass became one of the first to apply as a U.S. Army contract nurse. Ms. Maass requested that a physician she had-worked with at Newark German Hospital write a letter to certify that he had known her as a nurse. His letter stated that he had known her for 5 years and that she was a "dutiful, diligent, and conscientious nurse who recognized the responsibilities of her profession" (W. J. Roeber to Whom It May Concern, September 15, 1898). On her application to become a contract nurse, Clara indicated that she desired appointment in the Army rather than the Navy; could leave on October 1; had not had yellow fever; was a 1895 graduate of a training school for nurses; had no other hospital experience other than Newark German Hospital; but she had nursed continuously since graduation; had experience in invalid cookery with her private duty patients; was 22 years old, White, 5 feet, 4¾ inches tall, weighed 134 pounds; was single; had no tendency to disease; and had been successfully vaccinated in 1894 (Clara L. Maass, Application for Contract Nurse, Record Group 112, Entry 149). Her characteristic patriotism and love for adventure, which had been denied to her in childhood, or her quest to increase her earnings may have prompted her to apply. While she waited to be called, knowing that she would be leaving Newark German Hospital during a shortage of nurses and funds, she worked in excess of 12 hours a day without pay. Here was one of the first indications of her adult self-abnegation (Cunningham, 1968; Guinther, 1932; Herrmann, 1985).

Clara Maass signed her contract October 1, 1898, along with U.S. Surgeon General George M. Sternberg and received her first assignment as a contract nurse to the field hospital of the Seventh U.S. Army Corps in Jacksonville, Florida (Contract for Services as Nurse—Clara L. Maass, October 1, 1898). The fighting had ended when she arrived in Florida, but she nursed hundreds of wounded and diseased soldiers. Most were ill from malaria, dysentery, and typhoid fever. Soldiers who were febrile were prohibited from returning to their homes for fear that they would spread the diseases to those in their home state. Because typhoid fever was prevalent at Newark German Hospital, Clara Maass was familiar with the care of these soldiers and the requisite long, tedious hours. Three nurses from Pennsylvania shared her tent: Lucy Vandling from Williamsport; Utilie Scheerer, the eldest, and Minnie Lenox, both from Philadelphia. They named and labeled their tent with signs that read *Camp Cubra Libra* and *Potatoe Patch Tent*. They often teased the soldiers who guarded them from American and Spanish would-be suitors (Cunningham, 1968).

NURSING SOLDIERS WITH YELLOW FEVER

From Jacksonville, Clara was transferred to Savannah, Georgia, in November of 1898 and then to Santiago and Havana, Cuba, in early 1899, where she had her first brief exposure to yellow fever. The sailors there called this disease Yellow Jack, referring to the Navy's yellow quarantine flag, whereas the Spaniards dubbed it *el vomito negro* (the black vomit) for the blood secreted into the victim's stomach by breaking blood vessels. The U.S. and Spanish soldiers were ravaged by the uncontrollable yellow fever, but the Cuban soldiers were not as affected, as many had acquired immunity from frequent exposure (Iglesias, 2002). Clara Maas left Havana on January 21, 1899, and on February 5, 1899, Clara Maass was honorably discharged and her contract annulled (Clara L. Maass, Service Record, Record Group 112, Entry 149). She then returned home to New Jersey to resume her private nursing practice (Guinther, 1932). Within a week of arriving back in Newark, Clara wrote to Dr. McGee, director of the Army Nursing Service and acting assistant surgeon, requesting to enter the service again. She implored the director that she would go any place where she was needed, but if nurses were needed in the Seventh Army Corps in Jacksonville, Florida, she preferred to go with them, as she had just come from there. On February 6, 1899, she again wrote Dr. McGee stating that she had seen in the newspapers that the bill regarding the *corps* of nurses had been passed and that she wanted to enter her name as an applicant for a position in the service. She added that she would be willing to go to "any part to nurse" and had returned to this country from Cuba where she was in the service about 4 months (Clara L. Maass to Dr. Anita N. McGee, February 1, 1899; February 6, 1899). To support her case, Clara requested that Miss Carrie E. Rogers write a letter to Dr. McGee, a fellow member of DAR, on behalf of

a fine nurse, Miss Maass who is desirous of entering the regular
Army in that capacity. She has recently returned from Cuba
having been engaged as nurse there during the late war. Fifty
nurses were discharged and sent home, not long since. She being
among this number. She appeals to me as a D. A. R. to recommend
her to you. She was in my family for three months and we were
much attached to her, being faithful and lovely during the long
illness of my sister. Hoping you will be able to assist her.
(Carrie E. Rogers to Dr. Anita N. McGee, March 1, 1899)

Clara Maass was persistent in her efforts to become a member of the U.S.
Army Nurse Corps. In another letter to Dr. McGee, she wrote that she appre-
ciated her placing her name on the list of eligible nurses. She also reminded
Dr. McGee that she was "willing to serve at any time and any place" (Clara L.
Maass to Dr. Anita N. McGee, August 14, 1899).

Clara was neither ignorant nor naïve about her choice to continue her
perilous work nursing yellow fever victims. Newspapers in the 1880s carried official bulletins reporting the devastation caused by yellow fever epidemics in the southern states. Yellow fever terrified people throughout the
Western Hemisphere. In the United States, it had been recorded in New York
as early as 1668. In the 1790s, Philadelphians fled the city, as did the residents along coastal regions during the Civil War in the mid-1860s. In 1879,
much of the South was panic-stricken. When thousands fled the river city
of Memphis, Tennessee, 47 policemen were ordered to prevent looting and
all but seven died from yellow fever. Though tuberculosis, typhoid, and
dysentery were responsible for more deaths, yellow fever was more feared
because of its unique characteristics: high fever, muscle pain, backache, shiv-
ers, anorexia, nausea, and vomiting. It could create mild, flulike symptoms
lasting about a week or it could progress, as it did in 10% to 60% of cases, into
a period of *intoxication* wherein liver failure occurred, resulting in jaundice
and vomiting of dark, digested blood. Yellow fever spared no one, rich or
poor, young or old, clean or filthy. It disrupted everyday life, commerce, and
communication (Jusino, 2012).

Clara Maass nursed her patients diagnosed with yellow fever according to a regimen of universal rules consisting of strict bed rest in a supine
position to minimize exertion and to decrease bowel perforation. Sufficient
ventilation increased the antiseptic action of fresh air through an oxidation
process that occurred when interacting with noxious substances or organisms. As symptoms appeared, so did implementation of more specific
treatments. Purgatives were given at the onset of disease to rid the body
of systemic toxins; cold sponging, ice packs, baths, and ice water enemas
treated high fevers; rectal alimentation was given for vomiting; application
of mustard poultices relieved epigastric pain; and dry champagne, brandy,
or eggnogs were administered by tube to provide nutrition or to settle an irri-
table stomach. In addition to offering these treatments, nurses were expected

to encourage and soothe their patients while maintaining their own health and immunity to disease by their cleanliness, cheerfulness, and temperance (Herrmann, 1985).

Clara Maas had witnessed firsthand the consequences of yellow fever after the Spanish–American War and read the widely publicized reports of the returning soldiers who had contracted this disease. By 1899, J. C. Wilson's textbook, *Fever Nursing*, was in its third edition. Clara knew of and accepted the concomitant risks of her nursing practice abroad. She was fully informed of its all-consuming nature, leaving few opportunities for pleasure and exploration. Further, her bilingual competence in German and English were worthless in the countries where she chose to serve (Herrmann, 1985).

NURSING AMERICAN TROOPS IN THE PHILIPPINE ISLANDS

The 1898 Treaty of Paris officially ended the Spanish–American War and culminated in Spain's ceding the lands of Puerto Rico, Guam, and the Philippines to the United States (Herrmann, 1985). In 1899, American troops were stationed in the Philippines to quell an insurrection. Clara Maass continued her quest to serve as a nurse in the Philippines, writing in a letter to Dr. McGee dated September 1899:

> Dear Dr. McGee:
> You will think I am the bother of your life but really I do not want to trouble you and will try not to very much. But I should like to know, (if you can spare a few minutes to write to me) if I were to pay my transportation as far as Chicago, Ill., thus taking me farther west of here, if you would call me to go to the Phillippines [Philippines]. If it were necessary for me to pay it—further West—I think I could do it. I would like so much to go and hope I may go soon. Please let me know what you can do and how soon I would be called, if at all, and I will feel more settled. Hoping not to be disappointed I am Respectfully yours, Clara L. Maass. (Clara L. Maass to Dr. Anita N. McGee, September 22, 1899)

Dr. McGee responded to Clara Maass 4 days later, telling her that she was always glad to give the nurses information about prospects where it was possible, but that she was not able to foresee what the surgeons at different hospitals would do. Dr. McGee thought that it was probable that, early in the next month of October, the call for nurses would come for Manila, since most of the Western reapplicants had been appointed and those from the East would be sent next. She advised Clara Maass not to go to Chicago at that time as it might be an unnecessary expense (Anita N. McGee to Clara L. Maass, September 26, 1899).

Clara wrote yet another letter to Dr. McGee on November 1, 1899, informing her that she was "still very anxious to go to Manila and as I hear of so many nurses who were with the 7th Army Corps going, it makes me more anxious than ever." She requested to go with her nurse friend in Cuba, Miss Kane from Reading, Pennsylvania, on the *Logan* on November 20 (Clara L. Maass to Dr. Anita N. McGee, November 1, 1899). It is uncertain whether Dr. McGee suggested that Clara petition the surgeon general, or whether she chose to go over Dr. McGee's head, but on November 8, 1899, Clara Maass sent the following letter to U.S. Army Surgeon General George Miller Sternberg, in Washington, DC:

9 Sussex Ave.
Newark, N. J.
Sir:
I have the honor respectfully to request that my name be placed on the list of nurses sailing to Manila, PI from New York, and that I be sent on the first transport leaving.

Having served as contract nurse in the field hospital of the Seventh Army Corps continuously and with satisfaction from October 1, 1898, to February 5, 1899, I have been notified by Dr. McGee that I am eligible for service in the Philippines, and it is my desire to be sent there as I prefer a tropical climate to that of New York. I am in excellent health and I have a good constitution, and am accustomed to the hardships of field service.

Very respectfully, Clara L. Maass. (Clara L. Maass to George M. Sternberg, Surgeon General, November 8, 1899)

True to one who *challenges the process*, Clara Maass was relentless in her efforts to be sent to the Philippines as a contract nurse. Ten days later, she followed up her letter with a telegram to Surgeon General Sternberg: "Can I be sent with nurses on *Logan*. See application to Surgeon General November eighth recommended by Major Kilbourne. Wire answer my expense. Clara L. Maass" (Clara L. Maass Telegram to George M. Sternberg, Surgeon General, November 18, 1899). Surgeon General Sternberg responded by sending her a telegram at her mother's house in East Orange, New Jersey, summoning her to Manila, Philippines (George M. Sternberg to Clara Maas, November 20, 1899). Within 2 hours, she gathered a few belongings, took a train to Hoboken, ferried across the Hudson River, and taxied to the pier to board the Army ship, *Logan,* just as the last visitors were exiting the gangplank.

Once again in the capacity of a contract nurse, Clara Maass reported to Reserve Hospital in Manila on January 5, 1900. Most authors writing about Maass have based their information on the publications of Guinther (1932) and Cunningham (1968). They describe Reserve Hospital as one similar to the field hospital in Florida with its long rows of beds filled with soldiers sick and dying from typhoid fever, malaria, and the most mysterious yellow fever. They indicate that Clara was deeply affected by the heavy loss of life from yellow fever at Reserve Hospital (Burstyn & Women's Project of New Jersey, 1990; Chavez-Carballo, 2013; Cunningham, 1968; Guinther, 1932; Herrmann, 1985; Iglesias, 2002; Kyle & Shampo, 1980; Newcomb, 1975; Samson, 1990). Tigertt (1983), a retired general and researcher of communicable and infectious diseases in the military, argued many years later that yellow fever had never been recognized in the Philippines.

ANNULMENT OF NURSING CONTRACT AND RETURN HOME TO NEW JERSEY

After several months of strenuous nursing in the Philippines, the Army sent Clara Maass home to New Jersey in April 1900. The circumstances of her dismissal are divergent. Guinther (1932) and Cunningham (1968) wrote that, while in the Philippines, Clara Maass was stricken with dengue fever and hovered between life and death. They reported that, because her recovery was so slow, the Army sent her home to recover. Dengue (also called *break bone fever*) is characterized by agonizing joint and muscular pain and was considered to be highly contagious. Now we know that it is a virus transmitted by a species of the *Aedes aegypti* mosquito and that decreased pain and full recovery of former strength is a slow process.

The more likely version of Clara Maass's dismissal by the Army from her work as a contract nurse in Manila, Philippines, can be found in documents housed in the National Archives and Records Administration (NARA) in Washington, DC. There is no mention in any reports of her having contracted dengue fever while serving as a contract nurse in Manila. On March 21, 1900, Clara Maass wrote Colonel Charles R. Greenleaf, chief surgeon, Department of the Pacific and 8th Army Corps, requesting that her contract be annulled "on account of ill health" and that she receive transportation to the United States on the next transport (Clara L. Maass to Charles R. Greenleaf, March 21, 1900). On March 23, 1900, Major and Surgeon William R. Hall stationed at the First Reserve Hospital in Manila also sent a letter to Chief Surgeon Greenleaf informing him that if Miss Maass was unmarried, she should have her contract annulled. His letter explained that Clara Maass's roommate, Rose Kane, friend with whom she had requested to travel to the Philippines, had reported that Clara Maass had confided to her that "she was pregnant and that she would have an abortion produced," which she had done 3 days before on March 20, 1900. Hall reported that Clara Maass was "boasting that no one could prove it" and that was why head nurse McCloud compelled her to ask for an annulment of her contract. Hall also maintained that, at the time of his writing, Clara Maass was attempting to contradict her roommate and to force the head nurse to resign her position. He cautioned that Clara Maass, her "confederate," and the Army officer involved would attack the character of all who opposed them (William R. Hall to Charles R. Greenleaf, March 23, 1900). There can be no doubt that this behavior was *challenging the process*.

Three days after writing her initial letter to Chief Surgeon Colonel Greenleaf, Clara Maass wrote him a second letter to respectfully inform him "that after thinking the matter over and considering what a hot-bed for gossip this is, I have decided to ask for the *annullment* [sic] of my contract and receive transportation to take effect as soon as possible" (Clara L. Maass to Charles R. Greenleaf, March 24, 1900).

A week later, Colonel Greenleaf sent a letter to the U.S. Army Surgeon General George Miller Sternberg in Washington, DC, stating that he had the honor to transmit papers in the case of contract nurse Clara Maass, who would be sailing on April 1, 1900, on the transport *Sherman*, under orders to report by letter to the surgeon general on her arrival at her home for annulment of her contract. He added that after Clara Maass requested annulment of her contract, he was contacted by civilians who informed him that she had been charged with immorality and was forced by the head nurse to request that her contract be annulled. Thinking that this had the potential to become a public scandal, he had requested an official report from the commanding officer at the Reserve Hospital, W. R. Hall, which should be kept confidential. He assured Sternberg that he was looking into the matter and would report his findings at a later date. In the future, he was ordering that all matters and communications related to the conduct and discipline of the contract nurses be sent directly to himself (Charles R. Greenleaf to George M. Sternberg, March 30, 1900). Surgeon General Sternberg's response to Chief Surgeon Greenleaf's letter of March 30, 1900, clarified "that nurses about whom there was 'unpleasant gossip' should be ordered home at the earliest opportunity." He cautioned that there be no talk of this kind in regard to the Army nurses in the Philippines. Further, he directed that the "confederate" of Miss Maass should also be sent home if this had not already been done. He also supported the return of efficiency reports prepared by the chief nurses on a regular basis, quarterly, and when a contract was annulled. This would expedite the prompt return of nurses reported as unsatisfactory to the United States (George M. Sternberg to Charles R. Greenleaf, May 3, 1900).

Thus, according to a memo written by Surgeon William R. Hall at First Reserve Hospital and handwritten Service Record notes, Clara Maass left the Reserve Hospital in Manila on March 29, 1900, and proceeded on the transport *Sherman* to the United States (W. R. Hall to Charles R. Greenleaf, March 29, 1900). More details were provided in her Service Record that she arrived on April 30, 1900, at General Hospital in San Francisco, California; left San Francisco for New Jersey on May 5, 1900; and her contract was officially annulled "for cause" on May 7, 1900 (Clara L. Maass Service Record, Record Group 112, Entry 149). An undated note (author anonymous) accompanying vouchers for the final pay for Clara Maass was sent to Surgeon

General Sternberg indicating that she was sent home from Manila by Colonel Greenleaf and that the papers had been filed with Dr. McGee:

> She arrived in the U.S. about May 1. She delayed in San Francisco on her own account until May 5, and reached home (East Orange, NJ.) via Wash. D.C., May 13. She should have been home May 7th. The vouchers pay her to include May 7th, and annul her contract as of that date. Is this action approved by the Surg. Genl.? (Anonymous [Note to George M. Sternberg])

According to her Service Record, Clara Maass arrived at General Hospital in San Francisco after she left Manila. We do not know whether she was admitted as a patient but it is a logical assumption if she was recovering from an abortion as is reported by her Service Record documents and commanding officers' letters and reports.

A letter dated August 1, 1900, was sent by Dr. Anita Newcomb McGee, director of the Army Nursing Service and acting assistant surgeon in the U.S. Army in response to a letter written to her on July 26, 1900, by Clara Maass. This letter cannot be located; however, Dr. McGee informed her that her letter was received and that she would be glad to do all that was possible (Anita N. McGee to Clara L. Maass, August 1, 1900). It is noted that Dr. McGee's endorsement had been cited by Clara Maass to strengthen her November 1899 petition to Surgeon General Sternberg to serve as a U.S. Army contract nurse in the Philippines.

THE YELLOW FEVER COMMISSION IS ESTABLISHED IN CUBA

In 1897, the American Public Health Association (APHA) presented draft legislation to President William McKinley requesting that a scientific commission be formed to study the etiology of yellow fever (Guerena-Burgueno, 2002). Unfortunately, no congressional action resulted, so it was presented again the following year. While Clara Maass was still serving as a contract nurse in the Philippines, U.S. Army Surgeon General George Miller Sternberg, member of the APHA, renowned bacteriologist, and world authority on yellow fever, formed the Army Board of Medical Officers known as the U.S. Army Fourth Yellow Fever Commission on May 23, 1900. Its purpose was to pursue scientific investigations with reference to the infectious diseases prevalent on the island of Cuba, especially yellow fever. This Yellow Fever Commission was composed of surgeon members with assigned responsibilities: Major Walter Reed, American—head of affairs and U.S. Army contract surgeon; James Carroll, British—bacterial investigations; Aristides Agramonte, Cuban—autopsies and pathological work; and Jesse Lazear, American—mosquito work (Bean, 1983; Chaves-Carballo, 2013). Eventually, the Commission members decided to meet with Dr. Juan Carlos Finlay y Barres, known as Dr. Finlay, a Cuban scientist who had developed the theory that the *Culex fasciatus*, now called the *Aedes aegypti* mosquito, was the vector that transmitted yellow fever. Nineteen years earlier, in February 1881, the Spanish government had appointed Dr. Finlay to represent Cuba and Puerto Rico and to present his theory and experiences at the International Sanitary Conference in Washington, DC (Iglesias, 2002). He had tried to prove his mosquito theory for 20 years but, at that time, no one was trained in experimental medicine. Finlay did not control his subjects, prevent them from being bitten by other mosquitoes, or protect them from exposure to yellow fever (Bean, 1983). He was incorrect in maintaining that an infected mosquito bite could induce immunity without causing clinical yellow fever. Late in 1904, however, Dr. Finlay was elected president at the 31st meeting of the APHA and was honored at its meeting the following year in recognition of his scientific work with yellow fever (Guerena-Burgueno, 2002).

The Yellow Fever Commission began inoculating human volunteers on August 11, 1900, using mosquitoes harvested from larvae provided by Dr. Finlay. This was the first time in the modern era when written informed consent was obtained, and it was provided in Spanish and English (Chaves-Carballo, 2013). Subjects received an incentive of $100 in U.S. gold and an additional $100 in gold should they actually develop yellow fever. Nine inoculations by infected mosquitoes between August 11 and August 25, 1900, resulted in no cases of yellow fever. Though most of the Commission members were disillusioned, Dr. Carroll, a nonbeliever in Finlay's mosquito vector hypothesis, inoculated himself by being bitten by an infected mosquito. Five days later, he developed a severe case of yellow fever and never fully recovered. From that time, he was said to have been "a strangely embittered man" (Bean, 1983, p. 659). A second case occurred 5 days after a 24-year-old American soldier volunteer, Private William Dean, was bitten by the same mosquito that had bitten Dr. Carroll. Supporting Dr. Finlay's hypothesis, a second Commission member, Dr. Lazear, was supposedly accidentally bitten on the back of his hand by a stray mosquito at Las Animas Hospital on September 13, 1900, and subsequently died from a severe case of yellow fever. Dr. Walter Reed, deeply saddened by his colleague's death, realized the importance of these cases and received permission to present a preliminary note on the results of human experiments at the APHA's annual meeting held in Indianapolis, Indiana, on October 22–26, 1900. There was national and international celebration of the news of this significant discovery. Major General Leonard Wood hosted a banquet honoring Finlay in Havana, Cuba, on December 22, 1900. All of the Commission members attended except for Dr. Carroll who was still ill.

Six nonfatal cases of yellow fever were reported from mosquito bites to two American soldiers and four Spanish immigrants between December 5, 1900, and January 2, 1901. Between January 19 and February 7, 1901, four more cases of yellow fever resulted from mosquito bites to American volunteers. Four cases were reported from subcutaneous injection of blood or filtered serum from yellow fever patients. Five subjects volunteered for additional human experiments designed to disprove that yellow fever could be contracted from close contact with contaminated materials such as clothes and bedding of patients who had yellow fever. Between December 5, 1900, and February 7, 1901, experiments were conducted at a quarantine site established on November 20, 1900, near Camp Columbia at Los Quemados de Marianao. The site consisted of seven Army tents guarded by a military garrison and was named Camp Lazear in memory of the deceased Commission member (Chaves-Carballo, 2013). Before his death, Lazear had been responsible for raising the mosquitoes from eggs obtained from Finlay, each kept and meticulously labeled in separate test tubes (Bean, 1983).

The Yellow Fever Commission learned three things about yellow fever: (a) It was spread by the bite of a female *Stegomyia* mosquito that had sucked blood from a yellow fever patient within the first 3 days of the onset of the disease; (b) after biting the patient, the mosquito could infect another only after 12 to 20 days, and blood taken from the patient during the first or second day of the disease injected into a nonimmune person could also cause yellow fever; and (c) if a patient who developed yellow fever produced by a mosquito bite survived, he or she would develop immunity against a subsequent injection of blood from a yellow fever patient. Having completed his mission, Dr. Walter Reed left Cuba in 1901, leaving Major William Crawford Gorgas the work of clearing the mosquitoes out of Havana (Burstyn & Women's Project of New Jersey, 1990).

RETURNING TO CUBA TO NURSE YELLOW FEVER PATIENTS

On February 10, 1900, Major Gorgas, U.S. Army Medical Department, who was serving in the Military Government of Cuba, was appointed chief sanitary officer of Havana. He worked diligently for the rest of the year to clean up the city, believing that yellow fever was caused by poor sanitation. This did not influence the incidence of the disease in new arrivals. He also thought that vaccination might be the best measure to prevent the spread of yellow fever. Under the direction of Dr. Juan Guiteras, a Cuban pathologist trained in Philadelphia and a former professor at the University of Pennsylvania, Gorgas established an inoculation station at Las Animas Hospital. He expected that infected mosquitoes would bite those who were not immune, as in smallpox inoculations prior to the discovery of the vaccine. He also thought that all new arrivals to Havana would eventually contract yellow fever and that immunization under careful medical care would be preferable and less risky (Tigertt & Tigertt, 1983). He issued a call to nurses to care for the patients at Las Animas Hospital. Clara Maass, home in New Jersey, responded by sending him a letter offering her services. She received a telegram from Major Gorgas on October 14, 1900, urging her to "come at once." Even though she planned to marry "a certain businessman in New York," Clara sailed to Cuba, placing service to others above personal commitment (Cunningham, 1968, p. 42).

When Clara Maass arrived in Cuba, she was employed by the Sanitary Department of Havana, headed by Major Gorgas and paid by Cuban funds, not by the U.S. Army. Until the spring of 1901, Clara nursed patients at Las Animas Hospital, the primary hospital for yellow fever victims. Once diagnosed with yellow fever, patients were transferred to Las Animas Hospital. There, Drs. Guiteras and Gorgas alternated each month as visiting physicians. Their insistence that a strict therapeutic protocol be maintained resulted in the lowest mortality rates in yellow fever patients compared to all other Havana hospitals and private home care. Treatment was provided by Clara Maass and other "excellent corps of American female nurses" (Chaves-Carballo, 2013, p. 559). They ensured that this rigorous regimen was adhered to by offering constant bedside vigilance and accurately documenting temperature, pulse, and urinary output. Patients were placed on complete bed rest in a supine position, receiving no food during the active stage, progressing to clear liquids and cracked ice in 4 to 5 days. For the first few days, the only medication provided for headaches and muscular discomfort was phenacetin 5 mg or a similar analgesic. *External* applications, such as mustard plasters, or *internal* ones, such as ice chips, were given for stomach irritability. Saline enemas were administered if patients' urinary output fell below 500 mL in a 24-hour period. If temperatures remained at 103°F, cold water sponges were administered by the nurses.

CLARA MAASS VOLUNTEERS TO BE BITTEN BY INFECTED MOSQUITOES

Clara Maass had heard of the Havana Yellow Fever Commission. She had also heard about the experiments underway to determine the role of mosquitoes in transmitting yellow fever and to produce the disease in a controllable form so that immunization might be secured with minimum danger ("Clara Louise Maass," 1950). On her arrival in Havana, she initiated meetings with Commission members Drs. Finlay, Guiteras, and Albertini, and Majors Gorgas and Ross (Guinther, 1932). She witnessed their experiments and was impressed by their efforts to address the yellow fever problem (Burstyn & Women's Project of New Jersey, 1990). Dr. Guiteras told Clara Maass that they hoped their experiments would prove that the September 1900 death of 34-year-old Dr. Lazear had not been accidental. Between February 22 and August 24, 1901, in the Las Animas Hospital studies, 19 subjects were bitten by presumably infected mosquitoes on 42 occasions. Only one volunteer out of the first 28 inoculations developed a mild case of yellow fever. One half of the subsequent 14 experiments were positive for yellow fever with three fatalities.

Whether motivated to become immune to yellow fever to enhance nursing of her patients or to earn the $100 offered to volunteers by the U.S. Army to send home to her family, Clara Maass, the only American woman and nurse involved, consented to be bitten by infected mosquitoes. She was bitten on March 7 and 25; May 15, 16, and 27; and a date in June 1901 that some report as June 4 (Chaves-Carballo, 2013; Herrmann, 1985). Cunningham (1968) wrote that it was June 24, 4 days before her 25th birthday. He also stated that she developed a mild case of yellow fever from which she quickly recovered. Tigertt and Tigertt (1983) maintain that Dr. Guiteras, in his report, does not indicate that Clara Maass developed yellow fever as three others were bitten by the same mosquito and developed no symptoms. In a letter to her widowed mother, Clara wrote:

> I will soon send you $100. It will pay immediate debts and
> enable Sophia [her sister] to come to Cuba. I can get her a
> position as a nurse here at $50 a month. She can take my place,
> Mother, for—now don't be surprised—I am soon to be married.
> (Cunningham, 1968, p. 44)

The preceding letter was later printed in an article in the *New York World*, which described her fiancé as a "well-to-do New York businessman." Nothing more is known about him. In another letter to her mother, Clara implores her mother not to worry if she heard that Clara had yellow fever because it was a good time of the year to catch it and that most of the cases were mild. Also, if she did get yellow fever, she should be immune and not afraid of the disease in the future (Cunningham, 1968).

Neither Dr. Guiteras nor Clara Maass believed that she had developed immunity to yellow fever, in spite of her repeated exposure to infected mosquitoes. Thus, on August 14, 1901, Clara volunteered again to be bitten at 9 a.m. by four Alvarez mosquitoes. Juan Alvarez was a 13-year-old boy from Santiago, Cuba, who had experienced an extremely virulent form of yellow fever. These Alvarez mosquitoes were responsible for all three of the deaths from experimental yellow fever recorded at Las Animas Hospital. At the time she was bitten, Clara knew that two volunteers, Carro and Repressas, who had been bitten on August 8, had become ill on August 11. A third volunteer, Campa, was bitten on August 9 and became febrile on August 14 at 9 a.m. (Chaves-Carballo, 2013).

CLARA MAASS DEVELOPS YELLOW FEVER

Three days and 21 hours later, Clara Maass developed fever. She had chills, backache, headaches, and muscular pain, all dreaded symptoms of yellow fever. She wrote to her mother a last letter and by the time it arrived at East Orange, her family had learned that Clara was seriously ill:

Goodbye, Mother. Don't worry, God will take care of me in the yellow fever hospital the same if I were home. I will send you nearly all I earn, so be good to yourself and the two little ones. You know I am the man of the family, but do pray for me. (Cunningham, 1968, p. 44)

Clara's clinical chart indicated that her temperature rose to 104.2°F on August 19, 1901, and ranged between 103°F and 104°F on August 20; between 102.2°F and 103°F on August 21; between 101.4°F and 103°F on August 22; and spiked to 103.8°F on August 23. It plummeted throughout the day on August 24 before she died at 6:30 p.m. (Fever Chart for Clara Louise Maass, August 14, 1901).

Dr. Gorgas sent Clara's sister Sophia a telegram on August 20 that "Miss Maass has yellow fever" (Cunningham, 1968, p. 44). On August 24, Clara Maass's mother received a telegram stating that she was worse. The next day, her mother received a final telegram: "Miss Maas died twenty fourth six thirty pm Gorgas" (Cunningham, 1968, p. 44). Sophia arrived in Havana on August 25, unaware of her sister's death and she remained in Havana to attend her funeral. Clara Maass was buried in a lead casket within 24 hours of her death at Colon Cemetery in Havana, Cuba. Afterward, Sophia gathered her sister's few belongings and returned home to New Jersey.

The news of Clara Maass's death and human experimentation was sensationalized in some U.S. newspapers over the course of several days. Such headlines read "Girl Died for Mother;" "Miss Maass Braved Yellow Fever Because the $100 Was Needed," and "Sold Her Life for $100" (Chaves-Carballo, 2013, p. 560). The following editorial appeared on the front page of *The New York Times* on August 26, 1901:

The ethics of the Cuban experience would seem to depend a good deal upon the motive actuating the victims. In the case of Miss Maas[s], the young nurse who died on Saturday, it would seem to have been the very highest which could inspire a self-sacrificing woman to put her life in peril. She not only was willing to incur risk of infection if thereby she might assist in establishing a scientific hypothesis of first importance in the etiology of yellow fever, but she desired to make herself immune, to the end that her usefulness in her chosen vocation might be increased and her opportunities of service to those suffering from the disease enlarged beyond what should be possible in one liable to contract the disease. No soldier in the late war placed his life in peril for better reasons than those which prompted this faithful nurse to risk hers. Facing death on the battlefield does not call for the highest kind of courage. Thousands who would have rushed up San Juan hill with a shout would turn pale at the thought of facing less imminent danger in the quiet of the clinic, as the subjects of an experiment like that of a bite from an infected insect that might, or might not, be capable of imparting the disease he is supposed to carry.

The annals of medicine are full of the records of the noblest and most disinterested self-sacrifice for the sake of truth. Unmarked and forgotten graves are filled by those who have joined the army of martyrs and left behind as their legacy to humanity facts to assist in formulating the generalizations of medical science. (Cunningham, 1968, p. 46)

Dr. John Ross, the medical director at Las Animas Hospital, later wrote that "Miss Maass acted from a high sense of duty, and her conduct was truly heroic. I had warned her of the danger and advised her against it" (Iglesias, 2002, p. 12). Drs. Gorgas, Guiteras, and Agramonte shared the grief of Clara Maass's death with the Maass family. Guiteras was reported to have become despondent, refusing to discuss it in public. Even when he became chief sanitary officer in Havana, he would not endorse obligatory childhood vaccination programs in Cuba (Chaves-Carballo, 2013). Later, General Gorgas acknowledged the courage of Clara Maass by writing:

Miss Maass was a most excellent nurse. She died as the direct result of the mosquito bite. Large sums of money and many lives have been saved, and will yearly be saved, by this discovery of the manner of propagation of yellow fever. (Kyle & Shampo, 1980, p. 750)

POSTHUMOUS HONORS

On February 20, 1902, the U.S. Army disinterred the lead casket of Clara Maass and sent it to be buried with military honors in Fairmount Cemetery in Newark, New Jersey, a few miles from her birthplace (Newcomb, 1975). It was marked by a small Army stone. In 1904, the Army granted Clara's mother a pension of $12 a month in recognition of her daughter's service "of a military character at the time of her death" (Cunningham, 1968, p. 46).

Twenty-two years after Clara Maass' death, Leopoldine Guinther, a graduate from Philadelphia General Hospital, became superintendent of Newark Memorial Hospital. Though there was a portrait of Clara Maass above the mantle in the nurses' sitting room and the sickroom was named the *Clara L. Maass Memorial Room*, most of the nurses there knew little of Clara Maass except that she had been a former chief nurse. Miss Guinther became one of several champions to preserve the memory of Clara Maass. She contacted the living members of the early nursing school classes as well as Clara Maass's 80-year-old mother who was, by then, living in a nursing home.

She also searched for her weed-covered grave with the deteriorated, almost illegible headstone. Miss Guinther traveled to Havana several times seeking information about Clara Maass. During her first visit in the summer of 1927, the only assistance she received was from a fellow visitor to the American Consulate who had lived in Havana during the Spanish–American War and had met Dr. Aristide Agramonte, who had worked on the yellow fever experiments. After returning home, in a Philadelphia library she found his original yellow fever report to the governor of Cuba, which included Clara Maass's hospital record. Miss Guinther copied the entire report, written in Spanish, and took it with her the following year to Havana, determined to have it translated into English. On the cruise ship, she met a Cuban attorney who was so intrigued with the story of Clara Maass that he volunteered to translate Dr. Agramonte's report. Miss Guinther had raised funds so that in May 1930 she could dedicate a polished pink Milford granite headstone to replace the faded marker on Clara Maass's grave in Fairmont Cemetery. On it, she placed a plaque bearing an image of Clara Maass with a brief account of her part in the yellow fever experiments that led to her death. It ended with the words, "Greater Love Hath No Man Than This" (Cunningham, 1968, p. 76).

On September 28, 1936, Dr. Antonio Diaz Albertini, director of Las Animas Hospital and President of the Finlay Institute, made a presentation of memorial plaques for Clara Maass and Dr. Jesse Lazear to be placed within the hospital. His address included:

> Admirable lives of Miss Maass and Dr. Lazear who left us as a legacy the highest examples of abnegation, of sacrifice, and love of science, in which they offered their useful existence for the good and progress of medicine. . . . a tribute of remembrance and gratitude to the memory of Lazear and Miss Maass; placing in this hospital plaques which perpetuate the heroism of those cherished martyrs to science. (Translation [from Spanish] of speech by Antonio D. Albertini, September 28, 1936)

Five years later, on Palm Sunday 1941, Emma Maass, younger sister of Clara Maass, presented a memorial window to the Mountain View Methodist Church in New Jersey. It contained the same words on the plaque that Miss Guinther had placed on the headstone at her grave in Fairmont Cemetery: "Greater Love Hath No Man Than This" (Cunningham, 1968, p. 76).

Another long-time champion in perpetuating Clara Maass's memory was Reverend Arthur Herbert, pastor of the Holy Trinity Lutheran Church in East Orange, New Jersey, and trustee of the Lutheran Memorial Hospital, formerly the Newark German Hospital. Its name was changed on May 22, 1945, as a result of World War II sensitivities. In 1947, Pastor Herbert, also a philatelist, led the efforts seeking authorization from the U.S. House of Representatives to issue a stamp in Clara Maass's memory. No action was taken as there was a new U.S. Postal Service ruling that 50 years had to elapse following a stamp subject's death before a commemorative stamp could be issued. He was assured that her name would be kept on file and could be activated on August 24, 1951, the 50th anniversary of her death. Not to be squelched, Herbert put Clara Maass's name on the hospital's Christmas seals for the years 1948, 1949, 1950, 1953, 1955, 1957, and 1958. In the winter of 1949, *TIME* magazine published a story on yellow fever without a mention of Clara Maass. Pastor Herbert immediately sent a letter describing her role in the yellow fever experiments in Havana, a photograph of Clara Maass, and a plea that she be remembered as one who "symbolizes the sacrificial spirit, the best in young American womanhood" (Cunningham, 1968, p. 78). The magazine printed his letter and the photograph, which was followed on May 8, 1949, by *American Weekly* publishing an article selling over a million copies. Within weeks, the Clara Maass story was broadcast by Dr. Walter Maier in his *1949 Memorial Day International Lutheran Hour* to more than 1,100 stations in 50 countries and in 20 languages. She was portrayed in radio and television versions of "No Greater Love," on the *Cavalcade of America* series produced by E. I. DuPont de Nemours and Company. Also, in 1949, the Lutheran Memorial Hospital donated two $400 Clara Louise Maass Scholarships to Cuban girls aspiring to study nursing at the hospital. The director of Las Animas Hospital flew from Havana to New Jersey to accept them.

In 1950, Upsala College, where Lutheran Memorial Hospital nurses had been affiliated since the early 1940s, named a new dormitory the Clara Maass Hall; Las Animas Hospital dedicated a pavilion in her memory; and La Santisima Trinidad (Holy Trinity) Lutheran Church in Havana started a new college, Colegio Clara Maass. The American Nurses Association (ANA) Board of Directors, in its 1950 annual meeting, committed to securing a commemorative stamp recognizing Clara Maass's contribution.

Cuba issued 3 million 2-cent stamps on August 24, 1951, designed by the art director for the New Jersey Bell Telephone Company. On it were Clara Maass's portrait, a drawing of the old Newark German Hospital and Las Animas Hospital, and the inscription "For Science and Humanity–In Peace and War" (Cunningham, 1968, p. 81). Three of Clara Maass's sisters accompanied Pastor Herbert to Havana for the stamp's issuance and signing ceremonies. Herbert continued his campaign for a U.S. Commemorative Clara Maass stamp in meetings with Eleanor Roosevelt, Cardinal Francis Spellman, and President Harry S. Truman.

On June 19, 1952, the name of Lutheran Memorial Hospital was changed to the Clara Maass Memorial Hospital and relocated to Belleville, New Jersey, with a new building erected in 1955 to 1957. Now the Clara Maass Medical Center museum houses archives, preserving letters, documents, photographs, and publications to honor the memory of Clara Maass

(Chaves-Carballo, 2013). In 1956, the Public Service Advertising Council featured her photograph and story in advertisements for U.S. Savings Bonds that were carried in approximately 800 national magazines entitled "Young Miss Maass Bet Her Life" (Cunningham, 1968, p. 90).

After Pastor Herbert's death in 1969, the campaign to memorialize Clara Maass with a commemorative stamp was furthered by the Clara Maass Memorial Hospital's public relations staff and the editor of *RN* magazine. The target date was Clara Maass's 100th birthday. The nation's nurses were contacted by the media and leaflets distributed at professional meetings encouraging them to join the many interested citizens, health care organizations, and legislators in writing to the Citizen's Stamp Advisory Committee in Washington, DC. A stamp was designed by Paul Calle from Stamford, Connecticut, and on August 18, 1976, the first Clara Maass commemorative stamps were issued at ceremonies held at the Clara Maass Memorial Hospital. The large stamp had a light blue background with Clara Maass's profile in color wearing a black-banded white nurse's cap and uniform with her gold Newark German Hospital pin on the collar, and inscribed "She Gave Her Life" (Herrmann, 1985, p. 56).

Two other events occurring in 1976 commemorating the contribution of Clara Maass were her induction as an inaugural member into the ANA Hall of Fame and the Franklin Mint striking a Clara Maass metal.

MODELING THE WAY

Those who knew Clara Maass described her as one who was selfless and who lived courageously by her principles. Thus, she exhibited the exemplary leadership practice of *modeling the way* (Kouzes & Posner, 2012). From an early age, she demonstrated tenacity in her values and initiative by living and working outside of her home to lessen the burden of her care, to help others, and to contribute to her family's survival. Clara Maass intentionally chose a career of service, securing the education to guarantee that she would be a competent nurse and a leader and, at the same time, to continue providing financial support to her family. She could have remained securely in her head nurse position at Newark German Hospital but, instead, actively sought to nurse soldiers with tropical diseases in foreign locations. In this, she followed the lead of her idol, Florence Nightingale, and, in turn, modeed the way as a pioneer for others who would serve their country as nurses in the Army Nurse Corps. While nursing patients with yellow fever, Clara Maass investigated the yellow fever experiments being conducted in Havana, Cuba. Fueled by her value of service, she sought to contribute to the resolution of the controversy regarding the etiology of this horrific disease, to more effectively nurse her patients by developing immunity, and to offer ongoing financial compensation to her family by volunteering as a study participant to be bitten by infected mosquitoes.

CHALLENGING THE PROCESS

Though Walter Reed's Yellow Fever Commission had demonstrated that the mosquito was the vector of transmission of yellow fever, it was only after Clara Maass's death that some of Havana's civilians became convinced of this theory. Only then did they begin to accept the relationship between yellow fever and the *Aedes aegypti* mosquito. Her death was more "real" than the direct claims of the U.S. military leaders. The people of Havana were then willing to support General Gorgas' Department of Sanitation in wiping out yellow fever in a territory believed to be endemic for this disease. With success controlling yellow fever in Havana, the U.S. leaders gained enough credibility to continue implementation of its control efforts throughout much of Latin America (Jusino, 2012).

There are no records or firsthand accounts that explain precisely why Clara Maass sacrificed herself. Perhaps her behaviors suggest that she was a martyr, voluntarily and deliberately adhering to a tenet or cause at the risk of losing her own life. Her quiet, humble volunteering as a participant in the yellow fever experiments was congruent with the pattern of her entire life— a life based on principle. She possessed an abiding belief in her mission not only to alleviate suffering but also to preserve life itself. Clara Maass made a carefully thought-out choice to commit herself to a course of action to actualize her belief (Herrmann, 1985).

Clara Maass lived her brief life in service to others, putting the well-being of her family, community, country, and its territories ahead of herself. She was an exemplary and courageous leader, unafraid to *challenge the process*. Three times, in spite of fervent pleas of protest, she responded to calls for nurses brave, hardy, and hearty enough to care for U.S. soldiers in dangerous, distant locations. She was dedicated and undaunted in her quest to discover opportunities to be a catalyst for change. . . . *No greater love than this.*

TIMELINE

- June 28, 1876—Clara Louise Maass is born in East Orange, New Jersey, to a poor German immigrant family.
- 1888—Leaves home to become a live-in "mother's helper"; family moves for several months to a farm in Livingston, New Jersey; returns to East Orange and to job as mother's helper, working for room and board; attends East Orange High School.
- 1891—Begins a full-time job at Newark Orphan Asylum.
- 1893—Enrolls in the second class in Newark German Hospital's Christina Tref Training School for Nurses.
- October 1895—Graduates from school and receives her nurse's cap and pin; continues working as a staff nurse at Newark German Hospital.

- 1898—Earns a promotion to become head nurse at Newark German Hospital.
- October 1, 1898—Applies and is hired to be a "contract nurse" with the U.S. Army receiving a salary of $30/month.
- October 3, 1898—Reports to 2nd Division Hospital in Jacksonville, Florida, at the 7th Army Headquarters to care for wounded soldiers sent from Cuba; transfers to 1st Division Hospital in Savannah, Georgia.
- January 1899—Reports to 1st Division Hospital, Camp Columbia at Havana, Cuba, where she is first exposed to yellow fever.
- January 21, 1899—Leaves Cuba, honorably discharged and released from service.
- February 5, 1899—Nursing contract is annulled.
- November 20, 1899—Receives a telegram from the surgeon general summoning her to serve; reappointed as a contract nurse at $50/month; sails to Manila, Philippines.
- January 5, 1900—Reports for duty at the First Reserve Hospital in Manila, Philippines.
- March 23, 1900—Requests an annulment of her contract for "ill health."
- April 1, 1900—Sails on the *Sherman* to the United States.
- April 30, 1900—Arrives at General Hospital in San Francisco, California.
- May 5, 1900—Leaves San Francisco, California.
- May 7, 1900—Contract annulled by U.S. Army surgeon general "for cause."
- October 1900—Receives a telegram from Major William Gorgas to "come at once" to Las Animas Hospital in Havana, Cuba; employed as a civilian by the Sanitary Department of Havana, Cuba.
- March 7, 25; May 15, 16, 27; and June 24, 1901—Volunteers to be bitten by yellow fever–infected mosquitoes.
- August 14, 1901—Volunteers to be bitten by four Alvarez-infected mosquitoes.
- August 17, 1901—Develops a full-blown case of yellow fever.
- August 24, 1901—Dies at 6:30 p.m. from yellow fever at the age of 25.
- August 25, 1901—Buried in a lead casket in Colon Cemetery in Havana, Cuba.
- February 20, 1902—U.S. Army disinters and sends Clara Maass's casket to be buried with military honors in Fairmount Cemetery in Newark, New Jersey.
- May 1930—Leopoldine Guinther dedicates a new monument at Fairmount Cemetery to memorialize Clara Maass.
- September 28, 1936—Dr. Antonio Diaz Albertini, director of Las Animas Hospital, dedicates memorial plaques for Clara Maass and Dr. Jesse Lazear to be placed in the hospital.
- Palm Sunday 1941—Emma Maass presents a memorial window to the Mountain View Methodist Church to honor her sister Clara.
- January 1950—ANA Board of Directors endorse a plan to secure a Clara Maass commemorative U.S. postage stamp.

- August 24, 1951—Cuba issues a 2-cent Clara Maass commemorative stamp for the 50th anniversary of her death.
- June 19, 1952—Lutheran Memorial Hospital, formerly Newark German Hospital, changes its name to *Clara Maass Memorial Hospital.*
- June 28, 1976—Franklin Mint strikes a special metal commemorating the 100th anniversary of Clara's birth.
- August 18, 1976—U.S. Postal Service issues a postage stamp honoring Clara Maass (at the beginning of this chapter).
- 1976—ANA inducts Clara Maass as an inaugural member of the ANA Hall of Fame.

QUESTIONS FOR DISCUSSION

1. Even as a young child, Clara Louise Maass exhibited a vigorous desire to help her family and serve others without regard for herself. While nursing yellow fever patients in Cuba, she repeatedly *challenged the process* by volunteering to be bitten by infected mosquitoes. Do you believe self-denigration and sacrifice are essential to being a "servant leader"? Why or why not?
2. Clara Maass has been designated by some as a "hero" and others, as a "martyr." Which do you think she was and why? Can you identify present-day heroes or martyrs who are or have been "exemplary nurse leaders?"
3. Against repeated advice from her family and colleagues, Clara Maass insistently sought nursing assignments with military patients in distant locations, provided nursing care to yellow fever victims, and engaged in very risky yellow fever experiments. How are you *challenging the process* in order to adhere to your values and commitments?

REFERENCES

Application for Contract Nurse of Clara L Maass. National Archives and Records Administration (Record Group 112, Records of the Office of the Surgeon General-Army, entry 149—Personal Data of Spanish–American War contract nurses 1898–1939), Washington, DC.

Anonymous. [Note to George M. Sternberg]. National Archives and Records Administration (RG 112, entry 26, 7W2A 4/0/2/Box #303 File #52030 on Clara L. Maass), Washington, DC.

Bean, W. B. (1983). Walter Reed and yellow fever. *Journal of the American Medical Association, 250*(5), 659–662. doi:10.1001/jama.1983.03340050071035

Burstyn, J. N., & Women's Project of New Jersey. (1990). *Past and promise: Lives of New Jersey women.* Metuchen, NJ: Scarecrow Press.

Chaves-Carballo, E. (2013). Clara Maass, yellow fever and human experimentation. *Military Medicine, 178*(5), 557–562. doi:10.7205/MILMED-D-12-00430

Clara Louise Maass. (1950). *American Journal of Nursing, 50*(6), 343.

Contract for Services as Nurse—Clara L. Maass. (1898, October 1). National Archives and Records Administration (RG 112, entry 26, 7W2A 4/0/2/Box #303 File #52030 on Clara L. Maass), Washington, DC.

Cunningham, J. T. (1968). *Clara Maass: A nurse, a hospital, a spirit*. Cedar Grove, NJ: Rae Publishing.

Donahue, M. P. (1996). *Nursing, the finest art: An illustrated history* (2nd ed.). St. Louis, MO: Mosby.

Fever Chart for Clara Maass. (1901, August 14). Philip S. Hench Walter Reed Yellow Fever Collection. Department of Historical Collections and Services, the Claude Moore Health Sciences Library, University of Virginia, Charlottesville, VA.

Greenleaf, Charles R. (1900, March 30). [Letter to George M. Sternberg]. National Archives and Records Administration (RG 112, entry 150, Correspondence relating to the service of Spanish–American War contract nurses, 1898–1939 on Clara L. Maass), Washington, DC.

Guerena-Burgueno, F. (2002). The centennial of the yellow fever commission and the use of informed consent in medical research. *Salud Publica De Mexico, 44*(2), 140–144.

Guinther, L. (1932). A nurse among the heroes of yellow fever-conquest. *American Journal of Nursing, 32*(2), 173–176.

Hall, W. R. (1900, March 23). [Letter to Charles R. Greenleaf]. National Archives and Records Administration (RG 112, entry 150, correspondence relating to the service of Spanish–American War contract nurses, 1898–1939 on Clara L. Maass), Washington, DC.

Hall, W. R. (1900, March 29). [Memo to Charles R. Greenleaf]. National Archives and Records Administration (RG 112, entry 26, 7W2A 4/0/2/Box #303 File #52030 on Clara L. Maass), Washington, DC.

Herrmann, E. K. (1985). Clara Louise Maass: Heroine or martyr of public health? *Public Health Nursing (Boston, Mass.), 2*(1), 51–57.

Iglesias, M. A. (2002). Clara Louise Maass—Nurse (1876–1901). *Scalpel & Tongs: American Journal of Medical Philately, 46*(1), 11–14.

Jusino, M. A. (2012). *Nursing imperialism: Clara Maass, yellow fever and U.S. ambitions in Cuba, 1898–1901*. Unpublished thesis, Rutgers University Graduate School, Newark, NJ.

Kouzes, J. M., & Posner, B. Z. (2012). The leadership challenge: How to make extraordinary things happen in organizations (5th ed.). San Francisco, CA: Jossey-Bass.

Kyle, R. A., & Shampo, M. A. (1980). Clara Louise Maass. *Journal of the American Medical Association, 244*(1), 75.

Maass, Clara L. (February 1, 1899; February 6, 1899; August 14, 1899; September 22, 1899; November 1, 1899). [Letters to Dr. Anita N. McGee, Assistant Surgeon General]. National Archives and Records Administration (RG 112, entry 26, 7W2A 4/0/2/Box #303 File #52030 on Clara L. Maass), Washington, DC.

Maass, Clara L. (1899, November 18). [Telegram to George Miller Sternberg, Surgeon General]. National Archives and Records Administration (RG 112, entry 26, 7W2A 4/0/2/Box #303 File #52030 on Clara L. Maass), Washington, DC.

Maass, Clara L. (1900, March 21). [Letter to Charles R. Greenleaf]. National Archives and Records Administration (RG 112, entry 26, 7W2A 4/0/2/Box #303 File #52030 on Clara L. Maass), Washington, DC.

Maass, Clara L. (1900, March 24). [Letter to Charles R. Greenleaf]. National Archives and Records Administration (RG 112, entry 26, 7W2A 4/0/2/Box #303 File #52030 on Clara L. Maass), Washington, DC.

McGee, Anita N. (1899, September 26). [Letter to Clara L. Maass]. National Archives and Records Administration (RG 112, entry 26, 7W2A 4/0/2/Box #303 File #52030 on Clara L. Maass), Washington, DC.

McGee, Anita N. (1900, August 1). [Letter to Clara L. Maass]. National Archives and Records Administration (RG 112, entry 104, on Clara L. Maass), Washington, DC.

Newcomb, R. F. (1975). U.S. stamp to honor Clara Maass. *RN, 38*(9), 17.

Roeber, W. J. (1898, September 15). [Letter To Whom It May Concern]. National Archives and Records Administration (RG 112, entry 26, 7W2A 4/0/2/Box #303 File #52030 on Clara L. Maass), Washington, DC.

Rogers, Carrie E. (1899, March 1). [Letter to Dr. Anita N. McGee, Assistant Surgeon General]. National Archives and Records Administration (RG 112, entry 26, 7W2A 4/0/2/Box #303 File #52030 on Clara L. Maass), Washington, DC.

Samson, J. (1990). A nurse who gave her life so that others could live—Clara Maass. *Imprint, 37*(2), 81–89.

Sternberg, George M. (1899, November 20). [Telegram to Clara L. Maas]. National Archives and Records Administration (RG 112, entry 26, 7W2A 4/0/2/Box #303 File #52030 on Clara L. Maass), Washington, DC.

Sternberg, George M. (1900, May 3). [Letter to Charles R. Greenleaf]. National Archives and Records Administration (RG 112, entry 150, Correspondence relating to the service of Spanish-American War contract nurses, 1898–1939 on Clara L. Maass), Washington, DC.

Tigertt, H. B., & Tigertt, W. D. (1983). Clara Louise Maass: A nurse volunteer for yellow fever inoculations—1901. *Military Medicine, 148*(3), 252–253.

Translation (from Spanish) of Speech by Antonio D. Albertini. (1936, September 28). Philip S. Hench Walter Reed Yellow Fever Collection. Department of Historical Collections and Services, the Claude Moore Health Sciences Library, University of Virginia. Charlottesville, VA.

FURTHER READING

Leader, S. E. (1995). *Subjected to science: Human experimentation in America before the second world war.* Baltimore, MD: Johns Hopkins University Press.

PART V

Enabling Others to Act

Dorothea Lynde Dix: Privilege, Passion, and Reform

Barbara Ann Caldwell

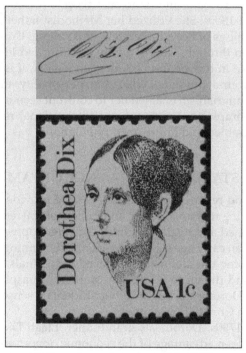

*U.S. postage stamp issued in 1983
honoring Dorothea Lynde Dix.*

•　•　•　•　•

To the General Assembly of the State of North Carolina (1848):

> I come not to urge personal claims, nor to seek individual
> benefits; I appear as an advocate of those who cannot plead
> their own cause; I come as a friend of those who are deserted,
> oppressed, and desolate. . . . I am the Hope of the poor crazed
> beings who pine in the cells, and stalls, and cages, and waste
> rooms of your poor-houses. I am the Revelation of hundreds of
> wailing, suffering creatures, hidden in your private dwellings,
> and in pens and cabins—shut out, cut off from all healing
> influences, from all mind-restoring cures. (Dix, 1848, p. 1)

Dorothea Lynde Dix (1802–1887) was born into an upper-class, highly educated, intelligent, and politically connected Bostonian family. These opportunities provided the foundation necessary to propel her into a leadership role as national and international advocate for the most vulnerable groups in the mid-1800s. She utilized her Methodist father's background to augment the teachings of her adopted religious calling, Unitarianism, which promises salvation through leading a pure and directed life. As we explore her leadership role in this period of American history, it is easy to see how her family background, pursuit of education, personality, and religious commitment to humanitarianism enabled her to confront seemingly insurmountable obstacles to implement national and international reform of care for psychiatrically disabled and imprisoned populations.

SETTING THE STAGE: THE INFLUENCE OF FAMILY

A short background regarding Dorothea Dix's life provides an understanding of the underlying religious, social, and philosophical tenets that emerged during her shortened and neglected childhood. Her appreciation for acquiring knowledge at an early age set the stage for her beginning role as a teacher. Teachers can become the lifeline of displaced individuals, assisting in providing a vision and dream to which any student can aspire. In her role as a young teacher, Dorothea brought to her students a sense of purpose and direction based on Christian principles.

During the 1790s, Dorothea's grandfather, Elijah Dix, was a wealthy doctor who had taken advantage of the economic opportunities of the Revolutionary War. He and his wife, Dorothy Lynde, settled in Worcester, Massachusetts, with the entire family clan, including a network of doctors, lawyers, and municipal officials. Her grandfather's life was an inspiration to Dorothea to make the most of the evolving economic and social life in Boston. In 1795, the family moved to Boston with other prominent families.

Her grandfather became an influential importer of European pharmaceutical products, chemicals, and appliances, which created the family fortune. As an entrepreneur, he developed local merchant institutions and diversified his investments. The Dix family mansion, built on Orange Street in Boston with its tailored botanical gardens, bespoke of the standards of the aristocratic community. Elijah Dix also transformed State Street into a city enterprise and erected chemical factories in South Boston.

Elijah and Dorothy Dix's rising influence was enhanced by their oldest son's graduation from Harvard Medical School under the tutelage of John Warren, the most prominent physician in Boston. Their daughter married a Harvard graduate who became a well-respected Methodist pastor in Dorchester. Their second son and Dorothea's father, Joseph, also attended Harvard, but as a result of erratic attendance, partying, and abuse of alcohol, was unable to apply himself to academic studies. In 1800, he married Mary Biglow, who, according to his father, Elijah Dix, was a step backward for the family's reputation compared to his daughter's choice of partner. As Elijah Dix's prestige and wealth grew, he invested in real estate, purchasing vast acreage in western Maine and developing a commercial center known as Dixmont, Maine. Because Joseph had not graduated from Harvard and made a place for himself in Boston, his father provided the couple with land in Hampden, Maine.

Dorothea was born in the small village of Hampden on April 4, 1802. Because of political events in 1807, an embargo halted the New England sea merchant trade and Elijah Dix's businesses failed. Shortly after, Elijah Dix died, leaving a small inheritance to his oldest surviving son and Dolly (Dorothea), his 5-year-old granddaughter.

Dorothea experienced an isolating and lonely childhood as a result of her mother's poor health during her pregnancies and her father's difficult temperament and alcoholic tendencies. In 1915, they then moved to Worcester, Massachusetts (Lightner, 1999). The birth of her brother was a difficult experience for Dorothea, aged 10, because it forced her into being the older sister, losing her role as an only child. Her parents began to rely on her to be more independent and self-sufficient, working with her father in his book-bindery business.

Her father was a fervent Methodist; Methodism, at the time, was practiced mainly by farmers and rural artisans. A new and more refined religious movement that attracted Dorothea was Unitarianism, a sect that evolved at a time when other religious movements were occurring. As an adolescent, Dorothea rejected Methodist teaching and embraced Unitarianism with fervor.

Dorothea's discontent with her place in her nuclear family, her mother's chronic illnesses, and her feelings of being abandoned by her parents, prompted her to leave home, seeking sanctuary with her grandmother in the Boston mansion. Her grandmother sent her home after 2 weeks. By the time she was 14, she again returned to her grandmother's home, but this time, her grandmother made arrangements for her to live in Worcester with the family of Sarah Fiske, whose husband was a prominent physician and a close friend and supporter of Dorothea's grandfather's initiatives.

In the early 1800s, age 14 marked the end of Dorothea's childhood and the beginning of early adulthood and independence for this adolescent girl.

Her early family experiences of feeling abandoned and alone shaped Dorothea's attitudes, personality, and future. She had a strained relationship with her grandmother, who had a similarly dominant personality; neither could easily relent under pressure. Dorothea desperately sought to find a replacement maternal figure. Seeking respectability for herself, she turned to older women in the community to serve as mentors and confidants.

Anne Heath, 5 years older than Dorothea, was able to fill this role as an older sister. Ann was one of six sisters and a devout Unitarian. The Heath family lived in Brookline, and this provided an active social environment for Dorothea. They often entertained recently ordained Unitarian ministers from Harvard Divinity School, thus affording Dorothea opportunities to meet eligible male companions. Dorothea, however, was not inclined to actively participate in Boston society. She was highly regarded as beautiful and articulate, but most of all, intelligent and resourceful, important qualities associated with an aspiring leader.

ENACTING NONTRADITIONAL FEMALE ROLES: EDUCATOR AND WRITER

Dorothea began to develop more fully as a nontraditional, independent woman. She was exposed to innovative ways of thinking about education and how change could be achieved. Dorothea was able to develop a self-reflective and goal-directed approach to daily life and began to ingrain these qualities in her students. She shared her talents and ideas through her published books. This, in turn, enhanced her social status. These actions set her apart from other women, but she continued to struggle to find an appropriate career path.

The traditional role of women in the 1850s was one of domesticity, benevolence, and education. Teaching became the exclusive profession available to single, respectable women who wanted to distinguish themselves in public life. Dorothea's moral compass was embedded in her new religious attraction to the teachings of Unitarianism in the churches of Boston. This attitude supported her ambitions to open a school. She believed that the poor and unfortunate were also entitled to be educated. So, at age 14, she convinced her grandmother to allow her to use a small portion of their home for her new school.

Dorothea, tall and elegant, projected confidence in her new role as a teacher. Contrary to the more traditional activities of needlework and sewing for women, as schoolmistress, her philosophy was that education should focus on developing ethical and religious foundations. She inculcated in her students a sense of self-control, perseverance, and goal directedness. Dorothea supplemented her own knowledge by attending lectures and classes at local schools, learning about horticulture, botany, and the sciences.

Dorothea Dix's reputation as a young educator grew in the Boston community. She was asked to lead an innovative educational initiative, developed by an English educator named Joseph Lancaster, dividing schools into smaller groups with older children teaching younger children. Initially refraining from accepting a position at the prestigious Boston Female Monitorial School because the focus was on needlework, she realized that she could influence more children through advocating her philosophy of moral teachings. The school's headmaster, William Bentley Fowle, introduced significant innovations into education by transforming the focus from discipline to learning, by using blackboards, maps, and written lessons. The school's prominence and innovative style enabled the development of an educational program designed to prepare women as teachers.

Dorothea was developing many new ideas about education and introducing change in large educational systems. In May 1824, at age 22, she published her first book, *Conversations on Common Things: Or Guide to Knowledge* (Dix, 1824), which was, ironically, a dialogue between a mother and her daughter on everyday knowledge and lessons on life. Publication was a major accomplishment for a woman at that time, and this greatly strengthened Dorothea's stature as an educator.

Traditionally, a young woman's role was to find a suitable husband, without which a woman would have to care for herself and make her own way in the world. In her early 20s, Dorothea's social life allowed her the hope of finding a young suitor in Ezra Stiles Gannett, a college friend of Ralph Waldo Emerson. Gannett was a graduate of Harvard Divinity School and Dorothea often attended his sermons. Gannett became interested in another Boston woman, Elizabeth Davis, but she married Daniel Webster's law partner. Dorothea's interest in Gannett faded as she became more convinced that she wanted to lead a productive and singular life. She also experienced a change in her relationship with Ann Heath.

The Heath family endured a significant tragedy with the death of Anne's 21-year-old younger sister, Mary. This tragedy brought the Heath family together and Dorothea's place in the family began to erode. Mary's death acted was a reminder to Dorothea of the unresolved loss in her life, activating her deep and hidden fears of abandonment, which she had never faced. She was beginning to come to terms with her fate in life as a single woman. As with most single women of her day, she moved into a boarding house in Beacon Hill.

FINDING MENTORS: RELIGIOUS AND EDUCATIONAL COMMITMENT

Dorothea continued her transformation with another mentor, William Ellery Channing, who translated his religious views into an action-oriented humanitarian program. Her time with the Channing family allowed Dorothea the opportunity to more fully expand her literary work. This was the time period of the American Literary Renaissance, which enabled expanded educational opportunities for women. Although Dorothea continued to be burdened by her difficult childhood, her quest for a moral imperative was coming into focus.

Mentors are a critical component in the development of exemplary leadership practices and behaviors. Mentors provide others with a role model to emulate. They do this not only in behavioral ways but also by providing opportunities for reflection on a potential leader's philosophical approach and career path. An important event in Dorothea's life was her meeting William Ellery Channing, who was considered one of the leading religious and literary leaders in the United States. His philosophy was known as Christian Humanism, which conflicted the prevailing Calvinist teachings of predestination (Howe, 2007). A Harvard classmate of Joseph Dix, Dorothea's father, and pastor of the Federal Street Church, William Ellery Channing was considered a very important intellectual and moral leader of his community (Howe, 2007). He requested that Dorothea lead a Sunday school class for his congregation.

As a result of her newest book, *Evening Hours* (Dix, 1825), Dorothea's reputation continued to expand in Boston. The book used a question-and-answer format for children to gain insight into the New Testament. Dorothea's compulsive work habits of taking on more than she could physically produce created health issues for her. She suffered from lung inflammation and chronic exhaustion as a result of her daily schedule (Brown, 1998). Because of ongoing health issues, she was forced to engage in intellectual pursuits rather than the more strenuous physical demands of teaching. She wrote another children's storybook series, *American Moral Tales for Young Persons* (Dix, 1832). In this book, she blended principles of Unitarianism with her own personal experiences to create moral-minded characters of poor and orphaned children. Around this time William Ellery Channing and his wife, Ruth, invited her to join their family in Newport, Rhode Island, and to take responsibility of their two children. Dorothea used this opportunity to network with other influential individuals, such as Sarah Gibbs, whose father had made his fortune in Newport. Like many wealthy people of the day, Dorothea decided to travel south to spend the winter in Pennsylvania (Brown, 1998). She stayed with Sarah Gibbs but found herself lonely and searching for emotional support. She subsequently reconnected with Anne Heath, who communicated with her by letters for the rest of her life.

Dorothea's moral underpinnings of Christian piety were further highlighted in another book, *Meditations for Private Hours* (Dix, 1828), a manual of daily devotional practices. Her religious perspective and continued involvement with Unitarianism was at odds with the more orthodox sects prevalent at that time in Boston. Her religious beliefs, which were founded on the Gospels, provided direction, she believed, for every good word and deed. Dorothea believed that for individuals, action, constant action, is life's true calling, not just the mere enjoyment of life. She felt strongly that women have a special place in society because women have a superior piety, benevolence, and morality.

Merging her religious commitment and literary talents earned Dorothea a reputation as an accomplished teacher and professional author. While in Philadelphia in 1828, she became the editor of a children's holiday book, *The Pearl or Affection's Gift: A Christmas and New Year's Present* (Dix, 1829). Such books were becoming popular as gifts in a prospering America. In this book, Dorothea told stories involving moral lessons for children. She also began to exercise her political thinking on topics such as the forced relocation of Native American Indian tribes and to support replacing jails and almshouses with new institutions for the insane.

Dorothea Dix's talents and reputation as an educator continued to grow, but her dogmatic religious principles and rigid thinking as an educational leader foreshadowed problems she would encounter as head of nursing during the Civil War. Boston was in the initial phase of an educational transformation for women. George B. Emerson, a headmaster of a leading private school for girls, believed that educated women "give a permanent impulse to the onward movement of the race" (Emerson, 1831, p. 25). Dorothea's mentors, besides Emerson, were Catherine Beecher who was headmistress at the Hartford Female Seminary, and Mary Lyon, who started the New England Female Seminary for Teachers, a project that founded Mount Holyoke College. Dorothea Dix proceeded to open a school for the wealthy families of Boston, requesting fees of $80 per 12-week quarter, not including room and board. This was considered expensive for the time, but allowed her the funds to support herself and finance the growth of more diverse academic programs offered at the school.

Her curriculum was innovative and included Unitarian religious services and bringing consultants in to teach French and the sciences. Dorothea's reputation continued to grow but, owing to her disciplinary rules and because of her continued strong-mindedness, students found the atmosphere of the school too rigid. By 1834, the conflict between her pupils and her rules continued. Many promising young, wealthy students left. Although stressed by these issues, she continued her commitment to teach and care for the young students. Nonetheless, she distracted herself with additional commitments, such as the development of charity schools for poor children, which were supervised by Nathaniel Hall.

Dorothea's inability to come to terms with her difficult childhood continued to haunt her. She was unable to clearly reflect and manage her life within normal boundaries. Working without giving any consideration to her own health, she soon became seriously ill. Dorothea was counseled by George B. Emerson to close her school. She was offered the opportunity to sail to Liverpool with the support of the Channing's friends, the Rathbones, a wealthy and influential British family. The Rathbones were responsible for launching the success of John James Audubon; they encouraged many

Bostonian families to visit London. Because of her continued health problems and the death of her grandmother, Dorothea decided to stay in England for several years. The turning point for Dorothea came when she returned to Boston. Her quest for a higher calling was revealed in a visit to the Middlesex County Jail and Boston Lunatic Hospital.

POLITICAL LEADERSHIP AND THE MORAL MOVEMENT

The 19th century was a period of rapid change in the United States, fueled by new and innovative ideas from Europe. The insane asylum reform movement, supported in England by the Religious Society of Friends, the Quakers, sought a gentle, patient, self-controlled approach to insanity. Thus, began the "moral movement" and institutional reform. Dorothea had arrived at the intersection of her religious beliefs and roles as educator and moral advocate. She was inspired by the fate of the most vulnerable, the mentally ill and imprisoned, and began her quest to understand the problems faced by the insane and to persuade others that they have a responsibility to support a new way of caring for this population. Her talent to *enable others to act* continued to expand. She understood, possibly by self-reflection, that collaborating and networking with political individuals who shared her vision required essential leadership skills and behaviors. She began to hone her talents in lobbying and partnering with superintendents of mental hospitals in order to bring her reform legislation forward. She began comprehensive data collection of the state's insane institutions in order to present the most accurate information.

In 1842, Dorothea Dix's interest in the most vulnerable was influenced by the writings of Edward Jarvis, a young physician who published *Insanity and Insane Asylums* (Jarvis, 1841). This book advocated for self-control versus violent coercion and was based on a philosophy from the European movement in France and England, known as the "moral treatment" approach. The word "asylum" means "haven," and, to Dorothea, a homelike place of calm and focused treatment. The "moral treatment" approach to the insane recommended a therapeutic milieu, a normal homelike environment where the insane would have a daily work schedule. Intellectual and social stimulation would be incorporated into the treatment setting. Dorothea, understanding best practices for the mentally ill, visited sites using this innovative method such as the Worcester State Lunatic Hospital, Boston Lunatic Hospital, and McLean Asylum of the Massachusetts General Hospital. She began to integrate the "moral treatment" model of care with her closely held religious doctrines, which would become the basis of her own reform doctrine.

Women had begun to participate in the presidential campaign in 1840 (Howe, 2007). In 1842, the Whig party, whose foundational cause was based on redemptive reform and positive government, had interests similar to

Dorothea's mission (Howe, 2007). The Whigs encouraged women to participate in political areas in an indirect manner by exerting influence on their
husbands. Seeking political connections, Dorothea understood that in order
to successfully achieve her goals for the mentally ill, she needed to keep her
agenda free of issues involving women's rights and slavery. In addition, she
needed to engage others in her vision.

Samuel Gridley Howe, a friend of Horace Mann, secretary of education in Massachusetts, was a major reformer for the blind. Dorothea Dix col-
laborated with him to launch efforts to expose the conditions of the jails and
almshouses in eastern and southern Massachusetts. They also persuaded the
editor of the *North American Review* to publish a commentary on the deplorable conditions of the insane, promoting the innovative "moral treatment"
movement. She began to collect data all across the state on all the town
and county institutions housing the insane. When Howe won the election
as a Whig member in the Massachusetts' House of Representatives, he had
Dorothea complete her report to be presented at the opening session of the
legislature.

Dorothea learned early that she needed to challenge the system in order
to accomplish her moral mission. Her report, *Memorial to the Legislature of
Massachusetts, 1843*, a 32-page comprehensive account, was considered one
of the most outstanding reports of the century. The report contained elements of political rhetoric, religious commitment, and eye-witness accounts
of the "cages, closets, cellars, stalls, pens that the insane are kept in" as well
as "the chained, naked, beaten with rods and lashed into obedience conditions found." This was her moment of awareness: This endeavor, uncovering
the horrible treatment of the insane and jailed, was to be her life's work, her
vocation, and would require her to enter public life, not a traditional life for
a 19th-century single woman.

She believed that the existing conditions were so horrific that only
new facilities could provide humane conditions. Dorothea did not focus on
the causes of insanity but rather on the duty that society had to respect,
protect, and care for those who could not care for themselves. Her views
reflected those of her early pastor and mentor, William Ellery Channing,
who preached that kindness was an essential part of human interactions
and the path to a more divine place. She appealed to the legislature's sense
of civil obligation to exercise its power and authority to take immediate cor-
rective action.

Dorothea proved to be a successful lobbyist. The *Memorial* report, not
unsurprising, was met with mixed reviews. Dorothea was not to be dis-
suaded. She used her capacity to network on behalf of the reform she was
seeking by soliciting letters from all of the superintendents of the mental
hospitals in New England in support of the construction of a new facility. She
became politically active by attending legislative debates and engaging legislators in her cause. As in all things political, a compromise funding bill was

adopted to enlarge the Worcester asylum to accommodate 150 more patients. With passage came the public acknowledgment that the government had a responsibility to care for the insane.

DEVELOPING LEADERSHIP EXPERTISE AND CAMPAIGNING FOR CHANGE

Dorothea embraced reform, continuing to expand her leadership base by collaborating with the superintendents of the various psychiatric hospitals and with politicians and ensuring that all reform legislation had the support of a board-based constituency. Using a team approach and sharing her vision in leading this transformation enabled her to garner support and *enable others to act*. She demonstrated her capacity to share her hard-earned power base with other prominent individuals by keeping her writings humble and direct, not filled with religious rhetoric. The important leadership strategies Dorothea used were her persuasive language skills and her ability to be available to meet and converse with powerful politicians and prominent professionals involved in the passage of much-needed reform legislation.

Dorothea Dix was a deliberate and intelligent woman who learned from her past experiences to enhance her new initiatives. Based on limited personal writings available, she concluded that the rehabilitation of the insane could be improved if the newly committed were separated from the more chronically afflicted, but ensuring separation would require new facilities. Even today, this model is the current evidence-based treatment strategy for individuals newly diagnosed with schizophrenia (Harder, Koester, Valbak, & Rosenbaum, 2014; Norman, Manchanda, & Windell, 2014). Individuals experiencing their first episode of psychosis are maintained in community settings with a treatment team and psychosocial interventions are delivered in day programs.

Dorothea Dix transformed herself into a reformer and advocate for the insane by continuing her visits to public insane institutions, almshouses, jails, and hospitals in Vermont, New Hampshire, Rhode Island, and Canada. She also widely distributed copies of her report *Memorial to the Legislature of Massachusetts*. Dorothea Dix's society background enabled her to network with wealthy donors who would be willing to support the reform movement for the insane. An example of the effectiveness of her social standing was her successful funding of an asylum in Rhode Island in collaboration with Nicholas Brown, Jr., the namesake of Brown University.

In the early months of 1848, Dorothea focused her energies on New York by engaging in a 10-week tour of all 60 counties to examine their almshouses, poorhouses, and insane asylums. The data she gathered was incorporated into a report similar to the one she had presented in Massachusetts. She delivered her new report to the New York legislature, seeking support from the former governor, William H. Seward, a strong supporter for a state asylum. Having learned from her previous experiences in Massachusetts, she deleted religious fervor from her text in favor of a strictly dispassionate, statistical account and objective evaluation of each facility she had visited. Her clear, straightforward narrative outlined a nonmedical model of care based on an approach used at Antwerp Hospital in the Belgium town of Geel. This outraged the medical community. As a result, in 1848, the Association of the Medical Superintendents of American Institutions for the Insane argued that all institutions should be controlled by physicians. Her "Memorial to the Honorable Legislature of New York" was rejected in New York (Dix, 1844; Wilson, 1975). Having met with failure, she learned an important lesson: Make sure that all the stakeholders are on board with any initiative and all opposition is neutralized.

With steadfast persistence, resilience, and a more refined sense of political savvy, Dorothea traveled to New Jersey and Pennsylvania. She traversed both states collecting copious amounts of data and field notes. She traveled by overnight stagecoaches so she could work during the day. Once again, she adapted to the resistance that had undermined her previous reports by placing the prevailing medical views in the forefront of her reports. She also incorporated a discussion of the cause of insanity as a condition of the brain rather than demons of the mind as had been championed by Philippe Pineal, reform advocate of the moral movement in Europe. She realized that in order to motivate others to join her cause, she needed to infuse the reports with concepts that physicians were willing to support: Prompt therapy cured most insanity; and the economics of building new hospitals administered by physicians would repay taxpayer investment by removing the newly cured from public assistance. This awareness is a perfect example of her ability to garner support and *enable others to act* by supporting her reform cause and legislative acts.

Her political acumen was demonstrated in her ability to exercise her leadership skills with the legislatures in New Jersey and Pennsylvania. Dorothea engaged the legislators in open dialogue concerning the dimensions of the moral treatment by infusing the meetings with her persuasive arguments. She met frequently with legislators, shuttling between Trenton and Harrisburg. In 1845, the passage of legislative funding allowed for the construction of state mental hospitals in both New Jersey and Pennsylvania.

Dorothea's fame in these extraordinary endeavors spread to other states. She was asked by William M. Awl, superintendent of the Ohio Lunatic Asylum, to support his efforts in launching a political campaign to fund a state asylum. At the same time, however, New Jersey and Pennsylvania officials requested that she act as design consultant to oversee the construction of their new state hospitals. Because Dorothea could not be in two places at the same time, she focused her energies on New Jersey and the construction of the first state psychiatric hospital in Trenton. Mindful of the necessity of establishing the best model for the new hospital, she visited the treatment facilities in Massachusetts, which were considered the premier national mental institutions employing the moral treatment model.

PRISONERS' LETTERS AND EXPANSION OF LEADERSHIP

Dix's reform successes for the insane expanded to prisoners. In her book, *Fifth Letter to Convicts in State Prisons and Houses of Correction or County Penitentiaries*, published for the prisoners, she states:

> The reforming man has truly to pass through fiery trials on
> his way to the Heavenly City; but each step forward, rightly
> planted, adds new force for making the next, and by and by
> the fearful rocks and precipices of the Hills of Difficulty are
> surmounted; the glittering gardens of sensual indulgences are
> passed, and the way becomes smoother, the air purer, the frame
> is braced to new efforts, the thankful heart finds peace and
> exceeding joy in serving God, and in believing and doing his
> commandments. (Dix, 1850, p. 6)

Dorothea's interests turned to the penal system in Pennsylvania, with a particular emphasis on the spiritual life of prisoners. She began by teaching Sunday school at the Eastern State Penitentiary, which gave her opportunities to preach self-discipline and redemptive work similar to her previous days as a schoolteacher. Ever the reformer, she evaluated the quality of treatment of prisoners based on two different models.

The first model, the "separate system," was developed at Eastern State Penitentiary, where solitary confinement was the main management system. The second model was the "congregate system" in which prisoners were isolated at night but during the day, were allowed to work and eat together in common areas. Based on her evaluations, she published *Remarks on Prisons and Prison Discipline in the United States* (Dix, 1845), which won her a place among the most prominent and well-respected women in America. Improvements in ventilation, lighting, heating, cleanliness, and security were the focus of Dix's review. Particular emphasis was on the need to have prisoners engage in work leading to the construction of "work houses" (Brown, 1998). America was seeking prestige in the area of moral leadership, and Dorothea Lynde Dix was able to achieve fame in moral leadership regarding the treatment of prisoners.

TRANSITION TO NATIONAL LEADERSHIP

Dix realized that she must change her role from state activist to national activist and attempt to have the federal government donate land for building state hospitals across the entire United States. She thus began a fierce campaign to get the U.S. Congress to pass her bill. She used all her political expertise to ensure that all influential politicians would support her bill. Although successful in achieving passage of this legislation, Dorothea's efforts ended with a presidential veto. Nevertheless, she was able to garner support for a public mental institution for residents and military personnel in Washington, DC.

In the winter of 1845, Dorothea, at the age of 43, continued her pursuit of moral treatment for the insane. She traveled to Kentucky to assist with the transformation of the Eastern Lunatic Asylum, proposing the need for a second hospital. Dorothea was not immune to the personal struggles of women of this age. She continued to experience an inner tension between being a moral crusader and her sense of being a proper 19th-century woman. This intense, private conflict was part of her continuing internal dialogue. Traveling as a single woman in untracked and dangerous territory, in itself was simply not done by respectable women of her time. But her commitment to the moral transformation of the treatment of the insane was not to be deterred. She traveled to the Southern states by steamboat, visiting Louisiana, Mississippi, Alabama, Georgia, South Carolina, Arkansas, and Missouri. She continued to visit state penitentiaries and insanity wards, tirelessly advocating for reform.

In May 1848, Dorothea demonstrated her innovative approach to exemplary leadership through one of her most brilliant ideas: to garner support to acquire federal government land for state mental hospitals, similar to the land-grant system in place for U.S. colleges. In 1848, Dorothea traveled to Washington, DC, with friends from Nashville, John and Jane Bell, to lobby for the procurement of an endowment for state mental hospitals. She had her eye on national public land being considered for sale to private purchasers.

The Louisiana Purchase and the end of the Mexican War had vastly increased land holdings of the United States. Dix intended to petition Congress to divide the land among the states for the purpose of using the funds from the sale to establish a perpetual fund for the care of the insane. She sought a sponsor, John Adams Dix, who was a New York business leader. He agreed to address Congress, but the proposal was transferred to a Senate Committee on Public Lands. In 1851, the politics in Washington were somewhat overwhelming, with opposition for the bill coming from the Southern Democrats and Westerners. Dorothea refused to be more flexible and make the necessary changes that would have given the bill more broad-based support. As in other cases, she believed that her way was the only way to proceed and resisted compromise.

Even though the bill was defeated, members of both political parties applauded her contributions and tenacity. Out of the ashes of the failure came an opportunity to establish a public mental hospital for residents and military personnel in the District of Columbia. Initially, she did not want to support the project because it reduced the likelihood that her own revised bill would be passed. But the government hospital bill was eventually passed. From this success, her national prominence led to her becoming a consultant to many of the state psychiatric facilities, hospital officials, and trustees. Dorothea was considered by all to be the knowledgeable expert who used her expertise to obtain positions for like-minded physicians as new superintendents. The scope of her stature and influence can still be seen today in the Dix Ward at McLean Hospital in Washington, a premier psychiatric facility.

No sooner had Dorothea succeeded in Washington than she turned her energies to Nova Scotia, Canada, to assist in the selection of a site for a new mental hospital there. Having become aware of the lack of support by the province's officials to provide lighthouses and rescue boats, she expanded her advocacy to aid the victims of shipwrecks.

On her return to Washington in December 1853, President Franklin Pierce was in office and her land-grant bill for the endowment for state psychiatric hospitals was passed by Congress. President Pierce, however, vetoed the bill based on his understanding of Jacksonian federalism, which had established a consensus that Congress could spend money only for the purposes specifically identified in the Constitution (Brown, 1998). Despite Dorothea's efforts, the veto was sustained.

INTERNATIONAL LEADERSHIP AND RECOGNITION

Dorothea's national prominence soared and she traveled to Europe to continue her moral reform mission. She found support and encouragement throughout Europe, Russia, and Scandinavia. She never missed an opportunity to learn about new ideas and wanted to visit sites established by Florence Nightingale, an important step in her subsequent appointment at the federal level.

In 1854, Dorothea left for Europe to spend time with the Rathbones. She obtained letters of introduction to the Earl of Shaftsbury, a prominent statesman who was successful in passing legislation creating a commission to oversee the treatment of the insane. During her time in England, she continued her networking by meeting with key women leaders, including Elizabeth Barrett Browning and Anna Jameson, popular British authors. She also traveled to Scotland and partnered with Dr. Hack Tuke, a prominent critic of the mental health system in Scotland. He wrote a book, *Chapters in the History of the Insane in the British Isles* (Tuke, 1882). One of Dr. Tuke's private letters to Francis Tiffany dated August 1888 from Hanwell, England, on his memories of Dorothea was as follows:

> Her long sustained exertions, undertaken from the highest
> motives, mark the untiring and irrepressible energy and
> fortitude which more especially struck me during our personal
> acquaintance. That these qualities must have exerted enormous
> influence in inducing others—especially young physicians—to
> engage in the humane treatment of the insane can easily be
> understood

Dorothea found conditions in Britain problematic, developed a comprehensive report on the horrible findings, and petitioned Parliament to set up a commission to investigate the conditions found in Scotland. This commission was eventually created in 1857. She then traveled to France and Italy, where she evaluated the treatment of the insane. She met privately with Pope Pius IX to share her accounts of the miserable conditions suffered by the insane in Italy. She received assurances that there would be a new asylum built with papal funds.

Dix's self-reliance and fearlessness continued in the face of the unknown. During her time in Europe, she was able to explore the work of Florence Nightingale, who was considered a "beacon of hope" during the Crimean War. Nightingale had, of course, established a hospital in Scutari, where she was able to ensure that nurses' duties and responsibilities were well executed. Dix studied the successful practices of Nightingale and used these as a foundation for her role as superintendent of nurses during the Civil War.

Dix traveled from Venice to Constantinople to visit hospitals and prisons. She visited Vienna and the major cities of Germany, as well as Moldavia, Walachia, and Serbia. In May 1856, she traveled to St. Petersburg and Moscow. She found that care of the insane in these countries was generally satisfactory, with little physical restraint used to manage patients. From Russia, she traveled to Scandinavia, finding outdated methods of treatment. She traveled to Belgium to see the famous Geel colony, a foundational model of moral treatment of the insane. She observed chronically mentally ill patients being cared for in an inexpensive, unrestrictive environment, engaged in daily active employment.

CAUGHT IN A POWER STRUGGLE

In the final phase of her career, Dorothea was chosen for a national role to lead nursing during the American Civil War, a role that she considered as within her scope of knowledge and skills. She was called on to perform an insurmountable job with little or no resources. Taking this opportunity, she launched the beginning of the nursing profession in the United States but was caught in the cross fire of physicians, surgeons, and nurses.

When she returned to the United States in 1858–1859, the nation was paying close attention to the Lincoln–Douglas debates. The magnitude of Dorothea's past successes allowed her to reflect on the direction her future should take. She decided to focus less on legislative action and more on direct improvement of her connections with individuals from North and South Carolina, Alabama, and Georgia. She was eagerly embraced and asked by the superintendents in these various states to visit and provide them with her recommendations to improve their hospitals for the insane.

After the fall of Fort Sumter, Dix became one of the first volunteers to respond to Lincoln's call to subdue the rebellion (Brown, 1998). On April 19, 1861, she gathered at the White House with the other volunteers and President Lincoln, committing herself to developing a volunteer army of nurses for hospital service. Dorothea became the commander of the army of nurses following Florence Nightingales' precepts, *Notes on Nursing: What It Is, and What It Is Not*, written in 1860.

Secretary of War Simon Cameron created the position of Superintendent of Women Nurses. Dix was authorized to organize the military hospitals by providing nurses and the collection and disbursement of Army supplies. Dix was the first woman to hold any position of federal executive authority in the United States. Dorothea was strategically positioned to be in charge of care for the wounded during the duration of the Civil War. She had extensive experience in hospital administration, had successfully lobbied and advocated for vulnerable populations, had actively been involved in national politics, and had established herself as an influential international woman leader. Dorothea was confronted with the almost insurmountable challenge of facing the outright animosity she received from the Army Medical Department and the disdain surgeons had for women volunteer nurses.

Hospital supplies were scarce, so Dix used her fund-raising experience and her own money to purchase supplies for Union hospitals. To overcome the even larger challenge of recruiting and training women volunteers for nursing, Dorothea worked with Elizabeth Blackwell, the first woman to graduate from an American medical school and established a training program for volunteer nurses. Dorothea recruited women in her own image: self-reliant, self-sacrificing, and self-controlled. Unfortunately, she was more concerned about the volunteers' moral and spiritual qualifications; women would need to pay, in part, for their own expenses, with no wage reimbursements (Brown, 1998).

The United States Sanitary Commission, under Henry Whitney Bellows, a Unitarian minister, sought to exert leadership in the promotion of the well-being and morale of both soldiers and civilians. Bellows was able to enlist the Medical Department, whose first mandate was to train 100 women nurses through the Women's Central Association of Relief (WCAR), considered young women from the New York elite. Dix asked that recruits be older than 30 years and present documents from doctors and clergyman verifying their character. This placed the younger women who were active members of the WCAR in conflict with Dix's policy. To add to the controversy, Dr. Blackwell's trainees were also under 30 years of age and had the appropriate knowledge and skill set. Dorothea's role and influence were greatly challenged. Again, her rigid thinking and clashes with recruits on what to wear, what to do with their off hours, and where the nurses could go in the evening, collided. Dix realized that the nuns were her principal rivals and instructed her nurses not to speak to the nuns (Brown, 1998). Her relationship with the surgeon general began to unravel over his support for the Sisters of Charity nuns, the moral agenda Dix was committed to, and the continuing conflict with the surgeons over decision making.

Chief surgeons were given the authority to dismiss any female nurse who was found to be incompetent, insubordinate, or in any way unable to carry out duties. In the end, the surgeons were allowed to choose their own nurses. As her influence waned, public criticism intensified. In 1863, the War Department abolished the office of General Superintendent of Nurses. At the time, Dorothea refused to resign, instead focusing her energies on caring for returning wounded soldiers.

In the summer of 1865, Dix finally resigned but continued to lobby and work in various states on issues related to care of the mentally ill. In 1881, by act of the New Jersey legislature, Dorothea was graciously given a place to live in the first hospital she had developed, the New Jersey State Lunatic Asylum in Trenton. She remained there, actively advocating for the vulnerable until her death, which occurred on July 18, 1887, while she was sitting at a tea table, of what her physician called ossification of the arterial membrane (Snyder, 1975).

TIMELINE

- April 4, 1802—Dorothea Lynde Dix is born in Hampden, Maine.
- 1814—Leaves home to live with grandmother in Boston.
- 1816—Opens girls' school in Worcester, Massachusetts.
- 1819—Returns to Boston, where she focuses on her own education.
- 1821—Grandmother allows her to use the Dix mansion to open up a charitable school for poor children.
- 1824—Publishes children's book, *Conversations on Common Things: Or Guide to Knowledge*.
- 1826—Experiences serious respiratory illness and forced to close school.
- 1827–1829—Publishes books: *Evening Hours, American Moral Tales for Young Persons, Meditations for Private Hours, The Pearl or Affection's Gift: A Christmas and New Year's Present*.
- 1830—Travels to St. Croix, Virgin Islands, with the William Ellery Channing family.
- 1831—Works with mentors: William Ellery Channing, George B. Emerson, Catherine Beecher, and Mary Lyon.
- 1836–1837—Travels to United Kingdom, stays with the Rathbones.
- 1841—Returns to Boston and teaches Sunday school at East Cambridge Prison.
- 1842—Visits state-of-the-art insane facilities in McLean Hospital, Boston.
- 1843—Presents *Memorial to the Massachusetts Legislature, 1843*.
- 1844—Conducts data collection in Rhode Island.
- 1845—Presents *Memorial* to the New Jersey and Pennsylvania Legislatures.

- 1845–1846—Data collection in Tennessee, Kentucky, Ohio, and Maryland.
- 1846–1847—Collects data and networks throughout Southern states: Louisiana, Alabama, Georgia, South Carolina, Mississippi, and Arkansas.
- 1848—Appeals to U.S. Congress for 5 million acres of public land to care for poor mentally ill individuals.
- 1850—Land-grant bill increased to over 12 million acres is passed by the U.S. House of Representatives.
- 1851—Land-grant bill is passed by U.S. Senate.
- 1853—Travels to Nova Scotia.
- 1854—Land-grant bill passes in both houses of Congress but is vetoed by President Pierce; sails to Liverpool, England.
- 1855—Conducts data collection and gives report in Scotland.
- 1856—Visits Italy and meets with Pope Pius IX; travels to Greece, Turkey, Austria–Hungary, Germany, Russia, and Scandinavian countries; returns to America.
- 1858—Continues reform efforts in Texas and throughout the Southern states.
- 1861—Appointed Superintendent of Female Nurses of the Union Army.
- 1861–1865—Assumes role and responsibilities as superintendent of nurses.
- 1867—Resumes role as reformer.
- 1881—Returns to the Trenton Hospital as a final home in apartment provided to her by act of the New Jersey State Legislature.
- July 17, 1887—Dies at the age of 85 in her apartment in Trenton Hospital, New Jersey.
- 1983—U.S. Postal Service issues a postage stamp honoring Dix (at the beginning of this chapter).

QUESTIONS FOR DISCUSSION

1. Dorothea Lynde Dix made significant contributions to improving the care and treatment of individuals with serious mental illness. What exemplary leadership practices did she use in leading mental health and psychiatric care policy change?
2. Dorothea Dix may be considered one of the first nurse leaders to use evidence-based practice principles to establish the philosophy guiding the newly constructed state psychiatric hospitals in the United States. What was her evidence-based approach to leading change in this important area of health care? How is this similar or dissimilar to the evidence-based practices of nurse leaders today?
3. Leadership was a central force in the life accomplishments of Dorothea Dix. What were some of her key leadership accomplishments in *enabling others to act* to transform the care and treatment for the seriously mentally ill and those who were imprisoned? How is her leadership legacy evident today in health care practices for the mentally ill and the incarcerated?

REFERENCES

Brown, T. J. (1998). *Dorothea Dix, New England reformer.* Cambridge, MA: Harvard University Press.

Dix, D. L. (1824). *Conversations on common things: Or guide to knowledge.* Boston, MA: Munroe & Francis.

Dix, D. L. (1825). *Evening hours.* Boston, MA: Leonard C. Bowles & B. H. Greene.

Dix, D. L. (1828). *Meditations for private hours.* Boston, MA: Munroe & Francis.

Dix, D. L. (1829). *The pearl, or affection's gift: A Christmas and New year's present.* Philadelphia, PA: Thomas T. Ash.

Dix, D. L. (1832). *American moral tales for young persons.* Boston, MA: Leonard C. Bowles & B. H. Greene. Munroe & Francis.

Dix, D. L. (1844). *Memorial, to the Honorable the Legislature of the State of New-York.* Retrieved from http://collections.nlm.nih.gov/catalog/nlm:nlmuid-66420620R-bk/

Dix, D. L. (1845). *Remarks on prisons and prison discipline in the United States.* Boston, MA: Munroe and Francis.

Dix, D. L. (1848). *Memorial soliciting a state hospital for the protection and cure of the insane-North Carolina.* Gloucestershire, UK: Dodo Press.

Dix, D. L. (1850). *Fifth letter to convicts in state prisons and houses of correction or county penitentiaries.*

Emerson, G. B. (1831). *A lecture on the education of females.* Boston, MA: Hilliard, Gray, Little & Wilkins.

Harder, S., Koester, A., Valbak, K., & Rosenbaum, B. (2014). Five-year follow-up of supportive psychodynamic psychotherapy in first episode psychosis: Long term outcomes in social functioning. *Psychiatry, 77*(2), 155–166.

Howe, D. W. (2007). *What hath god wrought: The transformation of American, 1815–1848.* New York, NY: Oxford University Press.

Jarvis, E. (1841). *Insanity and insane asylums.* Louisville, KY: Prentice and Weissinger.

Lightner, D. L. (1999). *Asylum, prison, and poorhouse.* Carbondale, IL: Southern Illinois University.

Norman, R. M. G., Manchanda, R., & Windell, D. (2014). The prognostic significance of early remission of positive symptoms in first treated psychosis. *Psychiatric Research, 218*(1–2), 44–47.

Snyder, C. M. (1975). *The lady and the president: The letters of Dorothea Dix and Millard Fillmore.* Lexington, KY: The University Press of Kentucky.

Tuke, D. H. (1882). *Chapters in the history of the insane in the British Isles.* London, UK: Kegan, Paul, Trench, & Co.

Wilson, D. C. (1975). *Stranger and traveler.* Boston, MA: Little, Brown.

FURTHER READING

Colman, P. (2007). *Breaking the chains: The crusade of Dorothea Lynde Dix.* New York, NY: ASJA Press.

Muckenhoupt, M. (2003). *Dorothea Dix: Advocate for the mental health care.* New York, NY: Oxford University Press.

Tiffany, F. (2012). *Life of Dorothea Lynde Dix.* San Bernardino, CA: Forgotten Books.

Lillian D. Wald: Pioneer of Public Health

Mary Ann Christopher, Regina Hawkey, and Mary Christine Jared

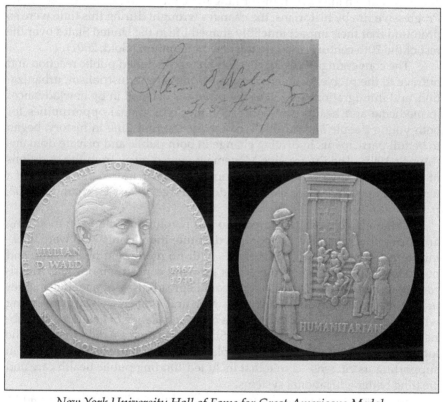

*New York University Hall of Fame for Great Americans Medal,
awarded in 1971, honoring Lillian D. Wald (front and back).*

Long credited as a pioneer of public health nursing in America, Lillian D. Wald (1867–1940) personified the attributes of exemplary leadership in a way that transformed not only the nursing profession but society as a whole. Visionary, innovative, inspiring, passionate, and tenacious, she viewed the circumstances of her time not as obstacles to be overcome but as compelling catalysts for positive change. By harnessing the conditions of the late 1800s and early 1900s as the driving forces of her professional journey, she charted a course that would irrevocably alter the lives of individuals, the circumstances of both local communities and the broader U.S. population, and the future of professional nursing itself.

AN AGE OF TRANSFORMATION

From the 1890s to the 1920s, an unprecedented amount of political, social, and economic change was transforming the United States. Trumpeted as the Progressive Era by historians, the changes wrought during this time were so profound that their impact indelibly shaped life in the United States over the rest of the 20th century and into the new millennium (Gold, 2001).

The converging forces driving this change included public reaction and outrage to the problems that accompanied massive industrialism, urbanization, and immigration, as well as the promises ushered in by new advances in medicine and health care and expanding educational opportunities for both young people and adults. Women, for the first time in history, began to be full participants in driving change in both public and private domains (Muncy, 1998). The Progressive Movement veered away from the traditions of the past and America's founding principles and "required the creation of a new order appropriate for the new Industrial Age" (West & Schambra, 2007, p. 1).

Other elements that factored into this revolution included a mounting anger over the treatment of poor and destitute immigrants who were flocking to the shores of the United States with no money, no health care, and no homes. Simultaneously, there was growing concern among the American elite that those living in poverty could spread diseases endemic in poor neighborhoods to anyone of any class. Men and women were also emerging who were uniquely motivated to take on the challenge of changing the fabric of society and leading the United States to become a nation in which the local, state, and federal government played a much more significant role in supporting its citizens—a role that included funding public health care and creating better educational systems.

One such person was the founder of public health nursing, Lillian D. Wald (1847–1940). Wald embodied a class of women who, because of their education, background, and social position, in combination with the cultural forces and changing attitudes of the Progressive Era, were able to make impressive contributions to "shaping public policy and creating public institutions" (Muncy, 1998, n.p.). Accomplished and often highly educated, these women were activists and leaders. These "new women," in the words of Lillian Wald's biographer Karen Buhler-Wilkerson, were "a revolutionary demographic and a political phenomenon." "The new woman was typically single, educated, economically independent, a champion of professional visibility for women and an advocate of economic and social reform" (Buhler-Wilkerson, 1993, p. 1780).

The framework within which Wald's contributions are perhaps best understood was captured poignantly in the words she herself offered to her staff in 1922: "The times call for the high spirit of the courageous pioneers among physicians, scientists, and nurses" (Buhler-Wilkerson, 2001, p. 113). A century before these concepts found their way into the health care landscape, Wald defined the criticality of patient and community engagement. In doing so, she distinguished herself first and foremost as a leader who enabled others to envision and create a better, bolder world. By *modeling the way*, Lillian Wald exhibited the attribute of exemplary leadership that creates and embodies standards of excellence, thus setting an example for others to follow. In Wald's case, her example established the visionary framework for community-based nursing practice that has underpinned the U.S. health care system for over a century (Kouzes & Posner, 2012).

EARLY LIFE

The seeds of leadership acumen can be traced to a childhood that, in many ways, was emblematic of the American experience. Lillian Wald was born in Cincinnati, Ohio, on March 10, 1867, the second of four children of German immigrants, Max D. Wald and Minnie Schwartz. Her parents were descendants of rabbis and merchants from Germany and Poland, although Wald, herself, was not raised in a religiously observant household. Her father, an optical goods dealer, moved the family to Rochester, New York, when Wald was 11 years old and she would, from that point on, consider Rochester her home (Feld, 2009).

The same restlessness and adventurous spirit that inspired her parents to emigrate from Germany to Cincinnati and then move on to Rochester pervaded Wald's personality. While she was afforded a private boarding school education and all the luxuries that money could buy during her childhood and adolescence, she also reacted to the shackles of a society that she felt offered limited opportunities for women. Rejected by Vassar College at the age of 16 because they considered her too young, Wald grew increasingly impatient with a life defined by the social circuit of Rochester (Lannon, 2006). Inspired by the home visit of a nurse to her then-pregnant older sister, Wald felt herself drawn to the care of the vulnerable and the sick. "In Lillian's eyes everything noble and magnificent was embodied in the trained nurse who came to the house at the time" (Smith, 1929, p. 32). The seeds were thus sown for her life's work.

Ambitious, intelligent, and talented, at age 22, Wald decided to leave her hometown to pursue a career in nursing. Given to rule breaking and risk taking, attributes often associated with exemplary leaders, Wald knew early on that she was called to a life not of privilege, but of serious work (Lannon, 2006). The same leadership attributes of taking risks and challenging rules would later characterize her approach to health care and societal reform. Ultimately, these leadership attributes would compel her to create the organizations that continue to carry on that tradition today—the Henry Street Settlement and the Visiting Nurse Service of New York (VNSNY).

Leaving Rochester in 1889, Wald enrolled in the New York Hospital School of Nursing. One year after graduation, following a discouraging stretch working as a nurse in a juvenile asylum in upper Manhattan, she enrolled at the Women's Medical College. While studying there, Wald was assigned to the Lower East Side of Manhattan—a defining event that would change her life course. "The lack of public health care for the growing immigrant population of the neighborhood prompted Wald and fellow student, Mary Brewster, to abandon medical studies and work full time in the service of New York's poorest residents" (Lannon, 2006, n.p.). A fundamental commitment to the poor would, in fact, always underscore Wald's community-based nursing practice.

Wald first dedicated herself to offering home nursing courses on the Lower East Side, with the purpose of improving the circumstances of child-rearing, stemming communicable diseases, and facilitating the assimilation of new immigrants into the community. Wald based her model of intervention on her belief that the nurses "would not carry the entire responsibility but rather were available for guidance concerning measures that might be taken to alleviate problems" (Buhler-Wilkerson, 1993, p. 1780). Through this model, she promoted a sense of client or patient empowerment and engagement—an approach that continues to resound in today's era of health care reform and health care delivery.

Quite serendipitously, Wald's role expanded from classroom health educator to that of home visiting nurse. While teaching, she was called to the home of one of her students by the woman's young child. Wald recounts following the child through "evil smelling streets," up "slimy steps," and into the sickroom. What she found there shocked her. "All the maladjustments of our social and economic relations seemed epitomized in this brief journey and what was found at the end of it," she later wrote. "The husband was a cripple . . . the family of seven shared their rooms with boarders . . . and the sick woman lay in a wretched, unclean bed soiled with hemorrhage two days old" (Wald in Buhler-Wilkerson, 1993, p. 1779). That single walk crystallized the vision, values, and framework for the field of nursing that would eventually constitute home- and community-based care and public health nursing. Catalyzed to action by what she had seen in that neighborhood and in that tenement, Lillian Wald and her nursing colleague, Mary Brewster, moved into the neighborhood, with Wald "rejoicing that her training in the care of the sick gave her an 'organic relationship' with the community" (Buhler-Wilkerson, 1993, p. 1779). This concept of grassroots connectivity continues to constitute a fundamental construct of visiting nurse services nationally.

Wald's bold shift in course evidenced the brand of creativity and imagination that differentiates exemplary leaders. This same quality allowed her to overcome a formidable societal knowledge deficit in pursuing her new direction. Wald had

> no theories about economics, sociology or politics, little knowledge
> as to how people outside her own social group lived . . . but she
> did have an imagination which enabled her . . . to put herself in
> other people's places. (Duffus in Buhler-Wilkerson, 1993, p. 1779)

This empathic competence facilitated her ability to establish the relationships that were critical to achieving health outcomes.

By exhibiting the adaptability, curiosity, and confidence to step from the classroom into the homes of patients, Wald displayed another attribute of exemplary leaders, one that creates a vision that is sufficiently flexible so that it is adaptable in a changing environment. A leader's vision should identify a common, mutually meaningful purpose and inspire hope, motivate people to become involved, and *enable others to act* in order to achieve a better future (Kouzes & Posner, 2012). This fundamental adaptability and flexibility continues as a requisite attribute of today's community-based nursing leaders, as the accelerated rates of change within health systems in transformation call leaders to mobilize staff, patients, and communities to a common, collective vision and goal in circumstances fraught with ambiguity.

Wald's embrace of this approach is reflected in her insistence on a model of patient and community empowerment, drawing on that attribute of exemplary leaders, which is exquisitely relationship oriented and which affirms the wisdom of actively involving others and investing in partnerships, trustworthy cooperative relationships, and team building (Kouzes & Posner, 2012). Wald nurtured personal strength and self-confidence in others and encouraged others in taking the initiative and having a sense of responsibility, thereby creating an atmosphere of trust, dignity, and empowerment (Kouzes & Posner, 2012). In all that she accomplished, she worked through people—philanthropists who sponsored her settlement house, immigrants who participated in developing the priorities for the Henry Street Settlement, and elected officials who endorsed public policy that promoted the public health.

BUILDING ON THE PUBLIC HEALTH AND SETTLEMENT MOVEMENTS

From the beginning, Wald was determined that her work would address the health of both the individual and of the public. Just as she was influenced by the Progressive Movement and the increasing role of women in achieving social justice, Wald was also significantly impacted by the public health movement. Initiated in the mid-1700s in Rhode Island with the enactment of legislation mandating that pub owners collect data on customers' infectious diseases, the movement expanded into nationwide, large-scale public health surveillance activities in the 1850s when "mortality statistics based on death registration and the decennial census were first published by the federal government for the entire country" (Thacker, Qualters, & Lee, 2012, p. 3). Systematic reporting of disease in the United States was introduced in the 1870s and, by 1893, all states were required to report infectious disease statistics to the federal government. The year 1893 is also when Lillian Wald and Mary Brewster moved into their tenement house on the Lower East Side of New York City in order to live among the people whom they would serve as public health nurses.

This relocation marked the beginning of Wald's work at the Henry Street Settlement. The fact that it occurred at this point in the evolution of public health surveillance and public health nursing is more than a coincidence. The timing was ideal for Wald's new endeavor: *Public health nursing* evolved in the late 19th century in the United States specifically to treat infectious disease in the home. The crowded, dirty, and densely populated tenements that arose in large urban areas during that period made for easy transmission of infectious organisms. Public concern from all levels of society drove historic change; community organizations mobilized and began sending nurses out into peoples' homes to care for the sick. With these efforts, nurses were "protecting the public from the spread of infectious disease" (Buhler-Wilkerson, 1993, p. 1779). Lillian Wald developed a nursing model during her tenure as a visiting nurse that "owed much to the Progressive Reform and Public Health movements" (Buhler-Wilkerson, 1993, p. 1778). But she took the practice of public health one step further, believing "that public health nurses must treat social and economic problems, not simply take care of sick people" (Fee & Bu, 2010, p. 1206). Wald addressed social problems, such as social isolation and boredom, by creating recreational programs in the settlement house, and she worked to optimize employment conditions through her sponsorship of labor unions, particularly to address the workplace issues of women.

Wald's decision to move to the Lower East Side was influenced by the settlement movement as well. This movement, which began in England in the mid-1800s and migrated to the United States shortly thereafter, encouraged educated and middle- to upper-class individuals to move into poor communities and live and work among those they served. Though the original intent was that the poor and uneducated would learn from their settlement benefactors, those managing the settlement houses also learned from those whom they served (Hansan, 2012). The movement became a mechanism for those who had never been introduced to the evils of poverty and the ramifications of its reach to see, firsthand, the horrible conditions in which the impoverished worked and lived. This understanding of a previously unknown, unacknowledged, or hidden reality spurred many settlement house owners to become advocates and activists for social change. Through this process, their immersion—once conceived of as a means of observing those in need, assisting them with health care services, and securing food and shelter for them—became a vehicle for long-lasting, sustained change and transformation, and a way to reach out to an entire population of people previously neglected or left behind.

It is also important to note that the settlement movement offered Wald and other women of her time a leadership opportunity and a chance to promote social change that was largely unavailable through other routes.

> One of the revolutionary characteristics of the settlement house movement was that many of the most important leadership roles were filled by women, in an era when women were still excluded from leadership roles in business and government. Approximately half of the major US settlement houses were led and staffed predominantly by women. Among the most influential leaders were Jane Addams, Mary Simkhovitch, Helena Dudley, Lillian Wald, Mary McDowell, Florence Kelley, Alice Hamilton, and Edith Abbott. (Harvard University Library Open Collections Program, 2014b, n.p.)

In 1895, Lillian Wald and Mary Brewster moved out of their own tenement house into a nearby house donated by financier and philanthropist Jacob Schiff, who had become very interested in the goals of the settlement venture and the mission of the work in which Wald and Brewster were involved. His decision to fund the purchase of the house at 265 Henry Street "provided Wald with the means to more effectively help immigrants and slum dwellers of every race and religion, whose care she made her life's mission" (Ruel, 2014, p. 2). In this new, larger space, the Henry Street Visiting Nurse Service continued to evolve into what would eventually be called the Henry Street Nurses Settlement.

As the following passage from Wald biographer Robert Duffus indicates, the organization's activities soon became well known enough to merit comment in one of the city's leading newspapers.

In 1898, *The New York Times* reported in an article titled, "A Modest Institution that Does Good in Many Ways on the East Side":

> A great deal of good is done on the East Side by an institution which is without an official name. It has come to be called "The Nurses' Settlement" and is the outgrowth of two young women, both trained nurses, to make themselves useful. . . . When the

two young women came downtown to begin their work, a little less than five years ago, they hired the top floor of a tenement and made their home there. Their work was at first chiefly the visiting of the sick. It grew, little by little, and now includes many forms of benevolence. (Duffus, 1938, p. 81)

Over the next decade and a half, the Henry Street Settlement continued to grow steadily. By 1901, it had 15 nurses attending to 3,000 patients. Five years later, in 1906, the settlement was employing 22 full-time nurses who attended to 5,500 patients, making 53,000 professional calls that year (Reznick, 1973) and operating out of 18 district centers (Feld, 2009). By 1910, the staff had grown to 54 nurses who ran convalescent centers, three country homes, a number of first aid stations, and a maternal–child health service. That same year, the staff made 143,589 home visits and administered 18,934 first aid treatments (VNSNY, 2014).

The Henry Street Settlement's development was rooted in Lillian Wald's personal philosophy that the nurse's "organic relationship with the environment should constitute the starting point for a universal service to the region" (Feld, 2009, n.p.). Wald saw this relationship between visiting nurses and their patients as key to helping society understand and empathize with the reality of how this entire population of people suffered, struggled, and tried to survive, as she described in her book, *The House on Henry Street* (Wald, 1915, p. 2):

Two decades ago the words "East Side" called up a vague and alarming picture of something strange and alien; a vast crowded area, a foreign city within our own, for whose conditions we had no concern. Aside from its exploiters, political and economic, few people had any definite knowledge of it, and its literary discovery had but just begun. The Lower East Side then reflected the popular indifference—it almost seemed contempt—for the living conditions of a huge population.

At the same time, Wald actively encouraged the city's public sector to assist in expanding her efforts. "In 1902, she arranged to have a Henry Street nurse provide full-time care to children in public schools. This program led the New York City Board of Health to organize the first public school nursing system" (Lannon, 2006, n.p.). Over the years, her advocacy came to have an impact on a national level as well: "As the Henry Street Nurses' Service drew national attention, it became the model for similar programs in cities throughout the United States. Public health nursing emerged as a profession as a direct result of Wald's work and ideas" (Lannon, 2006, n.p.).

EMPOWERING COMMUNITIES TO HELP THEMSELVES

As an exemplary nurse leader, Wald's approach was aspirational, broad, and visionary. She defined health in its broadest conceptualization. She embraced a philosophy that considered physical, emotional, social, spiritual, and environmental variables in the well-being of individuals and communities. A pioneer in the provision of holistic health care, Wald's methods encompassed what we now know as the biopsychosocial model of health care. This model recognizes that the psychosocial dimensions (psychological, socioeconomic, and cultural), along with the biologic aspects, contribute to an individual's functioning in the circumstances of disease or illness.

Although nursing services were a predominant focus of her settlement house, its scope also included housing, education, and social services. Within the Henry Street Settlement, Wald established boys' and girls' clubs, social events, classes in English, drama courses, and arts and crafts activities (Feld, 2009). In 1913, Wald described the settlement as having evolved into

> kindergartens, carpentry shops, dancing schools, gymnasiums, debating clubs, and literary societies. We started the experiment of house-keeping centers, we have story-telling hours, a Civic Forum, lectures on various subjects, from government to sex hygiene, a library and study, a place set apart from the sewing school, for the savings bank and for the cultivation of drama. There are clubs for boys and girls, which in their diversified form and method present concrete opportunities to teach self-government and civics; mothers' clubs; culture clubs for school teachers, for young lawyers, for the professional and laborer. A charmingly frank relationship exists, and the houses are used by the many with a very fair degree of propriety that guards the privilege of all without special advantage to any one over another. Around the tables many times in the seasons conferences are held or meetings arranged for bringing together diverging people. They do not always end in unanimity, but almost always in mutual respect for the other person's sincerity. (Duffus, 1938, p. 116)

This building of "community" was critically important to an immigrant population that was in many ways disconnected from the broader society.

Wald's broad view of health included standing up for social fairness. She "made sure that her Settlement Houses not only provided services, but also employment, for members of all racial and ethnic groups" (Jewish Women's Archive, n.d., n.p.). In 1909, her concerns over racial injustice led Wald to host "the National Negro Conference, a gathering held at Henry Street . . . [that] became the founding meeting of the National Association for the Advancement of Colored People [NAACP]" (Jewish Women's Archive, n.d., n.p.).

In 1944, VNSNY and the Henry Street Settlement separated into two distinct corporations. Today's Henry Street Settlement serves a new generation, primarily those of Asian, African American, and Latino backgrounds. With an annual budget of $35 million, the Henry Street Settlement now serves 50,000 individuals annually, supporting a range of programs that are reminiscent of those Wald founded. In the 2013 Henry Street Settlement annual report, which is posted on their website, a client's words are quoted that poignantly affirm Wald's continuing impact: "Henry Street changed my life for the better; all I had to do was walk in" (Henry Street Settlement, 2013, p. 7). This concept of neighborhood-based access continues to constitute a significant differentiator of effective community-based organizations.

In taking this broad approach, Wald's goal was to empower communities and individuals by giving them the skills and infrastructure to improve their own situation—thereby demonstrating the attribute of exemplary leadership that "enables people to do for themselves." To this end, Wald's model of care was distinctly focused on patient and community. Cognizant that the health of individuals and groups is significantly impacted by active participation, she mobilized the strengths and the assets of the community. When faced with the ponderous architectural and environmental hazards of the neighborhood landscape, she effected change by mobilizing people to "do for themselves."

Abraham Davis, who became acquainted with Wald as a small boy, recalled many years later at her memorial service: "She drew us into active cooperation with her and made us participants in her endeavors and thus fashioned our ideals, created our inspirations and stirred our ambitions" (Davis, 1940, as cited in Lannon, 2006, n.p.). When Davis first met Wald, he was attending the neighborhood boys' club. At her memorial service, he shared his memories of the discussions being held at that time about the widening of Delancey Street—recalling how, through Lillian Wald's lens, they began to view the possibility of a world no longer confined by narrow streets and congested pathways but instead filled with the advantages of broad thoroughfares, parks, and playgrounds:

> For the first time we became conscious of the narrow congested
> streets and then we wanted to bring about the widening of
> Delancey Street. She encouraged us to organize ourselves into
> groups and to list the number and extent of the encroachments
> on the sidewalks . . . the results were furnished to the
> appropriate authorities. In this way, we learned that parks
> and playgrounds and wider and more attractive streets were
> advantages to the people, the neighborhood and the City, and we
> gained experience in how to go about getting them. (Davis, 1940,
> as cited in Lannon, 2006, n.p.)

This concept of helping patients do for themselves grew out of Wald's initial step into community-based care, when she instructed young mothers in a classroom-like setting. In reflecting on the legacy of Lillian Wald, journalist Jean Hardin Farleigh recounted that while her work grew out of the needs of the people, "they have furthered it themselves. She prefers to be known as an educator" (Farleigh in Lannon, 2006, n.p.).

It is worth noting that Wald's vision of health education as the foundation of community-based nursing practice is increasingly emphasized in today's era of health care reform. Since her time, many factors have combined to largely deemphasize the educational role of visiting nurses and nursing in general—most notably, a public and private payer reimbursement system that has emphasized the technical over the teaching aspects of the nursing role. The result has been the long-standing perpetuation of a volume-based fee-for-service reimbursement system that has, in many ways, fostered client dependency. The current shift toward encouraging patient self-management of chronic conditions, however, is putting a renewed premium on the education and empowerment of patients and their families—a role that visiting nurses are ideally positioned to implement. This tradition of client and community empowerment has also remained a part of the fabric of VNSNY, the community-based health system that Wald founded with Mary Brewster more than 120 years ago. A prime example of this can be seen in VNSNY's community-based emergency response to "Superstorm Sandy" in 2012, which is described later in this chapter.

Wald's leadership style, a blend of the visionary and the practical, empowered those working alongside her as well. One of the most remarkable stories of the far-reaching effects of Wald's *leadership by example* is that of her protégée, Margaret Sanger, one of America's great pioneers in the fight to give women access to effective birth control. Kathryn Cullen-DuPont describes in her introduction to Sanger's autobiography how Margaret found her life's calling while working for the Henry Street Settlement:

After marrying William Sanger and securing nurses' training, Margaret began work with Lillian Wald's visiting nurse service. As she cared for New York City's impoverished women, it became clear that her mother's case was not an isolated one. Not only the women she tended in childbirth, but their friends and neighbors as well, pressed her for relevant information, pleading, "Tell me something to keep from having another baby. We cannot afford another yet." Their lives were overwhelmed by childcare, and their spirits crushed by the knowledge that they could not provide everything their children needed. Margaret despaired. As she writes in her *Autobiography*, these "were not merely 'unfortunate conditions among the poor' such as we read about. I knew the women personally. They were living, breathing human beings, with hopes, fears, and aspirations like my own, yet their weary, misshapen bodies, 'always ailing, never failing,' were destined to be thrown on the scrap heap before they were thirty-five."

At least one of her patients failed to live even to that age. Margaret cared for Sadie Sachs, the mother of three young children, as she lay ill with septicemia and other complications of a self-induced abortion. After a difficult recovery, Mrs. Sachs begged for contraceptive advice, only to have the attending doctor laughingly suggest that her husband sleep on the roof. Mrs. Sachs later died following another self-induced abortion. Margaret left the woman's deathbed and vowed to "change the destiny of mothers whose miseries were vast as the sky." She vowed to bring birth control to women. (Cullen-DuPont, 1999, n.p.; see Chapter 5 for more on Margaret Sanger's life and leadership)

The impact of Wald's leadership was not limited to younger reformers. Well-known activist Florence Kelley, 8 years Wald's senior, moved from Hull House in Chicago to New York City so that she could join forces with the Henry Street Settlement founder:

In 1899 [Kelley] became head of the National Consumers League (NCL), a position she held for over 30 years, and moved to Lillian Wald's Henry Street Settlement in New York City. Working for the NCL, Kelley organized local leagues and lobbied for better working conditions, a minimum wage, and shorter working hours for women, immigrant, and working-class laborers. (Harvard University Library Open Collections Program, 2014a, n.p.)

This community of women activists collectively changed the living circumstances of the populations of New York City.

MOBILIZING SOCIAL INSTITUTIONS TO IMPROVE THE HEALTH OF COMMUNITIES

In her work, Wald inextricably linked the care of patients and the community to the broader mission of social justice and to a policy agenda that addressed broader societal issues. Like many exemplary nursing leaders, Wald was an activist agent of change both for nursing and for society. As such, she embodied two other key leadership attributes—that of being willing to challenge established processes while also fostering cooperation among relevant organizations (Kouzes & Posner, 2012). Collaboration was so fundamental to her vision of community-based care that Wald "hardwired" it into the culture, training, and mentorship of the settlement nurses. She understood that it was only by mobilizing the assets of both formal and informal support systems that needs could be effectively addressed.

> Creation of cooperative relationships with organizations as varied as hospitals and newspapers allowed her to provide patients with ice, sterilized milk, medicines, meals and most importantly, jobs. As word of the nurses' work spread, hospitals, dispensaries, relief agencies, and private physicians became "believers" and referred neighborhood patients for skilled follow-up and teaching. (Buhler-Wilkerson, 1993, p. 1780)

In addition, Wald designed new roles for community health nurses in which they could practice more autonomously, thereby expanding access to quality health care for many more people in society. These new roles included school and industrial nursing, moving public health nursing into the countryside, integrating mental health care, and establishing public health nursing as an insurance benefit (Frachel, 1988).

The concepts of cooperation and collaboration continue to underpin VNSNY's practice model today, with visiting nurses functioning as coordinators of care, facilitating the linkage of formal and informal support systems to promote health, prevent disease, and provide support for advanced illness management of chronic diseases and the end of life.

Wald also demonstrated that assertiveness and political acumen were critical to enlisting the support of government institutions in achieving her public health aims. Recognizing early on that the care of children was dependent on a national solution to these issues, she and a fellow activist approached President Theodore Roosevelt in order to raise his awareness of the plight of America's children as evidenced in their health indices, living conditions, and child labor conditions. In 1912, her advocacy helped lead to the establishment of the federal Children's Bureau within the U.S. Department of Labor. In reflecting on Wald's ability to go from the concrete clinical example to the broader societal implication, Abraham Davis noted, "That is characteristic of her mode of thought. She starts with the concrete factor and works out to the general proposition" (Davis, 1940, as cited in Lannon, 2006, n.p.).

The Social Security Administration's official account of how that new federal agency emerged from a singular observation of Wald—and how this observation eventually turned into a national call for action—provides an ideal illustration of her remarkable ability to convert specific issues into broad causes:

> Lillian D. Wald . . . and her friend, Florence Kelley of the National Consumers League, were responsible for the idea and coined the name for a Federal agency to promote the health and

welfare of children. These two practical dreamers and fearless critics of the status quo met together for friendly conversation as often as their busy lives allowed in the years between 1903 and 1912. Very seldom did these talks end without suggestions for next steps needed to correct some of the social ills of the day. A firm operating principle was—the people must know the facts; influential leaders must be the spokesmen.

One day in 1903, while they were having their morning coffee at the [Henry Street] Settlement, two letters came in the mail. "Why is it so many children die like flies in the summer time?" one of these letters asked. "Is there something I can do to help matters?" The other was from a mother whose husband had died. She was troubled because now that she would have to go out to earn support for her children, she would have to place them in an institution.

"There must be thousands of mothers all over the United States in just such situations," observed Miss Wald. "I wish there were some agency that would tell us what can be done about these problems."

Miss Wald and Mrs. Kelley turned to the morning newspaper. The Secretary of Agriculture, the paper reported, was going south that day to find out how much damage the boll weevil was doing to the crops.

That gave Miss Wald an idea.

"If the Government can have a department to take such an interest in what is happening to the Nation's cotton crop, why can't it have a bureau to look after the Nation's crop of children?" she asked.

A friend of Miss Wald's, impressed with the idea, wired President Theodore Roosevelt. "Bully," the President wired back, "Come down and tell me about it." (Social Security Administration, 1962, n.p.)

Crucially, Wald and her colleagues were willing to put in the hard work required to turn visionary ideas into public policy. In this case, it would take 9 years of ongoing advocacy for her concept to be realized:

Seven years of nationwide campaigning by individuals and organizations helped to mobilize public opinion. The National Child Labor Committee worked unremittingly for the bills introduced in Congress between 1906 and 1912. Eleven bills, eight originating in the House and three in the Senate, met with failure although each one served the important function of developing a more positive acceptance of the necessity for a new

Federal agency. . . . The year 1912 brought to an end the long citizen campaign when the Congress passed the Act creating the Children's Bureau and charged it "to investigate and report . . . upon all matters pertaining to the welfare of children and child life among all classes of our people."

The United States led the world in a pioneering step when President William Howard Taft signed the bill on April 9, 1912, and the first appropriation of $25,640 became available in August of that year. Since then, the Children's Bureau has advanced the well-being of children in the Nation and the world along every path open to it. (Social Security Administration, 1962, n.p.)

ENLISTING PHILANTHROPIC AND BUSINESS INTERESTS TO PROMOTE THE PUBLIC'S HEALTH

Lillian Wald embodied another important attribute of exemplary leadership—that of a person who enlists others in a common vision by appealing to shared aspirations. Exemplary nursing leaders communicate their vision by involving others from the very beginning, thus creating greater support (Kouzes & Posner, 2012). As one historian noted,

> Wald's compassion and good humor drew admirers and
> supporters from individuals in the many circles in which
> she traveled. Her confidence, administrative talent, and
> understanding of the social causes of poverty, together with
> her membership in the neighborhood she had chosen to join,
> inspired her to link efforts with her network of women and work
> toward a vision of a unified humanity. (Feld, 2009, n.p.)

Wald exhibited this attribute with the multiple constituents with whom she interacted, relating as effectively with her donors and policy makers as she did with patients and staff.

> Although herself never possessed of great wealth she was a
> friend of some of the wealthiest people in the United States,
> and was able by the charm of her personality to divert some of
> this wealth to the uplift of the poor in whom she was always
> interested. (Social Welfare History Project, n.d., n.p.)

This leveraging of philanthropy underpinned Wald's early work. Her idea for a neighborhood-based health presence was initially supported by Mrs. Solomon Loeb, a member of New York's German Jewish elite and donor of the Sabbath school classes. It was Mrs. Loeb who had made the request that resulted in Wald's first engagement to teach young mothers on the Lower East Side. Recognizing the power of the Wald–Brewster enterprise, Loeb and her son-in-law, Jacob Schiff, a banker and philanthropist, agreed to underwrite their work for 6 months. This relationship played another important role when, "two years later, Schiff purchased the house on Henry Street, allowing Wald to have the space necessary to develop many of her unique ideas" (Buhler-Wilkerson, 1993, p. 1779).

Employing the leadership tools of transparency and empowerment, Wald was diligent about keeping her donors informed in detail on the mission they were funding and the impact their contributions were having:

In the detailed weekly reports that Lillian Wald wrote to the service's first sponsors, Jacob Schiff and Betty Loeb, she always started with an overall assessment of the situation and then described the individual cases that she and Mary Brewster treated. Here is an abbreviated example:

> Hon. Jacob H. Schiff
> Mrs. Solomon Loeb
> My dear Mr. Schiff and Mrs. Loeb;
> The month has brought the usual busy demands we expected and which we shall have for some time to come. Doctors agree that the diseases which follow a famine must come in the wake of a poorly nourished winter and though we are occupied with acute illnesses which care and attention will generally conquer, the fact is patients that have the anemic, consumption condition which is so general down here is beyond a hope of medicine or nursing. We cannot give them enough sunshine or space but we have been caring for many of the sick nevertheless and helped a few back to their poor lives perhaps— at least added something to their comfort.
> As I said, we do have the means of relieving the comparatively few that we meet and are grateful for that, to those who make some gleams of light, these dark days to our poor, helpless neighbors.
> Yours faithfully,
> Lillian D. Wald
> February 2, 1894 (Denker, 1993, p. 42)

Wald also embraced a tradition of using the power of a story to mobilize funding and support for her work. A contemporary description of her story-telling ability noted that

> much in demand among the possessors of great wealth . . . she is seen often at their houses, friendly, magnetic, disarming. Some quality in her dissolves, for the moment, the kinks and

complexes of people with whom she comes in contact. . . . Miss
Wald never asks anyone for money. Instead, with embroidery of
telling anecdote, she describes the need for more nurses. (Smith,
1929, p. 32)

Like other exemplary leaders, Wald used positive language and her
own personal energy to communicate a mutually shared vision that was
understandable to others by using symbols, graphics, word pictures, stories, examples, metaphors, and analogies (Kouzes & Posner, 2012). By
exuding her belief in her mission and communicating it in a way that was
compelling to others, Wald conveyed a vision that was authentic and lasting—one that is perpetuated to this day in the philosophy and operations
of VNSNY, one of the organizations that evolved from the original Henry
Street Settlement. Each year, the VNSNY annual report publication is distributed to the organization's multiple constituencies. The VNSNY relies
on mission-based reflections to garner support and understanding for its
work.

Cognizant that philanthropy alone was not sufficient to sustain community-based health care services, Wald later used this same methodology
to advance another revolutionary concept when she convinced the Metropolitan Life Insurance Company to fund visiting nurse services for their
policyholders. Supporting her proposal with data showing "that nursing
care saved lives," Wald was able to gain approval from the insurance company to implement her strategy (Buhler-Wilkerson, 1993, p. 1780). The program began in June of 1909, and within the first quarter of operation, it
was successful enough, in Wald's words, to "cover policy holders throughout the city" (Buhler-Wilkerson, 1993, p. 1780). Within another 2 years, the
services were opened up to patients throughout the entire United States.
The business grew exponentially until, by 1912, "three years after initiation
of the service, Metropolitan was paying for one million nursing visits each
year at an annual cost of roughly $500,000" (Hamilton, as cited in Buhler-
Wilkerson, 1993, p. 1781).

This innovative partnership represents one more way in which Wald
both anticipated and influenced the future of nursing. Today, VNSNY works
collaboratively with a broad range of public payers and private insurers to
provide a range of home- and community-based services and population-
based health care coordination.

EXEMPLARY LEADERSHIP IN ACTION: THE SPANISH FLU PANDEMIC OF 1918–1919

The settlement nurses' centrality to the health care system as curators of this
cooperative relationship between social institutions and guardians of the
public health was never more clearly in evidence than when the "Spanish

influenza" arrived in New York City in 1918. By then, Lillian Wald was long established as an important resource for public health, both in the city and nationally. The Henry Street Settlement had become the largest such organization in the nation in terms of its programming and reach into the community (Reznick, 1973). Wald had evolved the settlement model of care from one focused on care of the sick, a healthy diet, and care of infants and children to one that was also driving improvements in sanitation, food safety, and housing standards. She had combined a solid system of community-based care with a highly developed ability for administration and the communication of findings related to the health of the immigrant community.

During the flu pandemic, the Henry Street Settlement visiting nurses emerged as a critical resource. They had developed a system of care that included daily reports on care rendered to individual patients as well as findings related to the public health community. This information was already being used to develop files on the incidence of the prevalent infectious diseases of the time, such as meningitis, smallpox, typhoid, and tuberculosis. Wald established a system for cataloguing the data collected and reported by visiting nurses on current patients, prevalent diseases, treatments, and available medical resources, thereby creating a method for quick reference. This system enabled the Henry Street Settlement nurses to deliver effective care with a minimum of waste and duplication. The systematic collection of information was also used to shape the overall response to community need. Through these capabilities, the Henry Street Settlement was recognized in the first few years of its operation as contributing to the reduction in mortality resulting from tuberculosis, typhoid, and diphtheria (Reznick, 1973).

The assets of this high-performing community-based infrastructure positioned Lillian Wald to be a major force behind public health efforts to control the spread of influenza during the Spanish flu pandemic. The spread of influenza throughout the fall and winter of 1918–1919 had put an enormous amount of pressure on the health care delivery system of hospitals, dispensaries, and physicians who treated patients both in the office and in the home. Within days of the outbreak of influenza in major East Coast cities, hospitals were filled beyond capacity.

Accounts from those times indicate that when the influenza epidemic struck New York City in September, "the Henry Street Settlement visiting nurses, directed by Lillian Wald, were among the first to respond" (Keeling, 2010, p. 110). Like other institutions, they were overwhelmed at the start. Ongoing coverage by *The New York Times* of the number of flu-related deaths included the following item on January 29, 1919:

> The Henry Street Settlement, yesterday turned away applications
> for relief in broncho-pneumonia and double pneumonia cases,
> it was said, and a case was cited of a household of two families
> where seven of the eight persons were ill and no nurse available.

> . . . The visiting nurse service of the Henry Street Settlement, said
> Miss Wald yesterday, was overwhelmed with requests for nurses
> with demands for care in some cases of five, six and seven
> persons ill in a family. (*"Appeal for Nurses,"* 1919, p. 13)

By her own account, Lillian Wald recalled that, in the first 4 days, she and her staff received "calls from 467 diagnosed cases of pneumonia and influenza." In written communication to City Health Commissioner Copeland, she went on to recount, "Our entire staff is nursing influenza and pneumonia cases. . . . We are doing the best we can; nobody is hysterical. The supervisors themselves are carrying the bag" (Keeling, 2010, p. 110). Wald's reference to "carrying the bag" meant literally carrying needed supplies into patients' homes, including dressings, thermometers, alcohol for sponge baths, and other medications. Wald described a family suffering in upper Harlem. "The mother struggles with the flu; the father with lobar pneumonia; two children with the measles and a four week old infant." Wald described this situation as that emblematic of hundreds of homes throughout the city in which the family "had been without care of any kind until the case was reported to the visiting nurse" (Keeling, 2010, p. 110).

It is a testament to Wald's organizational leadership that, not long after this, "Henry Street Settlement cleared all cases of influenza and mobilized the efforts of thousands of volunteers" (Feld, 2009, n.p.). In large part, this was because of the 25-year experience of the visiting nurses from the Henry Street Settlement in caring for the sick and working to improve the public health on the Lower East Side. This allowed them to prepare a rapid response. This occurred in collaboration with communities with which the settlement had established close working relationships, including social service organizations, churches, and schools.

Mirroring Wald's approach, New York City's response to the epidemic was to draw on a robust system of resources long established to address the public health needs of the community. Most of New York City's public health responses to influenza were adapted from its previous campaigns against tuberculosis (Aimone, 2010). The existing public health infrastructure played a key role in shaping the city's practices and policies during the epidemic, and Lillian Wald and the Henry Street Settlement were an important part of this infrastructure. Wald's leadership and the work of the Henry Street Settlement's visiting nurses "was essential for influenza patients; in 1918 there was minimal understanding of the disease and no antiviral medications to inhibit its progression" (Keeling, 2010, p. 106). In fact, there was a mistaken belief in the medical community at the time that influenza was caused by a bacillus rather than a virus. Although they were unable to locate the cause of influenza, scientists and physicians did understand that influenza was spread through contact with droplets from the nose and throat of an infected person during coughing and sneezing.

In early 1919, Wald worked with the leadership of the Atlantic Division of the American Red Cross and other nursing leaders throughout the city to organize the Nurses' Emergency Council as a means of mobilizing resources to combat the epidemic. This coalition of nursing leadership created a safety net for the entire city by organizing motorcars from the Red Cross to transport nurses and move supplies. In addition to distributing linens and flu jackets, the visiting nurses brought "12,241 quarts of soup and 2,255 quarts of cereal, junkets and custards" (Doty, as cited in Keeling, 2010, p. 110).

Lillian Wald significantly augmented this response through the work she had done over the previous 20 years in establishing data collection as a critical component of visiting nurse practice. The long-standing practice of district nurses from the Henry Street Settlement delivering daily reports of the care they provided and the conditions they found in their communities became the template for the reporting of the Nurses' Emergency Council in 1919. Data gathered on daily rounds by New York City's many nurses and community workers were reported to the Commissioner of Health, contributing to the city's ability to control the spread of disease and evaluate the response to the measures that were being taken.

This reporting continued throughout the fall and winter of 1918– 1919 and included data collection done after the surge in the incidence of influenza had subsided. Organized by Wald, this evaluation consisted of a series of questions designed to collect data on the contributions of each settlement house during the epidemic. The questions ranged from the number of calls for assistance and individuals cared for to any knowledge of reports of profiteering by physicians (Influenza Encyclopedia, n.d.). This data-gathering effort reflected Wald's keen understanding of communicable disease risk among crowded immigrant enclaves, such as the Lower East Side, at a time when epidemiology was not yet an established scientific discipline.

Equally important as the care provided by nurses at that time was the Henry Street Settlement's well-established approach to public education. Lillian Wald had previously led campaigns to improve food safety through the regulation of pushcart vendors on the Lower East Side, improve the quality of the milk consumed by the immigrant population by establishing milk stations, and create safe playgrounds for immigrant children. Now she drew on that tradition in combating the flu epidemic. Responding to her advocacy and demonstrated effectiveness, on September 28, 1918, New York City's Board of Estimate approved an emergency appropriation to the Department of Health to fight influenza. The first and largest use of the appropriation went toward arming health department staff with health education materials. The second largest appropriation was used to hire nurses and health inspectors who could help the city count its sick. These initial appropriations are telling. When confronted with the prospect of an influenza epidemic, the Board of Estimate's first move was to increase its health education and surveillance capacities (Keeling, 2010).

In the aftermath of the epidemic, Wald and her organization were rec-ognized as having significantly catalyzed the city's response as a whole. In an interview with *The New York Times* after the epidemic subsided, New York City Health Commissioner Dr. Royal Copeland, commented that New York City "escaped" with a low mortality rate because of the city's health efforts over the previous 20 years. In a letter written to Lillian Wald, Dr. Copeland specifically referenced the consistent efforts of tuberculosis control to improve sanitary conditions, tenement house reform laws mandating good ventilation, and the constant effort to maintain clean streets and to keep the city clean and sani-tary—all causes for which Wald had fought. During the crisis itself, he added, "I found your organization alert to the necessities of the emergency and ready, day or night, to respond to the urgent calls for help" (Lannon, 2006, n.p.).

LILLIAN WALD'S LEGACY AS A LEADER—ALIVE AND WELL TODAY

One of the most telling attributes of an exemplary leader is the ability to con-tinue influencing policy and social thought beyond one's own lifetime. In this regard, Lillian Wald's leadership continues to be felt today, both organization-ally and philosophically. The VNSNY, which spun off from the Henry Street Settlement in 1944 to become a separate institution, now employs over 1,915 nurses with a staff in excess of 16,500. In 2013, 2,276,690 professional visits were provided by VNSNY's front-line staff. More than 120 years after Wald referred to "the high spirit of the courageous pioneers," her words still resonate throughout the meeting places of VNSNY staff (Buhler-Wilkerson, 2001, p. 113). Lillian Wald is continuing to inspire the latest generation of visiting nurses to approach their work with the dauntless optimism and resourceful experimen-tation that were her hallmark.

Today, as in Wald's time, the anecdote and story also continue to under-pin the work of VNSNY as much as the quantifiable and predictive analytics, scorecards, and benchmarked metrics. Internal meetings, from the board-room to staff meetings, start with "mission reflections"—personal, poignant, and often powerful stories that describe the outcomes achieved each day by VNSNY front-line staff. The organization's website highlights compelling patient anecdotes as well, many of them told in the first person, that draw friends and funds to the safety net mission of Lillian Wald's VNSNY. Front-line managers use this same technique of narrative reflection to identify and reflect the unique elements of management that pervade community-based care.

Like the Henry Street nurses in Wald's era, visiting nurses today are also assessing and drawing observations from the individual and commu-nity experience in order to eradicate disease, reduce health disparities, and promote the broader health of the community. In the process, the VNSNY is returning to other principles that Wald enumerated in powerful fashion over a century ago: To be historically grounded and concurrently fortified by the nation's call to empower the patient and community—not to do for them. VNSNY has recommitted itself to facilitating the broadest possible patient engagement through a model of transitional care and population health care coordination. This is manifested by establishing patient-centered goals, health coaching, telehealth, and the full use of social media and technology. Within both this historical and contemporary context, VNSNY nurses, in the tradition of Lillian Wald, are achieving best-in-class benchmarks in patient- and community-based initiatives. These initiatives are aimed at reducing health disparities, reducing unnecessary emergency room and inpatient admissions, and ameliorating the negative outcomes associated with acute exacerbation of disease.

A COMMUNITY IN CRISIS: VNSNY'S RESPONSE TO SUPERSTORM SANDY

Just as the response of the Henry Street Settlement to the Spanish flu in 1918 epitomized the leadership Wald brought to that organization, VNSNY's tradition of client and community empowerment came to the fore in the fall of 2012. This was the year the organization Wald founded was faced with the devastating impact of Superstorm Sandy. The work of VNSNY's staff during this natural disaster entailed a laser-like focus that centered on assets in the community and a belief in the power of people to heal and to mobilize on their own behalf.

In late October of 2012, Sandy ravaged the East Coast of the United States, with the shorelines of New Jersey and New York most significantly affected. When the storm ended, it was evident that the toll it had taken was enormous. Close to two million New Yorkers lost electrical power and 51 square miles in low-lying parts of New York City were flooded, including large sections of Manhattan, Brooklyn, Queens, the Bronx, and Staten Island. With buildings and other structures battered by high winds and rising waters, the storm forced companies, schools, hospitals, and stores to close, thus cutting residents off from vital services (Christopher & Goldstein, 2014).

VNSNY's response to Sandy began even before the storm struck, as the organization's staff reached out to the most vulnerable people in its care. This outreach was summarized by the VNSNY magazine *Frontline*, in a special post-Sandy issue, which described how calls were made to all patients to ensure that they were either evacuating to safer ground or, if staying at home, that they had sufficient supplies of medications, oxygen, and other essentials. The staff also called patients' family members to reassure them that their loved ones were being looked after.

> Anticipating the subway shutdown, many nurses worked
> Sunday to see patients who were scheduled for Monday.
> Partners in Care sent home health aides to move in with

high-risk clients so they would have food, medications, companionship and assistance with bathing and personal care throughout the storm and its aftermath. Many aides walked long distances, often leaving families at home, to stay at their clients' sides. (VNSNY, 2012, p. 1)

Following the storm, VNSNY mobilized large numbers of clinical workers and other employees to tend to the most pressing medical and logistical needs of patients and other community members—very much as Lillian Wald did over a century earlier. Some 5,000 nurses, rehabilitation therapists, home health aides, social workers, and other frontline staff took to the streets to check that patients were safe and had all the supplies they needed. With no working public transportation, they drove their own vehicles, took taxis, rode bicycles, or in some cases simply walked to their patients' homes, sometimes through knee-deep water. In addition to supplying medical care along with food, water, and batteries, these staff members provided an essential connection for patients who were marooned in their apartments, cut off from the outside world with no power and often no heat. They helped people move from flooded first-floor rooms to higher ground, brought cell phones to be recharged, and arranged for prescriptions to be refilled in cases where patients' usual doctors and pharmacies were unavailable.

Just as important, VNSNY also put long-term community empowerment programs into place in the areas hardest hit by the storm—again, much as Wald did in her day. As part of its massive relief effort across a much broader geography, VNSNY joined with the community of Gerritsen Beach, Brooklyn, in an outreach, based very much on the principles that Abraham Davis recounted at the memorial for Lillian Wald long ago.

Faced with a situation in which 90% of the homes in Gerritsen Beach, Brooklyn, were ravaged by the effects of the storm, the community's residents were forced to deal with temporary homelessness, disconnection from school, work, their worship sites, and health care delivery. In the tradition of Lillian Wald, VNSNY staff quickly recognized that the healing and restoration of this community rested on drawing upon the resiliency of the community members themselves. In the early weeks after the storm, occurrences of upper respiratory and gastrointestinal conditions skyrocketed as a result of the environmental effects of damaged and waterlogged housing, water supplies, and sewer systems. As the days and weeks stretched into months and many homes were still uninhabitable, tensions and desperation seeped in, and depression, substance abuse, and domestic violence increased. To address these challenges, VNSNY secured funding to build a strengths-based approach to community resiliency, pairing nurses and social workers who operated out of a makeshift office from the back of a storage unit, teaming with residents of the community who were trained as peer workers and coaches.

From their makeshift office on an abandoned roadside lot, the professional staff and peer workers went door to door to identify the vulnerable and to equip them to negotiate the convoluted steps to normalcy. During the 2 years that the program was operational, VNSNY staff knocked on 10,000 doors and ministered to over fifty-five thousand community residents. The outcomes of the effort were that every housing unit was restored, children were back in school, and all health measures—incidence of primary care illness, access to care, reported incidences of depression, substance abuse, and domestic violence—returned to pre-Sandy levels.

So effective was this effort that the American Red Cross funded it with $1,650,000 and featured it in their relief efforts nationally. In every venue in which VNSNY reported this effort—staff meetings, boardrooms, philanthropic tables, national and international conferences, and the local community—they continually referenced the words of Lillian Wald when she took that first walk through the Lower East Side:

> Over broken asphalt, over dirty mattresses and heaps of refuse
> we went. . . . There were two rooms and a family of seven not
> only lived here but shared their quarters with boarders. . . . What
> I had seen had shown me where my path lay. (Wald, 1915, n.p.)

As important as this symbolism was, Wald's leadership was also personally embodied by VNSNY's front-line staff. Just as Lillian Wald brought the promise of nursing care and intervention to the vulnerable residents of the Lower East Side in 1889, so did the VNSNY nurses of 2012. Within days of the storm, today's generation of visiting nurses followed in the exact footsteps of Lillian Wald on the Lower East Side as they conducted door-to-door canvassing of the homebound elderly, many of them trapped on high floors with no heat, no light, and no water. Like Wald's own personal example, their embodiment of her nursing legacy resonated with and inspired a watching nation—one more testament to her powerful leadership.

ABC World News correspondent Diane Sawyer shadowed one of the VNSNY nurses during her Sandy canvassing. Sawyer reported:

> They are out in the dark, the National Guard, City Meals on
> Wheels, carrying heavy loads up stair after stair in high-rises.
> . . . People like nurse Rosita Ortiz, one of the thousands of
> people who work for the Visiting Nurse Service of New York,
> checking on patients who have little food, little water, and no
> power. Seventeen stories later, we knock on the door. Carmen
> Wester and her daughter, homebound, her daughter on a walker,
> answer the door. "We want to know how you're doing." (ABC
> News, 2012)

There was no way Sawyer could have known how closely her report mirrored the words of Lillian Wald, written a century earlier—words that perfectly sum up the balance of inspirational vision and practical wisdom that served as an unerring guide not only for Wald herself but for all who joined Lillian in her journey:

> Enthusiasm, health, and uncommon good sense on the part of the nurse are essential, for without the vision of the importance of their task they could not long endure the endless stair-climbing, the weight of the bag, and the pulls upon their emotions. (Denker, 1993, p. 70)

TIMELINE

- March 10, 1867—Lillian Wald is born in Cincinnati, Ohio.
- 1877—Moves with her family to Rochester, New York.
- 1883—Applies to Vassar College and is not accepted because of young age.
- 1883–1889—Attends private French school and works.
- 1889—Wald enters New York Hospital School of Nursing.
- 1891—Graduates from New York Hospital School of Nursing; works for the Juvenile Asylum on 176th Street in Manhattan.
- 1891–1893—Enters Women's Medical College in Lower Manhattan.
- 1893—Moves to the Lower East Side of New York City with colleague Mary Brewster to live in the neighborhood and work as nurses there; begins using the term *public health nurse* to describe the role that she and the other visiting nurses exemplify.
- 1895—Expands her organization and moves into the building (purchased by her benefactor Jacob Schiff) that becomes the Henry Street Nurses Settlement.
- 1902—Starts the first program of installing nurses in public schools in the United States.
- 1904—Helps establish the National Child Labor Committee.
- 1905—Henry Street Settlement Nurses are seeing 4,500 patients per year.
- 1906—Henry Street Settlement Nurses begin seeing African American patients.
- 1909—First meetings to establish NAACP are held at VNSNY head-quarters.
- 1909—Metropolitan Life Insurance Company begins a nursing service for policyholders.

- 1910—Teachers College, Columbia University, creates the Department of Nursing and Health.
- 1912—The national Children's Bureau is created.
- 1912—Elected first president of the National Organization for Public Health Nursing.
- 1912—Awarded the gold medal for distinguished service to humanity by the National Institute of Social Sciences.
- 1918—VNSNY nurses provide services to New Yorkers during 1918 influenza epidemic.
- 1933—Retires to Westport, Connecticut.
- 1937—Awarded New York City's distinguished service certificate.
- September 1, 1940—Wald dies at the age of 73 at her home in Westport, Connecticut, after a long illness resulting from a cerebral hemorrhage.
- 1970—New York University admits Lillian D. Wald to their Hall of Fame for Great Americans and issues a medal honoring her as a humanitarian (at the beginning of this chapter).

QUESTIONS FOR DISCUSSION

1. Lillian D. Wald *enabled others to act* by emphasizing the relationship between the individual and the public's health. What are some of the public health interventions nurse leaders should be addressing today?
2. Within the context of population health care coordination, what are some of the emerging roles and sites of care for nurses within the health care delivery system? How can nurse leaders *enable others to act* in these new roles and within these new sites?
3. Increasingly, the international nursing community is being called on by organizations like the Institute for Healthcare Improvement and the Robert Wood Johnson Foundation to build a culture of health. Drawing on the leadership example of Lillian Wald, what are some of the innovative grassroots models within your community that *enable others to act* and foster a culture of health?
4. Lillian Wald modeled servant leadership as a pioneer in the public health nursing movement. How might you model servant leadership in the venues in which you participate?

REFERENCES

ABC News. (2012, November 5). *Hurricane Sandy relief: National guard delivers supplies to stranded senior citizens* [Video file]. Retrieved November 5, 2014, from http://abcnews.go.com/WNT/video/hurricane-sandy-relief-national-guard-delivers-supplies-stranded-17622268

Aimone, F. (2010). The 1918 influenza epidemic in New York City: A review of the public health response. *Public Health Reports, 125*(Suppl. 3), 71–79.

Appeal for nurses to fight influenza. (1919, January 29). *The New York Times*, p. 13.

Buhler-Wilkerson, K. (1993). Public health then and now: Bringing care to the people: Lillian Wald's legacy to public health nursing. *American Journal of Public Health,* *83*(12), 1778–1786.

Buhler-Wilkerson, K. (2001). *No place like home.* Baltimore, MD: Johns Hopkins University Press.

Christopher, M., & Goldstein, J. (2014). The visiting nurse service of New York's response to hurricane sandy. *American Journal of Nursing, 114*(10), 55–62.

Cullen-Dupont, K. (1999). Introduction. In M. Sanger (Ed.), *Margaret Sanger: An autobiography.* Lanham, MD: Cooper Square Press. Retrieved November 3, 2014, from http://www.womenandhistory.com/margaret_sanger__an_autobiography_9722.htm

Davis, A. (1940, December 1). "An inspiration to youth" Memorial Service. VNSNY Archives, Housed at Columbia University, New York, NY.

Denker, E. P. (Ed.). (1993). *Healing at home: Visiting Nurse Service of New York, 1893–1993.* New York, NY: Visiting Nurse Service of New York.

Doty, P. (1919). A retrospect on the influenza epidemic. *Public Health Nursing, 11,* 949–957.

Duffus, R. L. (1938). *Lillian Wald: Neighbor and crusader.* New York, NY: Macmillan.

Fee, E., & Bu, L. (2010). The origins of public health nursing: The Henry street visiting nurse service. *American Journal of Public Health, 100*(7), 1206–1207.

Feld, M. (2009). Lillian D. Wald. In *Jewish Women: A Comprehensive Historical Encyclopedia.* Retrieved October 9, 2014, from http://jwa.org/encyclopedia/article/wald-lillian-d

Frachel, R. (1988). A new profession: The evolution of public health nursing. *Public Health Nursing, 5*(2), 86–90.

Gold, L. (2001). *America in the progressive era, 1890–1914.* Austin, TX: Longman.

Hansan, J. (2012). The Progressive Era. The Social Welfare History Project. Retrieved October 5, 2014, from http://www.socialwelfarehistory.com/eras/progressive-era/

Harvard University Library Open Collections Program. (2014a). *Immigration to the United States, 1789–1930: Florence Kelley (1859–1932).* Retrieved November 5, 2014, from http://ocp.hul.harvard.edu/immigration/kelley.html

Harvard University Library Open Collections Program. (2014b). *Immigration to the United States, 1789–1930: Settlement house movement.* Retrieved November 5, 2014, from http://ocp.hul.harvard.edu/immigration/settlement.html

Henry Street Settlement. (2013). *Henry Street Settlement annual report 2013.* Retrieved November 3, 2014, from http://www.henrystreet.org/news/publications/hss-2013-annual-report.pdf

Influenza Encyclopedia. (n.d.). The American influenza epidemic of 1918–1919. In *Lillian Wald correspondence, 1919: Nurses emergency council.* Retrieved November 5, 2014, from http://quod.lib.umich.edu/cgi/t/text/idx/f/flu/0510flu.0016.150/2/--lillian-wald-correspondence-1919-nurses-emergency-council?page=root;rgn=subject;size=100;view=image;q1=Wald%2C+Lillian

Jewish Women's Archive. (n.d.). *Lillian Wald.* Retrieved November 5, 2014, from http://jwa.org/womenofvalor/wald

Keeling, A. (2010). Alert to the necessities of the emergency: U.S. nursing during the 1918 influenza pandemic. *Public Health Reports, 125*(Suppl. 3), 105–112.

Kouzes, J. M., & Posner, B. Z. (2012). *The leadership challenge* (5th ed.). San Francisco, CA: Jossey-Bass.

Lannon, T. (Ed.). (2006). *Lillian D. Wald papers*. Manuscripts and Archives Division. New York, NY: The New York Public Library.

Muncy, R. (1998). *Women and the progressive era*. Retrieved September 27, 2014, from http://www.nps.gov/nr/travel/pwwmh/prog.htm

Reznick, A. (1973). *Lillian D. Wald: The years at Henry Street*. Madison, WI: University of Wisconsin.

Ruel, S. (2014). Lillian Wald: A pioneer of home healthcare in the United States. *Home Healthcare Nurse, 32*(10), 1–4.

Smith, H. (1929, December 14). Profiles: Rampant but respectable. *The New Yorker*, pp. 32–35.

Social Security Administration. (1962). *It's your Children's Bureau*. Washington, DC: U.S. Department of Health, Education and Welfare (Children's Bureau Publication No. 357). Retrieved November 5, 2014, from http://www.ssa.gov/history/childb2.html

Social Welfare History Project. (n.d.). *Lillian Wald: Congressional tribute: Remarks of Hon. Samuel Dickstein of New York in the House of Representatives, Thursday, September 19, 1940*. Retrieved November 5, 2014, from http://www.socialwelfarehistory.com/people/wald-lillian-congressional-tribute/

Thacker, S., Qualters, J., & Lee, L. (2012). Public health surveillance in the United States: Evolution and challenges. *Morbidity and Mortality Weekly Report, Supplements, 61*(3), 3–9.

Visiting Nurse Service of New York (VNSNY). (2012). In the shadow of Hurricane Sandy: Bringing mission-driven care to a Storm-Ravaged city. *Frontline* (in-house publication).

Visiting Nurse Service of New York (VNSNY). (2014). *100 years in the community*. Retrieved November 3, 2014, from http://www.vnsny.org/community/our-history/100-years-in-the-community/

Wald, L. (1915). *The house on Henry Street*. New York, NY: Henry Holt and Company.

West, T., & Schambra, W. (2007). The progressive movement and the transformation of American politics (First principles series #12). The Heritage Foundation. Retrieved September 27, 2014, from http://www.heritage.org/research/reports/2007/07/the-progressive-movement-and-the-transformation-of-american-politics

FURTHER READING

Burke, T. (2010). Empiricism, pragmatism and the settlement movement. *Pluralist, 5*(3), 73–88.

Davis, A. (1994). *Spearheads for reform: The social settlements and the progressive movement, 1890–1914*. New Brunswick, NJ: Rutgers University Press.

Schneider, D., & Lilienfeld, D. (2008). *Public health: The development of a discipline: From the age of hippocrates to the progressive era* (Vol. 1). New Brunswick, NJ: Rutgers.

Smith, R. (2002). The biopsychosocial revolution: Interviewing and provider–patient relationships becoming key issues for primary care. *Journal of General Internal Medicine, 17*(4), 309–310. Retrieved October 10, 2014, from http://www.ncbi.nlm.nih.gov/pmc/articles/PMC1495036/

Tenement Museum. (2013). *Notes from the tenement museum*. Retrieved October 10, 2014, from http://www.tenement.org/blog/lillian-wald-and-giving-all-year-round/

Mary Breckinridge: Angel on Horseback

Denise M. Tate

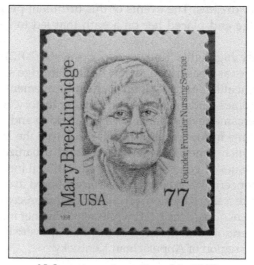

*U.S. postage stamp issued in 1998
honoring Mary Breckinridge.*

The easiest thing is to do, the next easiest
is to write, and the hardest is to think.
—*Mary Breckinridge*

•　•　•　•　•

Mary Breckinridge (1881–1965) is an iconic figure in the history of Kentucky and a woman who exemplified true leadership through her life's work. Praised as an "angel on horseback," she devoted over 40 years to building and sustaining the Frontier Nursing Service, an organization created to provide professional health care to one of the poorest and most rural regions in the Appalachian Mountains of Kentucky. From Mary's life experiences, one can glean the leadership qualities in her that make her stand out as a successful leader who has earned her rightful place among famous nurses in history.

Like other female activists of her era, Mary focused her drive and energy on addressing the concerns of motherhood and childrearing and believed that women were happiest in their traditional roles of wives and mothers. Deprived of these socially prescribed roles of her class by the deaths of her children and her first husband, she dedicated her life to the improvement of maternal–child health care (Goan, 2008). In this new role, she challenged prevailing social traditions and developed the skills and knowledge necessary to follow her dreams. The events of this turbulent period transformed Mary Breckinridge and placed her on a path that led to her life's work in eastern Kentucky.

This chapter highlights Kouzes and Posner's (2012) five exemplary leadership practices as a basis for a review of Breckinridge's contribution and service to public health, her dedication to the improvement of maternal and child health outcomes, and her impact on nursing history. It focuses on how Breckinridge overcame several barriers while working and living in the Progressive Era—a time in American history lasting from the 1890s through the 1920s—during which America experienced rapid urbanization and industrialization and issues of gender, class, and educational inequality became a greater societal concern. We examine how Mary labored in order to (a) model the way, (b) inspire a shared vision, (c) challenge the process, (d) enable others to act, and (e) encourage the heart while achieving her impressive success in the establishment of rural health care for the impoverished residents of a remote backwater region of Appalachian Kentucky.

NURSING LEADERSHIP

According to Kouzes and Posner (2012), leaders *challenge the process* as they search for opportunities and constantly challenge the status quo. They take risks and learn from their errors. They *inspire a shared vision* when they passionately believe that they can make a difference. They envision a future and through appeal and influence, they solicit the help of others to share in their vision. Leaders *enable others to act* by promoting collaboration as well as strengthening people by empowering them. They create energetic teams through shared respect, building of trust, and support. True leaders *model the way* via leading by example. They behave in ways that are in alignment with shared values and produce small wins that promote consistent progress and build commitment. Leaders *encourage the heart* by connecting performance and rewards and by celebrating and recognizing individual and/or team accomplishments.

Mary Breckinridge was an extraordinary nurse leader of her time. She epitomizes Kouzes and Posner's (2012) five practices of exemplary leadership as she articulated a vision of a better future, was passionate about working to make that vision a reality, was successful enlisting the help of others in the effort, was willing to take risks, accepted constructive feedback and suggestions, displayed great determination and drive, and was unwilling to accept the status quo.

The leadership principle, of enabling others to act (Kouzes & Posner, 2012), is clearly defined as a trait of leaders who promote collaboration and create strong, effective teams. They actively seek to involve others and make each team member feel skillful and empowered. Mary Breckinridge demonstrated this principle of leadership during the creation of her vision to bring home care to families and midwifery into the rural mountains of Kentucky, a region that had the highest infant and maternal mortality rates in the United States. To accomplish her dream of providing health care to this underserved population, Mary influenced foreign nurses to come to America, thus demonstrating her leadership ability to mobilize others to help accomplish her goals and got them not only to follow but also to be transformed in achieving Mary's shared aspirations.

Leaders *challenge the process* as they search for opportunities and innovate ways to improve the current situation (Kouzes & Posner, 2012). Along the way, Mary *inspired a shared vision* by engaging the help of many people to raise funds for her innovative plans. Mary's success was largely the result of her effectively speaking with others about how much better their communities would be in the future and creating a common vision by appealing to the local people to get involved. They, in turn, provided her with ideas and suggestions about how to improve living conditions and health care services in their region. Mary was known for her commitment and untraditional ways of improving health for women and children who had many barriers to accessible, affordable health care. She made her vision a reality and helped in *modeling the way* for many others. Like many good leaders, Mary was seen as one who took risks and made decisions.

This was a remarkable woman who turned her personal tragedies into a lifelong journey to help others. Mary's exemplary leadership practices had an important impact on nursing in her time that extends to nursing today.

FAMILY AND EARLY LIFE

Mary Carson Breckinridge was born into a prominent southern family in Memphis, Tennessee, on February 17, 1881. She was the daughter of Clifton Breckinridge, a U.S. Congressman from Arkansas, and the granddaughter of U.S. Vice President John C. Breckinridge, who served under President James Buchanan. Her mother, Katherine Carson Breckinridge, was the daughter of

Mississippi aristocrats. Mary had three siblings, a brother Carson born in 1878, a sister Lees born in 1884, and a younger brother Clif, born in 1895.

Growing up, Mary traveled extensively, living in various places and learning the cultural ways and lifestyles of others. As a young child, she lived on family estates in Mississippi, Kentucky, and upstate New York. As a teenager, she lived in Washington, DC; Russia; and Western Europe. Although she was an indifferent student, Mary enjoyed learning and school, and had a happy nomadic childhood (Breckinridge, 1952/1981).

In 1894, Mary and her family moved to St. Petersburg, Russia, when President Grover Cleveland appointed her father to serve as the U.S. ambassador to that country. Mary's first encounter with childbirth occurred when her younger brother was born in 1895. She was only 14 years old at the time, and although Madam Kouchnova (a Russian midwife) who attended to her mother and delivered her brother had made a great impression and taught her the value of a trained midwife, she, at that time, had no interest in nursing or midwifery. The Russian method of childbirth involved the birth of the baby delivered by the midwife while the physicians stood by in a corner in their white coats in case of an emergency (Breckinridge, 1952/1981). Because trained midwives did not exist in the United States during this time, it was undoubtedly Mary's first exposure to her future profession.

During their time in Russia, the Breckinridge family attended the coronation of Czar Nicholas II in Moscow; however, Mary was more impressed by her visit to a Moscow foundling asylum, which was founded by Catherine the Great, with her mother than the coronation ceremonies. She learned that the foundling asylum took in about 25 to 30 babies a day and kept about 3,000 babies at the asylum. These babies were either picked up from the streets or brought to the asylum by their mothers who would nurse them before dropping them off at the door. All of the babies were breastfed by wet nurses, two to a wet nurse (Breckinridge, 1952/1981). It was said that all of the "normal" babies were given away at 1 month of age to the local peasants who were paid for taking them in until they reached the age of 10, when their services would pay for their keep. It was then Mary realized for the first time that all children were not as lucky as she and her siblings (Ruffing-Rahal, 1991).

Mary was very lonely in Russia as she missed her American girlfriends and felt it largely in the evenings when her sister Lees and their two governesses would go to bed. She suffered physically and emotionally and demonstrated perhaps her first battle with depression. The family's physician recognized that she was unwell and limited her food intake believing that fasting could improve any condition. Over the course of 2 years of this treatment, Mary became weak and felt that she had no one with whom she could share her worries; she took up journaling and would sit for hours in her room and cover the pages of her diary with entries about her boredom and loneliness. She claimed that her journaling was the foundation for her autobiography and also helped her in learning to write and spell as no one taught her English grammar. Mary turned to books as an outlet, and admitted that

she had no aptitude for arithmetic and did not care to learn it. She did realize, however, that she had a real talent for intellectual pursuits and resented
her parents for failing to take her education seriously. Her older brother
attended the best schools in Washington, DC, before transferring to a European boarding school. Meanwhile at home, Mary and her sister Lees were
both educated by French and German governesses who spoke little English.
Mary's mother had been educated in this manner and wanted the same for
her daughters. The idea that her daughters may have to financially support
themselves one day never entered her mind. It was assumed that both girls
would marry appropriate gentlemen who would provide for them (Breckinridge, 1952/1981).

When she turned 15, Mary was overjoyed when she learned she would
attend the Rosemont Dezaley boarding school in Switzerland. During her
2 years of study there, she experienced a profound intellectual awakening.
The faculty scheduled frequent day trips that allowed the students to take
in the culture of nearby towns and the surrounding countryside, where the
girls were paired up and allowed to explore the streams and caves. Mary
later claimed that during her time at Rosemont she developed a strong affin-
ity to the mountains and their people. She excelled academically at school
but, true to Victorian thinking, her parents expressed concern that she was
working too hard and cautioned that she should consider her health. During
this period in history, a woman's pursuit of higher learning did not come
without conflict. Critics warned that higher education would physically and
emotionally damage delicate females, causing neuralgia, uterine disease,
hysteria, and other nervous system instabilities. When her father's assignment as ambassador ended, the family returned home to America, where
Mary finished her last 2 years of high school at Miss Low's finishing school
in Stamford, Connecticut (Breckinridge, 1952/1981).

Educated through private tutors and world travel, Mary still yearned
for more knowledge and viewed "serious study as a delightful thing"
(Breckinridge, 1952/1981, p. 30). Her conservative family did not approve
of higher education as suitable for women and encouraged their daughter
to follow the more traditional path of the times—to marry and have a family
(Ruffing-Rahal, 1991). After Mary suggesting several times that it would be
nice to do something with a purpose, Mary's mother finally permitted her to
attend a summer session at the University of Tennessee.

The social role of a woman during this time was at home—first in her
father's house until she married and then residing in her husband's home.
Mary knew that this life did not come without costs:

> [F]or a woman it meant she gave up her own ambitions, which
> she might cherish otherwise in the hope of their ultimate
> fulfillment, to embrace the career of the man of her choice.
> Marriage called upon a woman for renunciation entire and
> complete. (Breckinridge, 1952/1981, p. 48)

Societal pressures of the times demanded that women conform to these expectations, and those who deviated from this path faced disapproval from society and rebuke from family. For example, Mary's cousin, Sophonisba Breckinridge, trained as an attorney and social worker, but many family members regarded her departure from the norm as an unacceptable breach of societal expectations. Breckinridge's mother opposed higher education for her daughter. She focused on Sophonisba Breckinridge's education as an example of foolishness and the waste of education for young, single women (Breckinridge, 1952/1981).

After the summer spent at the University of Tennessee, Mary complied with her family's wishes; she relinquished her dream of furthering her education and made her choice to marry. In 1904, she married a lawyer, Henry Ruffner Morrison, whom she considered her soul mate. She described marriage as "an everlasting kind of thing and not entered into it lightly" (Breckinridge, 1952/1981, p. 48). They settled down in Hot Springs, Arkansas, and were eager to start a family. When no pregnancies occurred, Mary consulted with a New York doctor to find the cause of their infertility. Sadly, however, her husband developed appendicitis and died shortly after their first wedding anniversary (Goan, 2008). She rarely spoke of this marriage but wrote of it in her autobiography, "Of my own brief marriage I shall not write except to say it gave me all, and more than all, I had wanted in a friendship" (Breckinridge, 1952/1981, p. 49).

Morrison's death left her a widow at the young age of 24. She did not return to her family's home for fear of becoming an "object of their endless solicitude" (Breckinridge, 1952/1981, p. 51). Mary knew she wanted to provide care to others, not to receive it. Instead, she opted to travel to Banner Elk in the mountains of North Carolina. Here she spent a few months at Elizabeth McCrae Institute, a girls' settlement school. This was her first charitable work experience and introduction to Appalachia and its people. While there, Mary witnessed a child dying of typhoid fever and realized she could not offer assistance to the child or the child's mother. For the first time, Mary thought of training to become a nurse (Breckinridge, 1952/1981).

LATER LIFE

Devastated by her husband's death, Mary turned to nursing. In February 1907, after a little more than a year as a widow and with the help of a family friend, Dr. William Polk, she applied to and was accepted into St. Luke's Hospital Nursing School in New York City. It was one of the first schools to offer nurses' training and turned away hundreds of applicants each year. Her decision to study nursing allowed Mary to further her education in a socially accepted profession that welcomed women. Nursing was a career that allowed women to further their education in addition to the ability to display their nurturing and feminine characteristics. Nursing education was called "training" during this time period as in reality it was work—both physically and intellectually challenging as it required long hours of study in the classroom and 12-hour shifts, 6 days a week on the wards. Nursing students found themselves walking miles through hospital hallways and constantly lifting, pushing, and pulling patients and medical equipment. In return for their hard labor, the nursing students received free tuition, uniforms, textbooks, and room and board (Kessler-Harris, 2003).

Mary flourished in this environment and praised the education she received. During her 3 years at St. Luke's, she did well in her studies and graduated with a nursing degree in 1910. She passed her nursing examinations and received her nursing license shortly thereafter.

During her clinical rotations as a student, Mary experienced maternity nursing among the poor of the city of New York. There she encountered a sick child who profoundly impacted her eventual career path. She provided nursing care to a baby girl who had been abandoned at the hospital by her mother because the girl suffered from spina bifida, a birth defect that is caused by incomplete development of the spinal cord in the fetus. In the early decades of the 20th century, spina bifida was commonly fatal and few treatments were available. Mary developed an attachment to the baby and arranged to adopt her. She took the infant home and named her Margaret, thinking that the hospital approved the adoption. Upon her return to work, she was suspended from the hospital as they thought she had stolen the baby. Eventually it was sorted out, but from this incident, Mary acquired a distaste for bureaucratic maneuvering. Margaret died a few days later, and Mary paid the funeral costs, recognizing that all she could do now for the infant was save her from the further indignity of being buried in a pauper's grave. She completed her nursing education while dealing with the grief of her "little friend" (Breckinridge, 1952/1981, p. 57). After graduation, Mary returned to Arkansas to nurse her mother through a brief illness and attend to household affairs (Ruffing-Rahal, 1991).

In 1912, Mary married a second time, to Richard Ryan Thompson, a Kentucky native who, at the time, was president of Crescent College Conservatory in Eureka Springs, Arkansas. Different from her first marriage, Mary chose to pursue her own goals instead of helping to further her husband's career. Mary taught French and hygiene at the same college where her husband worked. She involved herself in the local community and helped create a nursing practice act for the state of Arkansas (Miller, 1988). She soon became pregnant with their first child and delivered a son they named Clifton Breckinridge "Breckie" Thompson, born in January 1914.

Mary devoted the next several years to caring for her son and working to advance the cause of child welfare. She used the latest scientific methods on childrearing and tracked her son's growth and development claiming that "the lives of few young children have been recorded in such detail" (Breckinridge, 1952/1981, p. 60). Breckie's growth and development was unremarkable and Mary had great hopes for her son. She imagined his future when she wrote that she believed he would be "in his manhood a leader of men, and would strike at the roots of poverty, vice and ignorance and rescue childhood" (Breckinridge, 1952/1981, p. 6). Mary again conceded to a social system that dictated she project her own ambitions onto her male child instead of pursuing them for herself.

In 1915, Mary became pregnant with their second child. This pregnancy was not easy, however, and she had to reduce the amount of time she devoted to her community work and focus on her pregnancy. In July of 1916, after a long premature labor, Mary delivered her daughter, Polly, who lived for only 6 hours (Breckinridge, 1952/1981).

If that was not enough grief, 2 years later, their beloved son, age 4, suddenly became ill and was hospitalized for a suspected intestinal obstruction. Breckie underwent surgery with his mother in attendance in the operating room. Mary was dismayed to learn that an infection had spread to his abdomen. He remained in the hospital for a week and eventually died from appendicitis. Mary was devastated and knew that, from that moment on, her life had changed forever.

Following these tragic events, which she claimed broke her marriage, Mary did the unthinkable and filed for divorce from her husband. She asked the court to take back her maiden name as she believed the Breckinridge name was more identified because of her powerful political family. Although she was entitled to use "Miss" Mary chose to use "Mrs." Breckinridge as she felt it provided her an acceptable place in society as a married woman instead of a single or divorced woman. She reasoned that her generation frowned on discussing a broken marriage and viewed it as a distasteful, embarrassing episode (Breckinridge, 1952/1981). She renounced marriage and the joys of motherhood and vowed never to love anyone or have anyone love her again (Pletsch, 1981).

CHALLENGING THE PROCESS

A leader *challenges the process* by taking the initiative to seek out and accept opportunities to change the status quo through experimentation and by taking risks (Kouzes & Posner, 2012). Examples that characterize this exemplary leadership practice include searching out opportunities to grow and innovate and to improve. Mary found herself in this situation when she needed a change to help her overcome the deaths of her children and her divorce. She was sad and lonely, but she did not feel sorry for herself. The loss of her children gave her the motivation and drive to help other children to live happy and healthy lives. She returned to nursing, and in 1918, after World War I, she joined the American Committee for Devastated France (CARD), where she organized a visiting nurse service in France. CARD provided nutritious meals for French children to help relieve the famine following the war. She rose quickly in the organization and was eventually responsible for a large district that contained 72 rural villages. She developed a community health nursing program for this area that provided health care, nutrition for children, and coordinated relief efforts. Because of a shortage of nurses, Mary used her prior experience in education and designed a professional nurses' training program in Paris (Campbell, 1984). She was recognized for her efforts and received the Médaille de la Reconnaissance française (Bullough, 1988).

This work set the stage for her future life's work of caring for the poor, especially children in Kentucky, and it was during her time in France that Mary again encountered midwives. Trained British midwives had volunteered for CARD and provided maternal and child health care in the homes of the local residents. She was unfamiliar with this type of nursing as America had "granny midwives" who were not professionally educated. As a result of this encounter she envisioned two goals: The first was to improve the health of rural American children and the second that nurses who are trained in the nurse–midwife model could meet the health care needs of the underserved population of the Appalachian Mountains (Breckinridge, 1981).

She wrote to her mother,

A decision has come to me and not of myself. Call it what you will—I definitely will follow it with the assurance that I am doing what is right. . . . I am to work directly with little children now and always—because that is the work I can do best, in which my health and enthusiasm and happiness do not fail. (Breckinridge, 1981, p. 73)

She considered this plan her life's calling (Pletsch, 1981).

Upon returning to the United States in 1921, she found there were no midwifery schools and planned to start one. To prepare for this undertaking, Mary studied public health nursing at the Teachers' College of Columbia University in New York City, and there she formed a friendship with Adelaide Nutting, who shared her beliefs. One course, in particular, taught her the importance of biostatistics as well as other descriptive techniques, which she often used in the gathering of data to support her vision for rural health care.

During the years following World War I, the public voiced concern about the high maternal and infant mortality rates. At the time, the national maternal death rate was 6.7 per 1,000 live births—one of the highest in the Western world. Women who were pregnant and living in rural areas had no alternative to care other than local "granny midwives" as physicians and hospitals were scarce. These women married young and, on average, gave birth to eight or nine children.

In the summer of 1923, Mary made a grueling trip on horseback to conduct a public health survey in Leslie County, Kentucky (West, 2013). She rode over 650 miles on horseback along rocky creek beds and unpaved roads to interview 55 "granny midwives" and evaluated the childbirth practices in the area. She learned that generally the midwives were elderly women with an average age of 60, who delivered an average of 19 babies a year. Most were wives of farmers, largely illiterate and untrained. As she talked with the "baby cotchers," it validated her plan that Leslie County would be the perfect place to start her nursing service. The granny midwives lived like the mountain people in one- or two-bedroom cabins with yellowing newspaper covering the walls to keep out the cold and dampness. If there was a window, curtains made from flour sacks were hung, and the same material was used to make dresses. But despite their obvious poverty, Mary learned that these were quite proud and well-mannered people (Dusek, 2006). Mary was quite distraught over the lack of prenatal care and found that these local lay mid-wifes would often use magic charms over the mother if she experienced any birth complications. An example of these practices is putting an axe, blade up, under the mother's bed in order to cut pain or complications (Breckin-ridge, 1952/1981).

In all of this massive mountain region, there were no hospitals, doctors, or nurses. No licensed physicians practiced in this remote area, which had the highest birth rates and infant mortality rates in the country. Doctors avoided underprivileged, isolated areas like Leslie County preferring larger regional areas or regions where coal camps were located. These preferences were based on economic concerns, as areas that lacked the ability to pay for medical services did not attract medical providers. Mary viewed this as an advantage in support of her plan.

Compelled to help, she rode to the mountain people every day and, because blacksmiths were scarce, she carried extra horseshoes in her saddle-bag. Her days were long and often she was too tired to ride home. She would sleep in a crowded cabin of a hospitable mountain family and, at times, would even share a bed with the whole family. She was very disciplined in her approach in dealing with such difficulties and in her efforts to change the rugged conditions that she encountered. Characteristic of her behavior was her commitment to cleanliness during these strenuous horseback travels. It was common for her to wash herself and to wear clean underwear that she washed the evening before (Breckinridge, 1952/1981).

At summer's end, Mary said good-bye to the mountain families to begin her plan to become a midwife and train others to care for the Appalachian Mountain families that she had grown to love. She chose the rural Kentucky Mountains as her model site for a number of reasons. First and foremost, she believed that rural pregnant women ran a higher risk of developing complications and maternal death than urban women. In addition, she also had close personal ties to the state as her great-great grandfather, John Breckin-ridge, had served as U.S. senator from Kentucky. In selecting Kentucky over other areas, she was determined to develop a program that would demonstrate the efficacy of nurse-midwives in remote underserved areas, thereby gaining public support for nurse-midwifery. Also, she thought that by placing the program in an area that was so remote, accessible only by foot or horse and without electricity or telephones, the model could be reproduced without difficulties in less isolated regions. In addition to building a database from her fieldwork, Mary also took the opportunity to get to know the community stakeholders. These were the landowners, schoolteachers, and people from prominent families who would become informants, committee members, and coactivists with her in helping form a unique model of rural health care (Breckinridge, 1952/1981).

At age 43, Mary returned to England to study midwifery at the British Hospital for Mothers and Babies in southeast London. She was already a nurse, so her coursework lasted 4 months and included delivering 20 normal births under supervision and attending complicated deliveries performed by a doctor. After receiving her midwifery certification, Mary toured the Scottish Highlands and Islands Medical and Nursing Service among remote rural areas and outer regions of the Outer Hebrides, terrains very similar to the Appalachian Mountains. Nurse-midwifery was founded by Sir Leslie MacKenzie and his was clearly the model on which she built the Frontier Nursing Service (West, 2013).

In 1925, she returned to Leslie County, Kentucky, and declared her intention to start a visiting nurse and midwifery service in that section of Appalachia. She had made a point of collecting facts about the people residing in the Kentucky Mountains. She contacted the chief of the Bureau of Vital Statistics of the State Department of Health regarding the need to collect statistics and, as a result, the chief made interview forms available to nurses in order to document births, deaths, and marriages. Mary challenged the status quo by providing statistics that measured the positive outcomes the nurses were achieving that ultimately resulted in Kentucky's health commissioner's approval of Mary's license to practice midwifery.

INSPIRING A SHARED VISION

Leaders passionately believe that they can make a difference when they envision the future and breathe life into a shared vision of future potential (Kouzes & Posner, 2012). Mary Breckinridge *inspired a shared vision* by breathing life into her plan of providing midwifery care to the mountain people and ventured out to share it with others. She was passionate and enthusiastic and spoke with such conviction that it inspired people to believe in her new model of care. Mary knew that the mountain people needed her services and believed that the mountains had a scenic appeal that would make it easier to raise necessary funds.

In fact, Breckinridge proved to be a talented fund-raiser. It was through her social networking and her family name that she influenced affluent Kentucky residents to provide financial support. She also demonstrated personal commitment by pledging money from her inheritance to build and financially support the Kentucky Committee for Mothers and Babies for the first 3 years of its operation.

In addition to money, she needed help, especially that of nurse-midwives. The contacts she made during her graduate training in England and Scotland enabled her to recruit qualified nurse-midwives (Pletsch, 1981). Advertising in the *Glasgow Times*, April 7, 1925, she enticed new nurse-midwife graduates with the promise of an adventure and was able to recruit six trained midwives (Wells, 1998).

ATTENTION! NURSE GRADUATES

With a sense of adventure! Your own horse, your own dog,
and a thousand miles of Kentucky mountains to serve. Join
my nurses' brigade, and help save children's lives. Write to:
M. BRECKINRIDGE, Hyden, Kentucky, U.S.A. (Wells, 1998, p. 23)

Through her persuasion, Mary inspired the English and Scottish nurse-midwives to leave their homelands, travel to Kentucky, and provide maternal–child care. She paid their way to America but this payment was contingent on their staying for 2 years. Those few who opted out before the contract term had to pay their own way home (Wells, 1998).

Scholarships for training in England were offered to American nurses with equestrian experience who were interested in becoming midwives. These full scholarships included housing, tuition, food, and transportation for the 6-month midwifery program. Because the nurses made their rounds on horseback, Mary required those without equestrian skills to take a minimum of five riding lessons before beginning work (Dusek, 2006).

At first, the "granny midwives" were jealous of the nurse-midwives and claimed that the "outsiders" would turn the babies into bears. But soon the mountain people realized that not only did the midwives not turn the babies into bears but they actually saved the lives of many of the mothers and infants (Dusek, 2006).

By the 1930s, these nurses provided family health care in addition to maternity care and midwifery for over 1,000 mountain families (West, 2013). They were respected and accepted by the locals, who often showed their gratitude with gifts of food, crafts, livestock, and hard work.

THE CREATION OF WENDOVER

It was during one of her many rides that Mary first saw and fell in love with a stretch of land that faced the great North Mountain, along the Middle Fork of the Kentucky River, just a few miles from Hyden.

When I raised my eyes to towering forest trees, and then let them
fall on a cleared place where one might have a garden, when

> I passed some jutting rocks, I fell in love. To myself and my horse
> I said, "Someday I'm going to build me a log house right here."
> Two years later I did. (Breckinridge, 1952/1981, p. 121)

She engaged local workmen to build a large log cabin that became her home and was named Wendover, also referred to as the "Big House" by her Aunt Jane. She asked a contractor from Hazard, New York, to oversee the building of the two-story Big House but local workmen completed the actual construction. By Christmas of 1925, the Big House had a roof and Mary's father dedicated the building to her two deceased children, Beckie and Polly, with a bronze plague on the living-room chimney. ·

Wendover became inhabitable in the spring of 1926, and the next several years it served as not only a residence but also a community-based nursing organization, originally known as the Kentucky Committee for Mothers and Babies. In 1928, it was renamed the Frontier Nursing Service. Because of unreliable roads and no means of transportation, the Service featured nurses on horseback who were able to reach even the most remote areas in all kinds of weather. They became known as "angels on horseback." The Frontier Nursing Service charged only $1 to cover an entire year of a family's health care, and $5 was the fee for a birth. As cash was scarce, a barter payment system in the form of goods or services was accepted and no one in need was refused care. Breckinridge recalled,

> Thousands of people have traveled to Wendover since it was
> first built and know the character of the house it is. What
> they can never know is how crowded it was until we built
> Hyden Hospital. For the first three years Wendover was used
> as a cottage hospital, and often overflowed with sick people.
> (Breckinridge, 1952/1981, p. 187)

Wendover was also known for other services, as it contained two of the five bathtubs in the county. It was said that the downstairs bathtub received so many visitors that Mary was going to place a guest book bound in blue-and-white linoleum in the room (Breckinridge, 1952/1981).

The Wendover barn was built to accommodate the horses that were the mode of transportation for Mary and her nurses when summoned for a mother in labor or a sick child. From the start, the Wendover Big House was, and continues to be, the focal point of the Frontier Nursing Service. People from the community, state, and nation met in the living room to plan ongoing rural health care in the United States and to plan educational programs for nurse-midwives and nurse practitioners. Mary wrote, "Wendover's long breezy dogtrot, its bathtubs and the shade of its giant beeches were refreshing spots to anyone who had spent a summer's day in the saddle" (Breckinridge, 1952/1981, p. 323). Today, the Big House serves as a bed-and-breakfast that is filled with displays of heroine nurses and the barn contains Frontier Nursing memorabilia and crafts made by the local people (How the FNS Began—Frontier Nurse Service, n.d.).

ENCOURAGING THE HEART

Leaders *encourage the heart* of those on their teams by visibly recognizing their contribution to the shared vision and celebrating the accomplishments of an individual and/or the team (Kouzes & Posner, 2012). As the community accepted the services of Mary and her nurses, the program's reputation grew, and it received large donations that enabled her to build a small hospital. In June of 1928, Hyden Hospital, Leslie County's first 12-bed hospital and health center, opened its doors. It was built atop Thundersticks Mountain that overlooks the quaint little town of Hyden, Kentucky. It made perfect sense that Mary invited Sir Leslie MacKenzie to come over from the Scottish Highlands to dedicate Hyden Hospital, as his work had done more than any other to make "regions, rugged, road less, and mountainous" safe for women and children (Breckinridge, 1952/1981, p. 221). She also thought to invite Lady MacKenzie to accompany him and represent the pioneer wives who crossed the ocean and rode with their men through rugged terrain to found Kentucky. The hospital dedication ceremony took place on the hospital's veranda and Sir Leslie's address was published in *The Lancet* of London. He strayed from the written words many times, as the occasion moved him deeply (Breckinridge, 1952/1981). In his conclusion, Sir Leslie recited the following: "This hospital is the radiating center of the nursing service in these mountains. The maxim of the trained nurse is: 'You need me? I am ready.' The hospital is a temple of service where the lamp never goes out" (Breckinridge, 1952/1981, p. 225).

Generous contributions allowed for the hiring of a medical director who was trained in obstetrics and for establishing a number of outpost centers. From 1927 to 1930, Mary and her staff opened nine nursing centers that were 9 to 12 miles apart. Designed around the hospital and employing one physician, each center had a waiting room for patients and two assigned nurse-midwives. Between Wendover and Hyden Hospital, care was provided within reasonable distance for all 700 square miles of the Frontier Nursing Service region (Breckinridge, 1952/1981).

Several years later, a charitable gift made it possible for the hospital to expand to 18 beds with eight bassinets. It grew again in 1949, to hold 25 hospital beds and 12 bassinets. Hyden hospital was known for many reputable things but one, in particular, was the opening of the first tonsillectomy clinic in 1930. Dr. Kobart performed 151 operations over a 2-day period. All but 19 of the surgeries were tonsillectomies (Appalachian Regional Healthcare, n.d.).

In addition to delivering babies, the nurse-midwives treated common illnesses of the day such as tuberculosis. It was during one of her rides to provide care that Mary fell from her horse and suffered a crushed vertebra in her lower back. For over a year, she was unable to ride and the accident left her having to wear a steel brace for the rest of her life.

Through the Great Depression and World War II, the Frontier Nursing Service changed with the changing times. The state constructed a paved road between Hyden and Hazard, Kentucky, and built Highway Route 80, which included concrete bridges over the Kentucky River that permitted safe crossings for cars and ferry service.

Electricity reached the county in the 1930s although it did not become available at Wendover until 1948. Telephone lines followed shortly thereafter, and by mid-century, most of the county's local people had access to electricity, telephone services, and paved roads (Breckinridge, 1952/1981). The new and improved roads and facilities brought good fortune to Leslie County and enabled a coal boom that changed the economy in the late 1940s and 1950s. The Ford family was one of the largest landowners and lessors of mine properties in the county, and Mary became good friends with the family. Edsel Ford of Detroit presented the Frontier Nursing Service with a reconditioned Model A Ford that Mary and her staff lovingly named "Henrietta."

ENABLING OTHERS TO ACT

Enabling others to act is another exemplary leadership practice that became evident in Mary Breckinridge's life's work. It is the practice of leaders to build teams with spirited cohesiveness and shared ideas, and to develop collaborative relationships among them (Kouzes & Posner, 2012). It entails two guarantees on the leader's part, namely, promotion of cooperative goals and mutual trust and the strengthening of others.

One might ask, how it was that Mary *enabled others to act*? She did so when World War II broke out in 1939 and the British nurse-midwives of the Frontier Nursing Service wanted to return to their homeland. Wartime made it impossible to send American nurses overseas to London for training. Mary saw this as an opportunity rather than a setback, and, as a result, she put her plan into action to build a midwifery school. On November 1, 1939, the Frontier Graduate School of Midwifery opened, the first of its kind in America, with just two students. It housed a faculty who shared the common goals of educating a much-needed workforce of midwives. The school has been in continuous operation since that time. Graduates of the midwifery program have provided care all across the country and even in foreign developing countries.

In response to the changing health care landscape of the 1960s, the Frontier Graduate School developed a curriculum, offering the first certificate program for family nurse practitioners. In 1970, the school changed its name to the Frontier School of Midwifery and Family Nursing, and in 2011, the name changed to Frontier Nursing University to reflect its master's and doctoral program offerings. These innovative programs are tailored for nurses who want to become nurse-midwives, family nurse practitioners, or women's health nurse practitioners. Distance education has strengthened enrollment and now enables students from all over the United States and even foreign countries to pursue the goal of becoming a midwife. This allows the curriculum to be delivered from the historic location in Hyden, Kentucky, where nurse-midwifery originated in the United States.

MODELING THE WAY

Leaders who *model the way* hold to high standards and values and lead by providing an example that followers can emulate. When Mary Breckinridge penned her autobiography in her 1952 book, *Wide Neighborhoods: A Story of the Frontier Nursing Service*, she told the story of her early life and detailed life events that influenced her interest in nursing and her efforts to establish health care for women, children, and families in rural Kentucky. It reflected the exemplary leadership practice of *modeling the way* and illustrated examples of her behaving in ways that are consistent with shared values. Her journaling depicted her life in Wendover and described her love of the Frontier Nursing Service and the achievement of her many small wins since its establishment in 1925. She was equally proud of the Frontier Graduate School of Midwifery, today known as Frontier Nursing University, and the hundreds of graduates it has produced.

In her writings, Mary compared the Frontier Nursing Service to a banyan tree, a metaphor that aptly described the organization's unwavering and loyal "roots" in the isolated mountains of eastern Kentucky. During the years covered in the book, nearly 9,000 babies were delivered by the Frontier Nursing Service—all delivered by nurse-midwives and born at home in their cabins. It is a proud fact that, in the next 55 years and nearly 19,000 deliveries, the Frontier Nursing Service lost only 11 mothers and, since 1951, not one mother was lost in childbirth. By 1979, the infant mortality rate was zero. Clearly, Mary Breckinridge carried out her plans, expressed in her life story "like the banyan tree of the forest yielding shade and fruit to wide neighborhoods of men" (Breckinridge, 1952/1981, p. xvii).

THE PASSING OF MARY BRECKINRIDGE

Shortly before her passing, Mary Breckinridge told a reporter, "If you are able to take the unborn child as a focal point you will soon be led to a broad program of public health" (Crowe-Carraco, 1978, p. 179). In this concise statement, Mary encapsulated over five decades of public service. On the day before she died, she was busy editing the manuscript for the Frontier

Nursing Service's *Quarterly Bulletin*. It was well known that, following a fall from a horse in 1931 in which Mary broke her back, she ran the Frontier Nursing Service from her bed at Wendover until her death.

On May 16, 1965, Mary Breckinridge died at the age of 84 surrounded by her loyal friends and employees. She is buried alongside her two children, Breckie and Polly, in a cemetery located in Lexington, Kentucky. Newspapers across the United States eulogized her and referred to her as the "Angel of the Frontier, and the most illustrious Kentucky woman of all time, certainly of her own time" (*Courier-Journal*, 1965, n.p.).

MARY BRECKINRIDGE HOSPITAL

Many changes have taken place in the Frontier Nursing Service since its early beginnings. New government health care programs provided funding for indigent and elderly patients. It was decided shortly after Breckinridge's death that a fitting memorial to her would be a new hospital. In October of 1970, a groundbreaking ceremony was held, and in 1975, a new 40-bed, state-of-the-art hospital that included a pharmacy, laboratory, physical and respiratory therapy programs, and delivery and operating rooms, was dedicated. No longer needed as the primary medical facility, the Hyden Hospital became the home for the Frontier School of Nurse Midwifery and Family Nursing and the Primary Care Clinic (Breckinridge, 1952/1981).

Today, Mary Breckinridge Hospital continues to meet the challenges that confront a small rural hospital and an ever-evolving health care system. The nurses have traded in their horses for jeeps, and patients receive treatment in a modern hospital. The Mary Breckinridge Hospital provides primary care for the local community, employs over 100 medical residents, and is the second largest employer in Leslie County (How the FNS Began— Frontier Nurse Service, n.d.).

BRECKINRIDGE HONORED

In 1926, Mary Breckinridge was awarded the Harmon Fanton Prize for her contributions to the field of public health work, and in 1961 she received the Mary Adelaine Nutting Award for Distinguished Service, the highest honor of the National League for Nursing.

In addition, she was recognized for her lifework and inducted into the American Nurses Association's (ANA's) Hall of Fame in 1982. The ANA applauded her vision in introducing a rural model of health care delivery, and women's health, family, and community health nursing services. Accolades were given for the nursing care Mary had provided to the underserved mountain people in the Appalachian region of Kentucky. Thanks were given for lowering the maternal and infant mortality rates in Leslie County, Kentucky, from the highest in the nation to well below the national average.

Credit was given to the Frontier Nursing Service that nurse-midwives were no more than 6 miles from any of their patients and for the nurses who continue to serve this area today.

Furthermore, the ANA praised Mary and staff members of the Frontier Nursing Service who formed the American College of Nurse Midwives in 1929. The American College of Nurse Midwives recognizes Breckinridge as the first to bring nurse-midwifery to the United States and the Frontier School of Midwifery and Family Planning as "a leader in nurse midwifery in the United States and a tribute to her accomplishments and her contemporaries" (Dusek, 2006, p. 28).

On November 9, 1998, the United States Post Office issued a 77-cent postage stamp to honor Mary for founding the Frontier Nursing Service. She was recognized as a nursing figure in the Great American Series, a series of postage stamps that began release on December 27, 1980, and is known by stamp collectors for its simplicity and elegance (Smithsonian National Postal Museum, 2014).

At their 2011 commencement ceremony, the Frontier Nursing University presented honorary doctorates to five nursing leaders who shaped Frontier Nursing University. First among the awardees was Frontier Founder, Mary Breckinridge, who was recognized with a posthumous doctor of humane letters for her tireless efforts and documented success in transforming health care for rural and underserved populations.

MARY BRECKINRIDGE'S LEADERSHIP LEGACY

Mary Breckinridge devoted her life to creating a legacy much larger than herself. Many lives in rural America were saved because of her dedication and vision. During her career with the Frontier Nursing Service, 14,500 babies were delivered, over 50,000 people were treated, over one quarter million vaccines were given, and the rate of maternal and infant mortality decreased dramatically. In addition, Mary amassed $10 million through her fundraising efforts. She is one of the most famous nurse leaders in history.

Today, the Frontier Nursing Service continues with six health care clinics as well as the Mary Breckinridge Hospital and Mary Breckinridge Home Health Agency. People come from all over the world to study the example of rural health care that Breckinridge founded. The Frontier School of Midwifery and Family Nursing is still in existence and offers excellent educational opportunities for nurses and nurse practitioners.

The year 2014 marked the 75th anniversary of the Frontier Nursing University. The university is the longest operating nurse-midwifery program in the country. It continues to graduate qualified, competent, caring nurse-midwives who practice in Kentucky, all over the country, and the world.

It is clear that Mary Breckinridge is a nursing leader who not only influenced people in a small remote corner of Kentucky, and nurse-midwives from afar, but was also an exemplary leader in public health nursing. She succeeded in fulfilling her vision of creating a health care model to deliver low-cost care to an underserved population of rural America. It appears that her quote, "The easiest thing is to do, the next easiest is to write, and the hardest is to think" (Breckinridge, 1952/1981, p. xiv) does not apply to its author, as Mary Breckinridge "thought out of the box," she wrote about how she succeeded in accomplishing her plans, and enlisted the help of others to do what needed to be done.

Mary Breckinridge recognized a group of people in need of access to health care and used all of her available means to create and implement an efficient and effective health care model to improve their well-being. Does this sound like anything different from what we are still trying to accomplish to this day?

TIMELINE

- February 17, 1881—Mary Breckinridge is born in Memphis, Tennessee, into an affluent Southern family; her father was a U.S. ambassador to Russia and her grandfather served as vice president under President Buchanan.
- 1907—Enters nursing school at St. Luke's Hospital in New York City, where she trains for 3 years and eventually becomes head nurse of an infant's ward.
- 1918—After World War I, volunteers to work with CARD where she distributes clothing, food, and supplies to people in remote areas of France; in addition, she cares for the sick, especially children, and becomes acquainted with the midwives in France and Great Britain.
- 1921—Returns to the United States with a plan to provide health care to people in rural America; takes courses at Teachers College in New York City where she meets Adelaide Nutting who agrees with Breckinridge's vision.
- 1923—Conducts a public health survey in the mountains of Leslie County, Kentucky, where she interviews all the granny midwives she can locate; learns that many are elderly, largely illiterate, and have no training in nursing.
- 1924—Leaves for training in midwifery at the British Hospital for Mothers and Babies in Woolwich in southeast London.
- 1925—Returns to Leslie County, Kentucky, obtains state license to practice as a nurse-midwife, and establishes the Kentucky Committee for Mothers and Babies, later renamed the Frontier Nursing Service, to provide maternity care and childbirth services to the underserved rural women and children in eastern Kentucky.
- 1928—Hyden Hospital is dedicated.

- 1939—Establishes the Frontier Graduate School of Midwifery, the first rural-based nurse-midwifery school in the United States.
- 1952—Publishes her autobiography, *Wide Neighborhoods: A Story of the Frontier Nursing Service*, where she writes about midwives who rode on horseback in order to reach and provide care to women and children in the Appalachian mountains.
- May 16, 1965—Breckinridge dies at age 84.
- 1970—Frontier Graduate School of Midwifery offers the first family nurse practitioner program in the United States.
- 1975—The Mary Breckinridge Hospital is dedicated.
- 1982—ANA inducts Breckinridge into the Hall of Fame for her contributions to the nursing profession in women's health, community, and family nursing, and rural health care delivery.
- 1998—A U.S. postage stamp is issued in her honor as part of the "Great American Series" (at the beginning of this chapter).
- November 1999—Frontier Nursing Service celebrates its 60th year of nursing service; it is estimated that a quarter of all certified nurse-midwives graduated from this school; one of the most famous babies delivered by a Frontier Nursing Service–trained midwife is Tim Couch, quarterback for the Cleveland Browns.
- 2005—The school adds the Women's Health Care Nurse Practitioner Program.
- 2014—November 1, 2014, the school celebrates its 75th anniversary.

QUESTIONS FOR DISCUSSION

1. By *modeling the way* and *enabling others to act*, Mary Breckinridge led change in improving rural health, women's health, and midwifery education and practice. What are some of the new and emerging health care specialties that will benefit from nurses' leadership by enabling nurses and others to act?
2. Mary Breckinridge traveled far and wide from her childhood home to Leslie County, Kentucky, to focus on and meet the health needs of a specific population, namely, rural women and children. What specific populations can you identify that have unique health needs today? Where are they located? How can nurse leaders have an impact on addressing their needs?
3. Thanks to the pioneering efforts of Mary Breckinridge, we now have many women's health nursing education programs. How can nurses lead change in higher education and *enable others to act* in preparing nurses and other health care professionals to address the unique health needs of specific populations?

REFERENCES

Appalachian Regional Healthcare. (n.d.). *Mary Breckinridge Hospital.* Retrieved November 7, 2014, from www.arh.org/locations/Mary_Breckinridge/our_history.aspx

Breckinridge, M. (1981). *Wide neighborhoods: A story of the frontier nursing service.* Lexington, KY: University Press of Kentucky. (Original work published 1952)

Bullough, V. L. (1988). Mary Breckinridge. In V. L. Bullough, O. M. Church, & A. P. Stein (Eds.), *American nursing: A biographical dictionary* (pp. 46–47). New York, NY: Garland.

Campbell, A. G. (1984). Mary Breckinridge and the American Committee for Devastated France: The foundations of the Frontier Nursing Service. *Register of the Kentucky Historical Society, 82*(3), 257–276.

Courier-Journal. (1965, May 17). Louisville, Kentucky.

Crowe-Carraco, C. (1978). Mary Breckinridge and the Frontier Nursing Service. *Register of the Kentucky Historical Society, 76*(3), 179–191.

Dusek, K. H. (2006). Angel on horseback. *Child Life, 85*(4), 28.

Goan, M. (2008). *Mary Breckinridge: The Frontier Nursing Service and rural health in Appalachia.* Chapel Hill, NC: The University of North Carolina Press.

How the FNS Began—Frontier Nursing Service. (n.d.). Retrieved from https://www.frontiernursing.org/Source/s-howFNSbegan.shtm

Kessler-Harris, A. (2003). *Out to work: A history of wage-earning women in the United States* (pp. 116–117). New York, NY: Oxford University Press.

Kouzes, J. M., & Posner, B. Z. (2012). *The leadership challenge* (5th ed.). San Francisco, CA: Jossey-Bass.

Miller, E. L. (1988). Arkansas nurses, 1895–1920: A profile. *Arkansas Historical Quarterly, 47,* 154–171.

Pletsch, P. K. (1981). Mary Breckinridge: A pioneer who made her mark. *American Journal of Nursing, 81*(12), 2188–2190.

Ruffing-Rahal, M. A. (1991). Ethnographic traits in the writing of Mary Breckinridge. *Journal of Advanced Nursing, 16,* 614–620.

Smithsonian National Postal Museum. (2014). *Great Americans issue (1980–1999).* Retrieved from http://arago.si.edu/category_2037993.html

Wells, R. (1998). *Mary on horseback, three mountain stories.* New York, NY: Dial Press.

West, E. (2013). History, organization and the changing culture of care: A historical analysis of the frontier nursing service. *Journal of International Women's Studies, 14*(1), 218–235.

PART · VI

Encouraging the Heart

Edith Louisa Cavell: Courage in the Face of Duty

Barbara J. Patterson

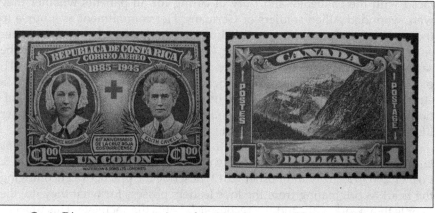

Costa Rica postage stamp issued in 1945 honoring Florence Nightingale and Edith Cavell (left). Canadian postage stamp issued in 1930 honoring Mount Edith Cavell (right).

• • • • •

The Germans arrested Edith Cavell on August 5, 1915, on charges of harboring Allied soldiers and organizing their escape across Belgium to neutral Holland. Despite the efforts of the American ambassador, Brand Whitlock, to obtain a mitigation of her sentence, Cavell was executed before a firing squad at 2:00 a.m. on October 12, 1915. Her last words are reported as

> I have nothing to regret. If I had to do over again, I would do just
> as I did. . . . I was very tired and so pressed with a multitude of
> petty things that life brings that I have not had time for many
> years for quiet and uninterrupted meditation. It was a welcome
> rest for me—before the end. I know now that patriotism is not
> enough. I must have no hatred or bitterness toward anyone.
> (Judson, 1941, p. 281)

As a nurse during World War I, Edith Louisa Cavell (1865–1915) was faced with the challenge and duty of caring for all patients whether they were wounded Allied soldiers or Germans. Her commitment as a nurse to the care of every person transcended patriotism; it was who she was at her core. Edith has been quoted as saying, "I can't stop while there are lives to be saved," which captured her conviction to help anyone in need (Judson, 1941, p. 236). Although some accounts of her nursing leadership portray her as a strict and dour matron, Cavell's actions reflected her vision and the recognition of others. These actions to *encourage the heart* were characteristic of her life and they continue after her death.

Edith Cavell exemplified the leadership practice of *encouraging the heart*. The word *encouragement* literally means to give others heart (Kouzes & Posner, 2003). Kouzes and Posner (2012) describe the practice of encouraging the heart as originating from the love leaders possess for what they do, the people they work with, and the accomplishments they achieve. This practice requires leaders to exhibit courage.

Courage is how leaders inspire others to reach their common goals. In facing the evil of war, Edith had the courage to assume the role of a nurse leader during a dark time in the history of the world. Brown (2007, p. 8) described Edith's courage as "not simply a matter of perseverance," but also as her duty and dedication, as a nurse, to relieve suffering for all. Edith also expressed the courage and strength of character to assume the risk of changing nursing in Belgium, not an easy task for a woman in the early 20th century. She had a strong sense of social justice and made a difference as a nursing leader.

Edith's journey to becoming a leader in nursing was a relatively brief one, but it had tremendous impact across several continents. Born on December 4, 1865, Edith Louisa Cavell spent her childhood in the English village of Swardeston in the county of Norfolk on England's east coast. She was the first-born child of Reverend Frederick and Louisa Cavell.

ASSUMING HER DUTY TO HUMANITY

For Edith Cavell, the decision to become a nurse had its origin in her upbringing in a Victorian English household. This was a time when women had tremendous constraints on occupational choices beyond becoming a governess or nurse. Edith grew up in a house with a strict orthodox upbringing. Her father was a vicar of an Anglican church and was the person who took charge of her educational trajectory (Batten, 2007). His manner was strict, demanding, and firm, thus setting the stage for her future and creating an expectation of hard work. There was routine with little change for those who lived in the English countryside.

Under a shadow of duty, it was during Edith's early years that she acquired her social values and a worldview of serving others in need, those who were less fortunate. This became her moral standard. Roots for a common treatment of humanity were deeply established within Edith. Her Christian belief system to *encourage the heart* was well established as a young girl and provided the foundation for her future endeavors. Likewise, Edith was credited with *challenging the process* in her early teenage years when the need for a parish Sunday school building became apparent. Without her parents' support, she wrote directly to the Bishop of Norwich, asking for financial assistance. Although initially not supported by the Bishop, undeterred, Edith ultimately acquired the money necessary to build the school (Judson, 1941). These values formed the foundation for her future work. Her unprivileged beginnings instilled in Edith the quality of humility, later exhibited as a leader in her years as a matron of nursing.

Reverend Cavell provided most of her primary education in the family home and, at the age of 16, he sent Edith to London and western England to three different boarding schools in order to broaden her knowledge and exposure to the arts (Souhami, 2010). Given Edith's social class, this education was designed to prepare her for a life of marriage or, if not marriage, respectable employment as a governess. Alternatively, she could become a nurse, an occupation of mixed regard at the time.

In 1889, Edith Cavell traveled on holiday to the Bavarian province in Germany and had her first sense that nursing might be the profession for her (Batten, 2007). She visited an institution that offered free medical care, the Free Hospital. This experience had a lasting impact. The compassion she felt for others contributed to her selfless sense of duty (Walker, 2003). Edith was quoted as saying to her cousin "Someday, somehow, I am going to do something useful. . . . I don't know what it will be, but it must be something for people" (Grey, 1960, p. 16).

Over the next 8 years, Edith was a governess for several different families. It was her last post with the François family in Brussels that introduced Edith to life in Europe. In Belgium, she was able to perfect her French. Culturally, she experienced a refined lifestyle, unlike her life at home in Swardeston. It was during her time with the François family that Edith demonstrated independence and the courage to stand up for her beliefs, another quality that she would demonstrate throughout her professional nursing career. There occurred an incident when Paul François offered a rude comment about the Queen of England, and despite the fact that he was her employer, Edith had the character to voice indignation in defense of the monarch (Batten, 2007). Reflecting on these times as a governess, Edith has been quoted as saying, "How little did I realize at the time that particular experience would be so valuable, but it was just what I needed to help me with the work I was to do later" (Judson, 1941, p. 29).

Life as a governess took a turn for Edith Cavell in 1895. Nursing, as a career path, was validated by the experience of caring for her father. Despite Edith's two sisters being nurses, she left Brussels and her governess's position to return home to care for her father when he became ill. The personal satisfaction she felt with this episode brought her thoughts of being a nurse once again to the forefront. Her desire and perceived destiny to help others became a reality with her choice to pursue nursing.

Fortunately, the social profile of being a nurse in England in the mid to late 19th century was beginning to improve through the efforts of Florence Nightingale (Souhami, 2010). Nightingale had raised the standards of nursing as a profession, and nurses were making a difference in patient care. For nurses and nurse leaders at this time, Nightingale *modeled the way* in the education and preparation of nurses to be dedicated professionals. It was also during this time that the suffragist movement was emerging in urban settings, such as London, and women's roles were beginning to change.

To achieve her professional goal, at age 30, Edith Cavell applied to become a probationer or student nurse at the London Hospital in Whitechapel. The London Hospital was where Edith trained as a nurse in accordance with the Nightingale educational model. The demands of being a probationer nurse were significant. The hours were long and arduous with little financial compensation. The community in which the nurses worked contained mostly destitute and underprivileged individuals (Souhami, 2010). Edith accepted these challenges, and she believed nursing would lead to the social reforms that were desperately needed during this time.

Eva Lückes, a disciple of Florence Nightingale, was the matron of the London Hospital and introduced many reforms into the education of nurses (Souhami, 2010). She embodied the five leadership practices of Kouzes and Posner during her time as matron. She was considered a strict disciplinarian and served as a role model for Edith Cavell. A leader in early nursing education, Matron Lückes envisioned a training school for nurses where they had lectures from physicians and students took examinations. She created a structured educational program, which included anatomy and physiology. Fighting for better working and training conditions for her nurses, Lückes told the hospital board "The best way to predict the future is to create it—and you create it by strategy, structure, and resources" (Souhami, 2010, p. 15). The resources were her probationer nurses. The school was recognized in

England for its reputation of training competent nurses. *Inspiring a shared vision*, Lückes has been described as having "possessed vision, the vision to see in the future the trained nurse—an intelligent woman of more than average education, working under fair and comfortable conditions and thereby giving more efficient care to her patient" (Judson, 1941, p. 44).

Under Lückes's leadership, the London Hospital acquired recognition throughout Europe as a model of nursing education (Judson, 1941). The London Hospital, grounded in Nightingale's philosophy of nursing care, provided Edith Cavell with the context for developing her leadership skills under the exemplary role model of Eva Lückes. Setting the example and *modeling the way* for nursing education, the leadership exhibited by Matron Lückes was admired and respected by Edith for many years.

It has been noted that, apart from Edith's mother, Lückes made the greatest impression on Cavell (Judson, 1941). She spoke of her training experience with fondness, describing her feelings about the school, "No place will ever be to me what the 'London' was nor any Matron like the one under whom I trained" (Judson, 1941, p. 48). Lückes wrote an annual Christmas letter to her nurses, *encouraging the heart* and maintaining a sense of community among the nurses. Lückes would correspond with graduates individually regarding advances in patient care (Judson, 1941). From the time Edith started her school of nursing in Brussels in 1907 and her death in 1915, she remained in contact with Matron Lückes.

In 1901, a new opportunity to teach nursing arose for Edith Cavell. Edith was ready for a change and new challenges; she accepted the position of assistant matron at Shoreditch Infirmary. The matron at Shoreditch described Edith as someone with "hidden resources within her. Her reserved manner in another person would have appeared to be snobbery, but in Edith Cavell, it was a grave dignity that filled her associates with deep admiration for her" (Judson, 1941, p. 73). She supervised and taught a nursing staff of 120. Setting an example by visiting children in their homes after discharge from the infirmary, she was a role model for her senior probationer nurses through her personal behavior. The nurses looked up to Cavell as their leader.

Edith Cavell's sense of duty, responsibility to humanity, and desire to advance the nursing profession established standards that were emulated by her students. She led by example and never sought personal praise or attention. Humility was a virtue deeply embedded within Edith. Her seriousness did, however, influence her interactions with others. Edith lacked a sense of humor (Judson, 1941). Whether it was the influence of her puritanical upbringing or a personal limitation, she had difficulty in appreciating the humorous aspects of day-to-day life. This quality never appeared to impact Edith's work and dedication to others; however, as a leader it may have influenced her ability to *encourage the heart*.

By 1906, Edith Cavell had been in nursing 10 years and she expressed a desire to have a greater impact. She felt it was her moral obligation. There remained an internal unrest within her. She left her position at Shoreditch and traveled abroad several months for a much-needed rest and exploration of her own desires. In correspondence with her former matron, Eva Lückes, Edith expressed concerns about the challenges of securing another position upon return from holiday (Souhami, 2010).

Returning from abroad, Edith applied for various teaching positions and she received multiple rejections (Arthur, 2011). Edith had vast experience in nursing but she had not received strong recommendations from others. She was discouraged and frustrated. Her age, quiet demeanor, and retiring style may not have served her well at this time. Although somewhat disheartened, she ultimately secured a temporary position as a district nurse and remained there until she received the offer to start a school of nursing in Belgium. Edith felt she had more to give during her lifetime than what she had already accomplished. During these years, her letters reflected her passionate desire and capacity to help others, without an emphasis on ambition and self-advancement (Brown, 2007). Her resolve and personal qualities of humility, courage, and compassion provided the framework for her leadership.

The opportunity to make a difference arrived in a letter, which changed Edith Cavell's life dramatically. She was asked to start the first training school for nurses in Belgium. This was the challenge Edith most wanted and she was well suited for it. Dr. Antoine Depage, a leading surgeon in Brussels, was a medical visionary who sought nurses trained like those under the Nightingale model in London (Souhami, 2010). Edith had all of the characteristics Dr. Depage desired, an English nurse trained in a leading London hospital, fluent in French, and familiar with the Belgian way of life. Edith recognized this position as both a challenge and an enormous undertaking. Her desire to make a significant contribution to humanity and to implement her leadership skills by establishing a training school for nurses was now a reality. She accepted the offer and left for Brussels with all of the zeal and energy needed to change nursing practice in Belgium. Her life journey to make a real difference had started.

ENCOURAGING THE HEART: CHANGING NURSING IN BELGIUM

Having been trained under the Nightingale educational model in England, Edith Cavell experienced the shift felt in the early years toward a positive regard for nursing from the English people and an accompanying sense of professionalism. Although nursing was a relatively young profession in England, there was a respect and acknowledgment of nurses' training. Arriving in Belgium in late 1907, Edith encountered a culture in which professional nursing was unknown and the training of nurses mirrored conditions as they had been in England before Nightingale's influence. In recognition of her nursing skills, teaching abilities, and leadership qualities, she was chosen by a leading physician in Belgium to be matron of the first nurses' training school at the Berkendael Institute, a progressive teaching hospital in Brussels. Nursing in Brussels presented challenges Edith did not anticipate.

Reforming and setting the standards for nursing in Belgium was not an easy task. When Edith arrived in Belgium, the Catholic Sisters managed the care of the sick. These devoted women "were absolutely untrained in modern methods of nursing; rather they were imbued with the medieval routine prevalent in the Convent, and were wholly ignorant of the progress achieved since the time of Florence Nightingale" (Judson, 1941, p. 97). Introducing modern nursing to the care of the sick resulted in major conflicts with deeply held traditional attitudes. Having lived and worked in Belgium as a governess proved invaluable in making the changes crucial to nursing and ultimately to patient care. Nevertheless, "even her energy and courage were solely taxed amid the confusion, the lack of organized leadership, and the general attitude of irresponsibility" that Edith encountered in the first few years in trying to change the practice of nursing (Judson, 1941, p. 103).

Within a few days of her arrival in Brussels, Edith Cavell was interviewing prospective nurse probationers. Five students comprised the first class. *Inspiring a shared vision*, Edith wrote to Eva Lückes, "It is pioneer work here and needs much enthusiasm and courage and intelligence, as there are many looking askance at it. It will also require great tack. I hope to pull through this and soon have a model school" (Arthur, 2011, p. 62). Edith spoke with conviction to the probationers about how important it was for nursing to be recognized as a profession. To Edith, this meant nurses were to be treated with dignity and respect and not as a servant for the physician. There was a deeply ingrained stigma about nurses being little more than maids that had to be overcome (Batten, 2007).

Challenging the process, Edith set out to transform four dilapidated buildings into a school to train nurses. She would need to make decisions about classroom space, equipment, living accommodations, and an educational curriculum. The school was being built from scratch. This transformation required convincing the Ladies' Committee that nurses needed to understand anatomy and physiology in order to provide the best nursing care for their patients. The nursing curriculum Edith proposed was rigorous and, for some, it was threatening. The training was far more advanced than most nursing programs of the time. Edith's vision was to see the role of nursing change dramatically. In her leadership, she set a personal example of her expectations of the probationers to accomplish this goal. Although her conviction fueled this opportunity, it was also a risk. This would be just one example of a pattern of risks she assumed throughout her entire life.

To change the public perception of nurses, Edith Cavell mandated a change in uniforms for her nurses. The Sisters wore heavy, drab black uniforms. Edith envisioned her nurses wearing crisp blue cotton dresses with starched white collars, cuffs, and aprons with a simple cap (Arthur, 2011). Exhibiting a professional appearance was a first crucial step in securing this new future for nursing; the difference in clothing was described as "a contrast of the unhygienic past with the enlightened present" (Batten, 2007, p. 37).

Recruiting new probationers in Brussels was a challenge for Edith Cavell. Belgians believed that for a woman to become a nurse was "tantamount to sacrificing her place in society" (Arthur, 2006, p. 31). Nevertheless, Edith refused to lower her standards just to increase enrollment in her school. In 1908, to advertise the accomplishments of the school and attract new trainees from other countries, Edith published an article about the school in London's *Nursing Mirror*. She shared the objectives of the training of the school's nurses as "first to create a profession for women; secondly to forward the cause of science; thirdly to provide the best possible help for the sick and suffering" (Souhami, 2010, p. 104). Additionally, Edith shared her vision of nursing through public lectures about the school in Brussels. As part of a Belgian nursing delegation to the International Congress of Nurses in London, she shared the school's progress and its mission and goals. Edith met with success; by 1909, there were 23 probationers enrolled in the training program (Souhami, 2010). The school and its matron were gaining an international reputation.

One recruit, who responded to the *Nursing Mirror* article, was Sister Elizabeth Wilkins. She applied to the school to be an assistant matron to Edith Cavell. Sister Wilkins spoke French and was very well qualified for this position. She described her ambitions as a nurse to be similar to that of both Florence Nightingale and Cavell herself. She was devoted to nursing and shared in her interview with Edith that she had much to learn and stated, "I strongly believe my destiny is in Brussels, working under your leadership" (Arthur, 2011, p. 77). Sister Wilkins remained loyal and supportive of Edith throughout the remainder of Edith's life.

Edith Cavell hired Sister Wilkins for the position of assistant matron. Edith had grown and matured as a leader during this period of growth for the school. As the matron, she had the authority and power to accomplish much. For Edith, however, leadership was not about power and control; she remained focused on her duty to humanity and was confident and secure in her own reserve. By *enabling others to act*, "Exemplary leaders build an environment that develops both people's abilities to perform a task and their self-confidence. . . . Leaders significantly increase people's belief in their own ability to make a difference" (Kouzes & Posner, 2012, p. 243). Sister Wilkins was the individual who Edith enabled, strengthened, and involved in making important decisions about the school.

ENCOURAGING THE HEART: THE MATRON

The atmosphere Matron Cavell created in the school was one of high standards and a professional sensibility. As articulated by Kouzes and Posner (2012), a leader needs to be clear about goals and expectations. Edith Cavell's goals and values set the course of action for her as she *modeled the way* for the probationer nurses. There was nothing Edith would expect her nurses to do that she herself did not do. She set high standards for her nurses and was portrayed as a firm, strict disciplinarian. Starting with her first class of five students, she said, "We expect you to bring passion, determination, perseverance, and a strong sense of commitment to the profession. . . . To do this work, you must study hard" (Arthur, 2011, p. 66). The probationers had to be women of suitable character with professional qualifications.

Edith Cavell inspired her nurses through her courage and hopes for the profession. She was a very private, solitary person, and praising others did not come easily. However, her love for others and the work they were doing together provided recognition of their accomplishments. As a leader, her encouragement would energize the nurses. Edith demonstrated *encouraging the heart* by creating a sense of community among the nurses. Weekly tea parties and musical evenings were customs that Edith brought from her own training with Eva Lückes. Additionally, Edith had informal interactions with the students that focused on nursing within the "philosophical context of service, vocation, duty, pride, honour, and professionalism" (Brown, 2007, p. 13). It was within this educational environment that the probationers described the school as a place where they were family (Batten, 2007).

Even after imprisonment, in a letter to her nurses, Edith continued to *encourage the heart* and communicate to them what they could accomplish. She wrote:

> It is necessary that you should study well, for some of you must shortly sit for your examinations and I want you very much to succeed. The year's course will commence shortly, try to profit from it, and be punctual at lectures so that your professor need not be kept waiting. In everything one can learn new lessons of life. . . . To be a good nurse one must have lots of patience. . . . Your devoted Matron. (Brown, 2007, p. 31)

Nursing was Edith Cavell's world. Being a reserved individual, she was uninterested in meaningless interactions. In her private life, Edith remained single with few friends. She acquired a stray dog, Jack, who was her devoted companion and followed her throughout the school and clinic. Despite her sometimes cool and aloof demeanor, she was committed to the nurses and patients. Edith was driven by her vision to help others, including her nurses; "If her nurses were ill, she did all she could for them" (Souhami, 2010, p. 115). She provided them with the social support they needed, a strategy that is good for both mental and physical health (Kouzes & Posner, 2012). As the possibility of war emerged, Edith perceived her duty to be with her nurses.

If Edith Cavell was discouraged by her probationers and their difficulty understanding nursing, "she never showed it; and she always told us that we must have more patience" (Judson, 1941, p. 133). Instilling the meaning of the profession into the young nurses was one of the more significant challenges Edith encountered. Serving as a role model and teaching a sense of duty was difficult. Edith used examples in her day-to-day encounters with the students to convey professional duty. One commonly shared example was when a probationer attempted to kill a large spider in the classroom; Edith said, "Nurse, do not kill; take it outside. A nurse gives life; she does not take it" (Judson, 1941, p. 123). She hoped this example would assist them in understanding their duty to care for others, even if a spider. Kouzes and Posner (2012) contend that "it's this kind of personal dedication and involvement that earns leaders the respect and trust of their teams. It's what builds credibility and loyalty. It's also what develops an engaged and productive workforce" (p. 318).

In the summer of 1914, 7 years after her arrival in Brussels, construction of a new school building to train the nurses was underway. Under her leadership, she had accomplished so much for the nursing profession in Belgium. Her vision was to prepare more matrons like herself to train nurses across the country. She was shaping the nurses of the future. Unfortunately, the nature of the world and Belgium would dramatically change before the year ended.

With the German occupation of Brussels in August 1914, Edith Cavell recognized the fear being experienced by the nurses. Nevertheless, she reinforced the nurses' duty to care for any wounded soldier since "each man was a father, husband or son" (Souhami, 2010, p. 144). Both German and Allied soldiers received equal care at the Institute. The day the Germans marched into the city, the staff expressed feelings of doom. Edith courageously refused to leave her post, even when the fall of the city was imminent. Maintaining some sense of control over a situation in which she had no control was Edith's way of supporting the staff and nurses. In one instance, acknowledging the worry and concern for their lives, she remained calm and unexpectedly started to play the piano (Arthur, 2011). She kept them busy and in a state of readiness. The safety of the nurses was a priority, no matter what their nationality.

In order to achieve a sense of order in her life, Cavell wrote an editorial for *Nursing Mirror* in 1914. Edith felt the nursing community needed to be aware of the deteriorating situation in Brussels. She lamented, "I can only feel the deep and tender pity as a friend within the gates, and observe with sympathy and admiration the high courage and self-control of a people enduring a long, terrible agony" (Arthur, 2011, p. 137).

There was little activity in the clinic in 1914; there were few patients and the number of student probationers had decreased. However, always ready for the care of the wounded, Edith and the nurses spent hours making clothes for refugees and planning a Christmas party for the children (Batten, 2007). The children's Christmas party was a way to put aside the reality of war. It was during mid-December 1914 and mid-January 1915 that the clinic began to hide French and British soldiers (Batten, 2007). Edith connected with these soldiers and provided encouragement while, simultaneously, feeling the strain regarding the safety of the nurses and clinic staff at the hands of the Germans. Despite the risks she assumed, the courage and hope she displayed with her nurses exemplified her leadership ability and sense of duty for humanity. She continued to *model the way* during a terrifying chapter in world history.

Even as the war surged throughout Europe, Edith Cavell was frustrated and worried about completion of the new school, as well as the reform of nursing standards. Although her vision of duty to humanity never wavered, there was new meaning in helping the fugitive soldiers. She *challenged the process* and remained hopeful that her nursing work would continue after the war, since hospitals were depending on the availability of trained nurses. During this time, she saw in the Belgian people and the resistance workers,

> the qualities she had tried to apply in her nursing life and to
> inspire her students: altruism, courage, attention to detail,
> working for others without counting the cost. The difference was
> the context: the civilized structure of peacetime, as opposed to
> the madness and squalor of war. (Souhami, 2010, p. 209)

Over the next year prior to her execution, in October 1915, Edith Cavell helped hundreds of Allied soldiers escape to freedom and safety. Gordon Brown, former prime minister of the United Kingdom, in his book on courage (2007) wrote:

> People of courage will always be loved, because they ennoble
> the human race to which we all belong. We are drawn to them
> and revere them because through their actions they open up
> the possibility of hope in time of cynicism, dignity in times of
> degradation, and purpose in times of despair. . . . They raise our
> sights and challenge us to be all that we are capable of being.
> (p. 237)

The courage Edith Cavell embraced captured Brown's (2007) description of altruistic courage. It was more than physical bravery; it was a "sacrifice and determination for a higher purpose; the courage that endures and prevails; and eventually dignifies all humanity. It was an expression of both strength of character and strength of belief" (Brown, 2007, p. 1). Unwavering, Edith exhibited these strengths throughout her life. She was, and remains, a leader and role model for nurses worldwide.

Edith could have left Brussels at the start of the war, but she felt it was her duty to stay for the nurses, patients, and school. She consciously chose to remain in Belgium and, therefore, in harm's way. Even within the context of numerous injustices, Edith never refused to help anyone in need. Her humanitarianism gave purpose and meaning to her life. The nursing profession was the vehicle through which she put her values and ideals into practice.

Brown (2007) has argued that one must not define Edith Cavell's "courage simply as the courage to perform her duty as a nurse no matter what the circumstances. . . . nursing and her clandestine wartime activities proved to be arenas in which she could put these greater ideals into practice" (p. 18).

Edith Cavell's last words prior to her execution, "I must have no hatred or bitterness towards anyone," reflected her ability to see humanity beyond the horrors of war (Brown, 2007, p. 32). In a final letter to her nurses, Edith wrote,

> My dear sisters, it is a very sad moment for me now that I write to you to bid you farewell. . . . When brighter days come, our work will resume its growth, and all its power for doing good. I have loved you all much more than you thought. (Brown, 2007, pp. 32–33)

Notwithstanding her reserved, private demeanor, she continued to *encourage the heart*.

LEADERSHIP LESSONS FROM EDITH CAVELL AND WORLD WAR I

The nursing profession saw significant change and advancement in the 19th century, from how nurses were educated to how they practiced nursing. The nursing leaders of the time encountered many challenges in the process. The problems that faced nursing leadership in the early 1900s may be more similar to than different from what leaders face today. For Edith Cavell, the nature of war, inadequate supplies and money, and the preparation of professional nurses were just a few of her challenges. Edith approached these challenges with the character of a leader and a strong sense of duty as a nurse. She believed in humanity and her values always guided her actions.

In 1941, a leader of nursing education in the United States, Isabel Stewart, then director of nursing education at Teachers College, Columbia University, gave a keynote address at the Forty-Seventh Annual Convention of the National League for Nursing, stating that it was important for nursing to "not only avoid the mistakes but to learn from the achievements of the nursing profession" (Stewart, 1941, p. 805). This address reflected what nurse leaders had learned from the nursing problems encountered during the First World War. She compared the profession's issues of 1917, when the United States entered World War I, with those of 1941 when the United States was positioning to enter World War II. The impact on nursing education and, thus, nurse capacity was huge. These were similar to the challenges faced by Edith Cavell in Belgium during World War I.

The historical significance of this address provides understanding of the leadership and legacy of Edith Cavell during the First World War, as what was happening to the profession in Europe had far-reaching impact across the Atlantic. After the United States entered the war in 1917, a self-appointed committee, comprising nursing leaders, met to design a plan of action to increase the number of nurses being prepared. Stewart noted that these leaders were challenged to consider

> what provisions had been made for war nursing in this country, what the situation was at that time in relation to the supply of nurses, and what authority and status the professional nursing group had in planning for military and civilian nursing needs in a great emergency. (Stewart, 1941, p. 806)

Comparing the status of professional nursing in the United States in 1917 to that of Great Britain, there were concerns about the number of untrained personnel diluting the numbers of trained professionals (Stewart, 1941). Nursing education leaders were pressured by "trustees and hospital administrators . . . to pull down the standards still further to service the constantly expanding hospitals" (Stewart, 1941, p. 808). These leaders reflected on stories from professional colleagues in Europe about their experiences with untrained war nurses and they resolved not to lower the standards of educational preparation in the United States. As a leader, Edith Cavell faced similar challenges as she struggled to maintain high standards for her nurses and the nursing profession in Belgium. In closing the address, Stewart asked, "Does anyone doubt the value of that experience of twenty-five years ago to us today? . . . Would nurses today be able to show equal resourcefulness and courage and intelligence in meeting them?" (pp. 814–815). Although these questions were asked of nursing leaders in 1941, even with additional assets, experience, and knowledge, these same questions could be asked of nursing leaders today.

Edith Cavell embodied many leadership qualities that nurse leaders today could learn from and embrace. She was an exemplary role model of humility. Kouzes and Posner (2012, p. 340) posit, "Humility is the only way to resolve the conflicts and contradictions of leadership." Edith's focus to help all others was her life goal. She did not want to be remembered as a martyr; however, her actions fueled others after her death and thus are indirectly *encouraging the hearts* of many. She had the courage to remain humble and unassuming. The motivation to lead requires love (Kouzes & Posner, 2012), which sustained Edith Cavell during the most difficult days of her life. The love for her nurses also extended to not endangering their lives. She chose to aid the Allied soldiers alone without identifying others in the role she assumed.

Edith Cavell had cared for soldiers who were in need of medical attention and supplied them with clothing, food, and money, which made it possible for them to escape Belgium to a neutral country. During her court martial, Edith said to the judge "My aim has not been to assist your enemies, but to help these men gain the frontier" (Brown, 2007, p. 35). She did not deny her actions and was sentenced to death under German Military Code. "For performing her duty as a nurse, she was tried for treason and shot" (Arthur, 2006, p. 30). She had the courage to stand for her professional obligation and treat all individuals in a nondiscriminatory, compassionate manner.

Unfortunately, arresting and imprisoning health care providers for doing their work is something that persists to this day, despite the Geneva Convention. Throughout the world, nurse leaders actively fight for medical neutrality. The principle of medical neutrality refers to

> noninterference with medical services in times of armed conflict and civil unrest: they must be allowed to care for the sick and wounded, and soldiers must receive care regardless of their political affiliations; all parties must refrain from attacking and misusing medical facilities, transport, and personnel. (Physicians for Human Rights, n.d.)

A violation of medical neutrality is considered a war crime under the Geneva Convention (Office of the High Commissioner for Human Rights, 1977).

In early 2011, one recognized nurse leader and her colleagues from the country of Bahrain were convicted and sentenced to jail for charges "including incitement to overthrow the Bahraini government, spreading false information, and participating in an illegal public gathering" (Human Rights First, 2014, para. 5). They were providing medical treatment to protesters during a prodemocracy uprising. Rula Al-Saffar, registered nurse, served as president of the Bahrain Nursing Society and as assistant professor at the College of Health Science in Manama prior to her arrest. She was sentenced to 15 years' imprisonment, with the conviction being overturned in 2012. Unable to practice nursing in her home country following the conviction, Rula Al-Saffir continues to fight for human rights internationally and to obtain the release of her health care colleagues.

EDITH CAVELL'S LEADERSHIP LEGACY

A "leader's unique legacy is the creation of valued institutions that survive over time" (Kouzes & Posner, 2012, p. 6). The legacy that Edith Cavell left for humanity and the nursing profession was profound. Most often, the writing of her story focuses on her fate and how she met the end of her life. But it is Edith's leadership that she should be most remembered for. She made many decisions throughout her brief life that influenced the nursing profession and changed the education and practice of nursing in Belgium against significant odds, always remaining true to her values. These exemplary leadership qualities were what she sought to instill in her nurses.

Reports of Edith Cavell's tragic death confirmed the strength of her humanitarian conviction. The decision to execute her was a serious propaganda mistake for the Germans (Shaddox, 1999). The Allied response was prompt and resolute. "Remember Edith Cavell" became a recruiting slogan throughout Britain. Her death was used as propaganda for military recruitment in the war effort. This heroic nurse had become a worldwide martyr (Clowes, 1996). Prime Minister Asquith told the House of Commons that Edith Cavell "has taught the bravest man amongst us the supreme lesson of courage" (Souhami, 2010, p. 342). The morale of the soldiers was strengthened and recruitment numbers doubled (Clowes, 1996).

Edith Cavell's life has been described as one of action over inaction (Brown, 2007). The actions of Edith Cavell were courageous even when her life was at risk. "It is an everyday requirement in our society, an essential weapon in the struggle against prejudice, racism, violence, discrimination and injustice, and in the creation of a good society" (Brown, 2007, p. 241). Edith had a strong sense of social justice and made a difference as a nursing leader. Her values and vision were ever present.

Finding the courage to lead requires leaders to have "the fortitude to reach inside and give your best even faced with great odds. . . . It involves a capacity to forcefully impart cherished values to the people who look to them for leadership" (Kouzes & Posner, 2003, p. xv). The leader needs to keep hope alive through setting high standards, being a role model, and allowing others to see the meaning in their work (Kouzes & Posner, 2003). Through some very challenging times, Edith Cavell kept the hope alive in her nurses—the hope that the future for humanity would be brighter.

Four words—*humanity, fortitude, devotion,* and *sacrifice*—capture her character and they appear on the granite statue of Edith Cavell that stands at St Martin's Crossroads in London. Numerous statues have been erected in her memory. Her story has been celebrated throughout the years in film, plays, books, postcards, and photographs. Authors have referred to Edith Cavell as "the other Nightingale," "the Florence Nightingale of Belgium," and "the poor man's Nightingale."

Inspiring nurses worldwide, tributes to Edith Cavell were vast and continue today. A beautiful mountain in Jasper National Park, Canada, and the most prominent peak entirely within Alberta was named Mount Edith Cavell in her honor. A glacier in Alaska bears her name. In honor of her valor, an annual memorial service is held on the Sunday nearest to the date of her arrest at the Anglican Church of St. Mary and St. George Jasper, Alberta, Canada.

In 1992, the New South Wales Nurses and Midwives' Association (NSWNMA) established the Edith Cavell Trust Scholarship to support nursing research and nurse education (NSWNMA, n.d.). In memory of Edith Cavell, Australians had raised these monies with the original intent to provide a rest home for nurses returning from World Wars I and II. The focus of the Trust changed in 1992 to a scholarship fund to support nursing students. This scholarship commemorates Edith Cavell and supports students applying for full-time study as registered nurses or midwives.

Edith Cavell was laid to rest at the Norwich Cathedral, just a short distance from her home. In London, there is an exhibit dedicated to her at the London Hospital where she attended school. The street where the hospital is located is named Cavell Street in her honor. In 2015, 100 years after Edith Cavell's death, the U.K. Royal Mint issued a commemorative £5 coin. Edith thought of herself as "just a nurse who did her duty," the duty she advocated for her nurses and her patients (Arthur, 2006, p. 35). She would be humbled by these recognitions.

The story of Edith Cavell *encourages the heart* of many. Her story is one that nurses should celebrate. She made a difference to the nursing profession and the soldiers whose lives she saved. *Modeling the way* for others requires a leader to take risks. Edith had the courage to assume risks by practicing what she believed. It was not simply risk taking. Her actions were based on her personal values and goals for nursing and they always remained at the forefront of her life's career.

Edith Cavell was not born a leader; she had strong character. She embraced strong beliefs that *challenged the process* to make the nursing profession a credible and respectable career in Belgium and to care for others, despite conditions of uncertainty and fear. Edith had an intense desire to succeed in advancing the nursing profession in a time of great peril. She communicated with conviction this higher purpose to *inspire a shared vision* for nursing and humanity.

All nurses can be leaders; leadership can be learned. Every nurse has this potential. Leadership is not about being a hero; "leadership is about relationships, about credibility, and about what you *do*" (Kouzes & Posner, 2012, p. 329). Leadership development is self-development and requires practice with deliberate intention, motivation, desire, and passion to do and be the best.

TIMELINE

- December 4, 1865—Edith Louisa Cavell is born in the English village of Swardeston, in the county of Norfolk on England's east coast; she is the first-born child of Reverend and Louisa Cavell.
- 1882–1884—Attends three different girls' boarding schools in England where she acquires competency in French.
- January 1887—Edith's father finds her a position as a governess in Essex County, south of Norfolk.

- 1889—Travels on holiday to the German province of Bavaria and visits the Free Hospital; Edith donates part of an inheritance to purchase new medical equipment.
- 1890–1895—In her fourth position as a governess, Edith travels to Brussels to work for the François family and their four children.
- Spring 1895—Reverend Cavell becomes ill and Edith returns home to care for him.
- September 3, 1896—At age 30, enters the London Hospital for 4 years of training as a nurse under Matron Eva Lückes.
- Autumn 1897—In her second year as a probationer, Edith is assigned to work in the town of Maidstone during a typhoid fever epidemic.
- 1899—During her third year of nurses' training, Edith attends to patients in their homes as part of London's private nursing staff.
- 1900—In her last year of training, Edith is appointed as a staff nurse in the hospital's Mellish Ward, a men's surgical and accident ward.
- January 1901—Is appointed to her first nursing position as a night superintendent in the St. Pancras Infirmary in London, an infirmary dedicated to serving destitute people of the community.
- 1903—Is appointed as an assistant matron at the Shoreditch Infirmary and stays for 4 years.
- September 1907—At the age of 41, Edith is appointed the first matron of the 'L'École Belge d'Infirmières Diplômées, a training school for nurses, based in the Berkendael Medical Institute in Brussels, Belgium; there are five students.
- 1910—Edith begins a nursing professional journal, *L'infirmiere, documenting good nursing practice and professional standards*; Edith's father, Reverend Cavell dies in June; Jack, a German shepherd mix stray dog, arrives at the school and becomes Edith's close companion.
- 1912—Edith is training nurses for three hospitals, 24 communal schools, and 13 kindergartens; 60 nurses are training under Matron Cavell; at the International Congress of Nurses in Cologne, in the opening address, Dr. Antoine Depage reports the first school of nursing in Belgium to be a success.
- 1914—Edith is giving lectures to both physicians and nurses.
- July 28, 1914—World War I (*The Great War*) begins.
- August 1, 1914—While visiting her mother in Norwich, Edith receives a telegram from a senior nurse at the clinic warning her that war in Belgium seems imminent; Edith returns to Brussels.
- August 13, 1914—Writing as the war correspondent for *Nursing Mirror,* Edith reports on the wounded and the horrors of war.
- August 20, 1914—Brussels becomes an occupied territory of Germany; the clinic is functioning under the International Committee of the Red Cross.
- August 5, 1915—Edith is arrested by local German authorities for aiding the escape of Allied soldiers from Belgium to neutral Holland.

- October 12, 1915—At 2:00 a.m., wearing her nurse's uniform, Edith, aged 49, is executed by two firing squads at a rifle range in Brussels.
- 1916—Mount Edith Cavell and Angel Glacier are named after Edith in Jasper National Park, Alberta, Canada.
- 1917—A rose variety bred in 1917 is named "Miss Edith Cavell."
- April 6, 1917—The United States enters the war.
- November 11, 1918—World War I ends with nine million military and seven million civilians having died as a result of the war.
- March 17, 1919—Edith's body is exhumed and returned to Norfolk, England.
- May 19, 1919—A memorial service is held in Westminster Abbey; Edith is again laid to rest near her birthplace in Norwich.
- 1920—A 40-foot statue of Edith is erected adjacent to Trafalgar Square.
- 1930—Canada issues a postage stamp honoring Mount Edith Cavell (see the beginning of this chapter).
- 1933—A play in three acts, *Nurse Cavell*, is written by C. S. Forester.
- 1945—Costa Rica issues a postage stamp honoring Florence Nightingale and Edith Cavell (at the beginning of this chapter).
- 1992—Establishment of the Edith Cavell Trust by the NSWNMA.
- 2012—The charity NurseAid is renamed Cavell Nurses' Trust to support the United Kingdom's registered nurses, midwives, and health care assistants.
- 2015—Edith is featured on a U.K. commemorative £5 coin issued by the Royal Mint to mark the centenary of the war.

QUESTIONS FOR DISCUSSION

1. Within the context of her time, Edith Louisa Cavell was a leader in nursing education. Examine the challenges that she faced as she tried *encouraging the heart* of nursing students and nurses. How can today's nurse leaders *encourage the heart* of nursing students, nurses, and others?
2. Discuss the values and behaviors that Edith Cavell embraced and exhibited to achieve her goals to advance the nursing profession. How did her values and actions directly and indirectly *encourage the heart of others*?
3. What were some of the internal and external influences on the leadership of Edith Cavell that impacted her ability to create a community for nursing students and nurses?
4. Apply the leadership style that Edith Cavell employed to the current nursing education and practice environments. Today, which of these leadership attributes would a nurse leader be able to transfer to his or her practice of nursing and nursing education?
5. Courage was an essential component of Edith Cavell's leadership. Who are some of today's nurse leaders exhibiting the courage to *challenge the process* in nursing practice and nursing education? How are they accomplishing this?

REFERENCES

Arthur, T. (2006). The life and death of Edith Cavell, English emergency nurse known as "the other Nightingale." *Journal of Emergency Nursing, 32*, 30–35.

Arthur, T. (2011). *Fatal decision: Edith Cavell WWI nurse.* Westport, MA: Beagle Books.

Batten, J. (2007). *Silent in an evil time: The brave war of Edith Cavell.* Toronto, Canada: Tundra Books.

Brown, G. (2007). *Courage: Eight portraits.* London, UK: Bloomsbury Publishing.

Clowes, P. (1996). A fanatically selfless sense of duty drove nurse Edith Cavell to harbor allied soldiers behind German lines. *Military History, 13*(3), 18–20.

Grey, E. (1960). *Friend within the gates: The story of nurse Edith Cavell.* New York, NY: Dell.

Human Rights First. (2014). *Stories from Bahrain's Crackdown: Dr. Rula Al-Saffar.* Retrieved from http://www.humanrightsfirst.org/blog/stories-bahrains-crackdown-dr-rula-al-saffar

Judson, H. (1941). *Edith Cavell.* New York, NY: Macmillan.

Kouzes, J., & Posner, B. (2003). *Encouraging the heart: A leader's guide to rewarding and recognizing others.* San Francisco, CA: Jossey-Bass.

Kouzes, J., & Posner, B. (2012). *The leadership challenge* (5th ed.). San Francisco, CA: Jossey-Bass.

New South Wales Nurses and Midwives' Association (NSWNMA). (n.d.). *The Edith Cavell Trust scholarship information.* Retrieved http://www.nswnma.asn.au/the-edith-cavell-trust-scholarship-information/

Office of the High Commissioner for Human Rights. (1977). *Protocol additional to the Geneva Conventions of 12 August 1949, and relating to the Protection of Victims of Non-International Armed Conflicts (Protocol II).* Retrieved from http://www.ohchr.org/Documents/ProfessionalInterest/protocol2.pdf

Physicians for Human Rights. (n.d.). *The principle of medical neutrality.* Retrieved from http://physiciansforhumanrights.org/issues/persecution-of-health-workers/medical-neutrality/

Shaddox, C. C. (1999). The martyrdom and myth of Edith Cavell. *Connecticut Nursing News, 72*(1), 7–9.

Souhami, D. (2010). *Edith Cavell.* London, UK: Quercus.

Stewart, I. (1941). Nursing preparedness: Some lessons from World War I. *American Journal of Nursing, 4*, 804–815.

Walker, M. (2003). Edith Cavell WWI nurse, hero, martyr. *Journal of Christian Nursing, 20*(4), 38–40.

FURTHER READING

Allen, T. (2014). *Edith Cavell on postcards: Picture postcards from the Great War 1914–1918.* Retrieved from http://www.worldwar1postcards.com/edith-cavell.php

Beck, J. (1916). *The case of Edith Cavell. A study of the rights of non-combatants.* New York, NY: G. P. Putnam's Sons.

Cook, R. (2013). Edith Cavell: "The poor man's Nightingale"? *British Journal of Community Nursing, 18*, 193–195.

Hoehling, A. A. (1957). The story of Edith Cavell. *American Journal of Nursing, 57,* 1320–1322.

Pettinger, T. (2010). *Biography of Edith Cavell.* Oxford, UK. Retrieved from http://www .biographyonline.net/humanitarian/edith-cavell.html

Roth, G., & Fee, E. (2010). A soldier's hero: Edith Cavell (1865–1915). *American Journal of Public Health, 100,* 1865–1866.

Van Maren, J. (2012). *Edith Cavell: The nurse who gave it all.* Retrieved from http://www .unmaskingchoice.ca/blog/2012/03/29/edith-cavell-nurse-who-gave-it-all

PART VII

The Future

Nurses Leading Change: The Time Is Now!

Susan W. Salmond and David Anthony Forrester

The domain of leaders is the future.
—*J. M. Kouzes and B. Z. Posner*

Health care is operating in a bewildering new environment characterized by rapid change with fast-paced innovations occurring in information and medical technologies along with new expectations for better care for individuals, better health for populations, and lower per capita costs (Institute for Healthcare Improvement Triple Aim, 2015). Within this lightning-quick, ever-changing environment, there is great complexity, even greater uncertainty, and tremendous opportunities for nurses to lead change. Just as it was for Florence Nightingale, Clara Barton, and all of the other nurse leaders profiled in this book, nurse leaders of today and tomorrow will have to be visionary, highly intelligent, and politically aware as they address the challenges of a new and rapidly evolving health care system and society. Being an exemplary nurse leader within this new context will require abandoning structures and processes from the current ineffective and fragmented system and shifting our focus from a profit-first industry to a quality-first healing enterprise. We must move to a new vision of a health care system that is universally accessible, coordinated across all points of care, marked by a focus on health and wellness, and the delivery of high-quality, safe care at an affordable price. Accomplishing this daunting task will require nurse leaders to leave behind hierarchical, top-down, command and control styles, common in organized health care. It will require courageous leaders who understand and embrace collaboration, team-based care, partnerships, and an unwavering focus on excellence and the patient experience. These are the skill sets of exemplary nurse leaders and this is the time to find our voice and take an active role in shaping the future of health care. It is time for nursing to lead the revolution and for nurse leaders to be activist agents of change.

Although there is a rich legacy of leadership, political activism, and policy development illustrated by the life stories of the great nurse leaders shared in the preceding chapters, the surprising reality is that few contemporary nurses have moved beyond an internal focus on advancing the professional status of nursing and nursing science to lead and advocate for broad health policy (Mechanic & Reinhard, 2002). Other factors contributing to this scarcity of nurses at the "health care revolution" policy table is the fact that, in spite of the distinguished history of nursing leadership chronicled in this book, the public generally does not view nurses as leaders. Instead of seeing nurses as strategic thinkers who make informed decisions and act independently, nurses have been viewed as "following physicians' orders" and it has been physicians who have been invited to the table. Creating a new future— a preferred future—for health care will require working hand in hand across professions with key stakeholders. The challenge of nurse leaders and other stakeholders will be to articulate a preferred future for health, health care, and society. Nurses, as the largest segment of the U.S. health care workforce, must be key contributors to this dialogue. In order to understand the importance and scope of this change and the need for nurses to take leadership roles, it is important to take a step back and examine the health care environment in which we have been operating.

AN UNSUSTAINABLE U.S. HEALTH SYSTEM: HIGH COST WITHOUT HIGH RETURN IN HEALTH OUTCOMES

Although many Americans believe that the U.S. health care system is one of the best in the world, the reality is something else indeed. An Institute of Medicine (IOM) report, *To Err Is Human: Building a Safer Health System*, released on November 29, 1999, shattered this misconception with the startling news that medical error was the eighth leading cause of death in the United States. In fact, it was estimated that between 44,000 and 98,000 people die each year from preventable medical errors (Kohn, Corrigan, & Donaldson, 2000). A major conclusion of the report was that this was not an issue of practitioner competence; rather, this represented an endemic system problem in which processes to prevent, recognize, and quickly recover from errors was lacking. The follow-up report, *Crossing the Quality Chasm: A New Health System for the 21st Century*, examined these systemic problems and concluded that "between the health care that we now have and the health care that we could have lies not just a gap, but a chasm" (IOM, 2001, p. 1). It reinforced that despite the best intentions of health care professionals, the system failed to reliably deliver efficient, high-quality care with a real focus on the patient. It asserted that improvements could not be achieved within the constraints of the existing system of care and that radical transformation of the health care system was needed. The report called for this revolution to be targeted toward six broad dimensions of health care performance: safety, effectiveness, patient-centeredness, timeliness, efficiency, and equity.

As a world leader in science and technology, we have invested our resources into an acute care model of health, treating highly specialized conditions *after* they have developed. We are known for our excellence in curative services, treating life-threatening emergencies that are acute exacerbations of chronic disease, and many routine health problems that require prompt action (Brownstein, 2014). This "disease care system," the most expensive in the world, spends more than double as much money per capita on health care as the average developed country spends. In 2013, the cost of U.S. health care was $2.9 trillion or 17.4% of our gross national product. Of this amount, approximately "95 cents of every medical care dollar went to treat disease after it had already occurred" (Brownstein, 2014, n.p.). Alarmingly, despite being number one in health care spending, the United States does not have significantly better health outcomes compared to other economically developed countries. In fact, the 2014 Social Progress Index rates the United States as the world's 16th most socially advanced country; however, when examining health and wellness specifically, the U.S. rank drops to 70th among 132 nations (Porter & Stern, 2015). A 2013 IOM report, *U.S. Health in International Perspective: Shorter Lives, Poorer Health*, ranks the United States near last among 17 high-income nations in several categories ranging from infant mortality and low birth weight to life expectancy. Similarly, the Commonwealth Fund analysis ranks the United States last among seven nations in health care and last among 16 developed countries in deaths that potentially could have been prevented by timely access to effective health care (2011). Clearly, U.S. citizens should be expecting a better return on investment than they are receiving.

Equally troublesome are the statistics on efficiency, variability, and waste. The United States scores "53 out of 100 on measures that gauge the level of inappropriate, wasteful, or fragmented care; avoidable hospitalizations; variation in quality and costs; administrative costs; and use of information technology" (The Commonwealth Fund, 2011, p. 9). The IOM report, *Best Care at Lower Cost: The Path to Continuously Learning Healthcare in America* (2012), highlights that 30 cents of every dollar spent on medical care in America is wasted, amounting to $750 billion annually. Components of this waste include inefficient delivery of care, excessive administrative costs, unnecessary services, inflated prices, prevention failures, and outright fraud. Moreover, it is estimated that between 40% and 78% of the medical testing, treatments, and procedures received are of *no* benefit—or are actually harmful (Prasad & Cifu, 2011).

The Dartmouth Atlas of Health Care clearly documents the variations in practice patterns/care, health care costs, and patient outcomes by individual practitioners, geographical regions, type of insurance coverage, and type of condition (http://www.dartmouthatlas.org/). Wennberg's (1984) classic article, "Dealing With Medical Practice Variations," showed that variations in children who underwent a tonsillectomy in the state of Vermont varied from a low of 8% in one community to a high of nearly 70% in another. In Maine, the variation in rates of women who underwent a hysterectomy by age 70 ranged from a low of 20% in one market to a high of 70% in another. These variations remain after adjustments are made for individuals' age, sex, income, race, and health status. And of critical importance, there is little to no correlation between spending and health care quality. Just as incomprehensible is how a cholesterol test in Dallas, Texas, could range from $15 to $343 for the *same* test. Making it more egregious is that the highest prices are typically reserved for those least able to pay, such as the medically uninsured (Skinner, Fisher, & Weinstein, 2014). The Blue Cross Blue Shield study of cost variations for knee and hip replacement surgeries in the United States (2015) found similar cost variability. Using Dallas to illustrate market variations, a knee replacement could cost between $16,772 and $61,585 (267% cost variation), depending on the hospital.

The burden of health care cost is undeniably being felt by us all. The unrelenting increase in health insurance premiums has resulted in employers cutting health coverage and consumers being faced with high-deductible plans. Thirty-three percent of Americans choose not to seek care because of the cost. Up to 35% of Americans report trouble paying their medical bills and a major cause of bankruptcy is linked with an inability to pay medical bills as a result of being uninsured or underinsured (Treas, 2010). Adding to the inequity of the situation is that medical debt impacts the poor and uninsured more severely because they are charged the full inflated price, whereas those with coverage have their costs radically reduced through prenegotiated lowered rates.

RE-VISIONING HEALTH CARE

Enter Health Care Reform

Continued skyrocketing of health care costs, less-than-impressive health status of the American people, safety and quality issues within the health care system, and nearly 50 million Americans uninsured and 40 million underinsured ushered in the *Patient Protection and Affordable Care Act* of 2010. This act, along with the *Health Care and Education Affordability Reconciliation Act*, are collectively referred to as the *Affordable Care Act* (ACA). This is certainly the most significant health care reform since Medicare/Medicaid in 1965. The ACA is more than insurance reform; it is health care reform with an intense focus on quality. A central aim of the ACA is to increase the value in health care by achieving quality while lowering health care costs and expanding access. To achieve this, new payment models, care models, technology, and other tools that will positively impact quality and reduce unnecessary spending are being introduced. The ACA has tasked the Centers for Medicare & Medicaid Services (CMS) to lead this transformation in strengthening and improving the nation's health care system to provide access to high-quality care and improved health at lower costs (CMS, 2013).

The Shift From Volume- to Value-Based Reimbursement

Historically, the U.S. health care system has used a fee-for-service payment model providing reimbursement for specific, individual services provided to patients. Consequently, there is an incentive to increase the number of high-cost services provided during each visit as well as the number of visits. There is no accountability for inadequate quality and little enticement to encourage "low-cost, high-values services, such as preventive care, coordination of care, or patient education" (Calsyn & Lee, 2012, p. 1). In contrast, the ACA ties payment reform to quality measures. Instead of asking, "How much did you do?" value-based reimbursement asks, "How well did the patient do?" (Berwick, 2011). A major goal for CMS is to provide better care (high-quality, coordinated, effective, efficient care) at lower costs and a key initiative to accomplishing this is to demand the move from volume-based care and payment toward patient-centered quality health care services that are accountable for outcomes achieved. Value-based reimbursement programs, such as nonpayment programs for "never events," bundled payments, the hospital value-based performance program, and the hospital readmissions reduction initiative are driving this change.

Although never events, which are serious adverse events that are largely preventable and should never happen in health care, were introduced prior to the ACA, the act prohibits federal payments to states for any amounts expended for providing medical assistance for health care-acquired conditions. The final rule published by CMS requires that states implement nonpayment polices for "provider-preventable conditions" (PPCs), including "health care-acquired conditions" (HCACs, such as stage III and IV pressure ulcers, falls, and trauma) and "other provider-preventable conditions" (OPPCs). OPPCs are intended for conditions more likely to occur in settings outside hospitals, such as outpatient or office-based surgery centers, skilled nursing facilities, and ambulatory/office practice settings (Haas, n.d.). Never events are publically reported and the health care facility is accountable for correcting systemic problems that contribute to the events (Haas, n.d.).

Value-based reimbursement approaches include bundled payments for care improvement. Rather than paying "per unit of care delivered," CMS will be paying for a "set of services"—the providers and/or health care facilities will receive payment for the full scope of treatment and care for a given condition (Porter & Lee, 2013). For an acute condition, such as a joint replacement, the bundled payment would cover the full care cycle, beginning prior to surgery and extending throughout recovery anywhere from 3 to 12 months after surgery. Bundled payment for primary or preventive care would be for a designated period of time (e.g., 1 year) for a specific population of patients (e.g., those with congestive heart failure). In this model, the provider receives a discounted payment, presets expected metrics, and assumes some of the financial risk for the cost of services. This incentivizes the provider teams to coordinate care, redesign care around patient need, and to innovate for maximal efficiency. As the providers' reimbursement amounts would depend, in part, on meeting quality and patient experience measures, the entire team of providers will be focused on redesigning care around patient need, assuring coordination of care, and improving quality.

The Hospital Value-Based Performance Program is another compelling program designed to improve quality, reduce inappropriate care, and promote better health outcomes and patient experiences during hospital stays (CMS, 2015). This is achieved through a system of incentive payments or fiscal penalties above or below their diagnosis-related group (DRG)–based operating payments. Fiscal year 2016 value-based performance scores will be calculated according to four weighted domain scores. The highest weighted domain, at 40%, is "outcome measures," which include data on inpatient safety indicators (e.g., 30-day mortality for acute myocardial infarction, heart failure, and pneumonia), and "patient safety indicators," including a composite score based on the incidence of eight potential complications, and specific patient safety indicators for the occurrence of central line-associated bloodstream infections, catheter-associated bloodstream infections, and surgical site infections for surgical procedures of the colon and abdominal hysterectomy. The domain of "patient experience of care," weighted at 25%, captures the patient's perspective of hospital care as measured by the Hospital Consumer Assessment of Healthcare Providers and Systems (HCAHPS) survey. The survey items are based on what patients perceive to be important to their satisfaction with the hospital experience and include questions rating communication with nurses and doctors, responsiveness of hospital staff, communication about medications, and discharge information. Also weighted at 25% is the domain "efficiency," defined as Medicare spending per beneficiary. The final domain, weighted at 10%, is "process of care measures." These are quality-of-care measures used to gauge whether practice is based on evidence and reflects guidelines or standards of care. Twelve process measures are tracked within this domain. Examples of process measures include blood cultures performed in the emergency department prior to initial antibiotic received in the hospital and fibrinolytic therapy received within 30 minutes of hospital arrival.

As CMS identifies ongoing fiscal and quality issues, it has the authority under the ACA to set regulations aimed at controlling or minimizing the problems and imposing penalties for health care organizations not meeting the set standards. An example of this is the focus on preventing hospital readmissions. As 25% of Medicare patients were found to be readmitted within 30 days, there was a concerted effort to set a Hospital Readmissions Reduction Program, which required CMS to reduce payments to "inpatient prospective payment system" (IPPS) hospitals with excess readmissions, effective for discharges beginning on October 1, 2012 (Boccuti & Casillas, 2015).

A new wave of change will accompany the implementation of the Improving Medicare Post-Acute Care Transformation Act of 2014 (the IMPACT Act) passed in September of 2014. This requires long-term care hospitals, skilled nursing facilities, home health agencies, and inpatient rehabilitation facilities to begin the reporting process of standardized patient assessment data with regard to quality measures and resource use. Similar to hospital reporting, this data will be transparent and available to consumers. Examples of the standardized domains include data on skin integrity, functional and cognitive status, medication reconciliation, falls, discharge to community, and preventable hospital readmission rates. The Act requires that CMS develop and implement quality measures around five of these quality-measure domains using standardized assessment data.

New Care Models to Improve Quality and Reduce Cost

A second major goal for CMS is to address prevention and population health. The expectation is that Americans will be healthier and their care less costly owing to their improved health status, a direct consequence of their use of preventive benefits and necessary health services (CMS, 2013). This goal will be achieved through a shift in focus from care paid and provided for a single individual for a single episode of care at single points in time to paying and providing care for discrete or defined populations. Population health is defined as the health outcomes of a group of individuals, including the distribution of such outcomes within the group (Kindig & Stoddart, 2003). These groups are often geographic populations, such as nations or communities, but can also be other groups, such as employees, members of a health plan, ethnic groups, those with a common set of needs, such as disabled persons, older adults, those with multiple chronic illnesses, or any other defined group. Population health management shifts resources from acute care or "after illness or disease has occurred" to "up-front things such as primary and preventive care and public health services—that have a much bigger effect on the overall health of the population" (Brownstein, 2014, n.p.). It is more than sick care; rather it systematically addresses the preventive and chronic care needs of every patient in the population. Its goal is to keep the people within the population group as healthy as possible, minimizing the need for expensive interventions such as emergency department visits, hospitalizations, imaging tests, and procedures. New models of care, such as patient-centered medical homes (PCMHs) and accountable care organizations (ACOs), are being structured to achieve the quality and fiscal goals associated with population health.

PCMH, a designation awarded by the National Committee for Quality Assurance, is aimed at transforming the organization of primary care with a greater emphasis on preventive care, wellness, care coordination, patient education, and communication. Similar to other programs, it is expected to prevent unnecessary hospitalizations and lead to higher quality, lower costs, and improved patient and provider experience of care. The PCMH is fundamental to the care within another program, the ACOs.

ACOs aim to eliminate or minimize the fragmentation in the health care system. In this model, a network of groups of health care providers (e.g., primary care providers, therapists, specialists) and hospitals share responsibility for coordinating lower cost, higher quality care for a group of patients. Through this integration of acute care with preventive and primary care, there is a coordinated health care system that fully encompasses all essential aspects of health care delivery and is likely to have a much bigger effect on the overall health of the population. For an ACO to share in any savings created, it must demonstrate compliance with 65 processes and outcome quality performance measures spanning five quality domains: patient experience of care, care coordination, patient safety, preventive health, and at-risk population/frail elderly health. Several of the proposed quality measures align with those used in other CMS quality programs, such as the Physician Quality Reporting System (PQRS), a quality-reporting program for professionals and group practices to report information on the quality of care to Medicare, the Hospital Inpatient Quality Reporting System, and the electronic health record (EHR) incentive program.

New Care Settings and New Technologies

The 21st century has brought a fundamental shift in where and how patients access health care services. In sharp contrast to the institutionalized health care systems advocated and innovated by Florence Nightingale and Dorothea Dix, health care is now moving well beyond the walls of hospitals and primary care providers' offices into communities and homes (Salmond & Atkins, 2015). This movement of health care from large institutions into the community would probably be very much embraced by Mother Mary Aikenhead, who in the early 19th century advocated for thoughtful, personalized, individual care for the sick and dying in their homes. Likely too, two activist agents of change in the early 20th century, Mary Breckenridge, an early advocate for rural health care and women's health, and Lillian Wald, a pioneer in public health, would understand the timing of and the need for this evolutionary change.

Payment incentives and new models of care are being designed to prevent hospital admissions and readmissions and to move care out of expensive acute care settings into ambulatory care, community, and home settings. Consequently, it is predicted that outpatient volume will grow 17% over the next 5 years, whereas inpatient discharges may decrease 3% (Herman, 2013). With this swing in care delivery site, the hospital of the near future will become reserved for the sickest of the sick. It will be like a large intensive care unit and a site for acute trauma care and highly complex service lines. Ambulatory or outpatient care will become the hub for most service across the continuum of care in a variety of settings. Settings would include, but would not be limited to, hospital-based clinics/centers, solo or group medical practices, ambulatory surgery and diagnostic procedure centers, telehealth service environments, university and community hospital clinics, military and veterans administration settings, nurse-managed clinics, managed care organizations, colleges and educational institutions, freestanding community facilities, care coordination organizations, and patient homes (American Academy of Ambulatory Care Nursing, 2011).

The move in core volume from inpatient to outpatient or postacute care necessitates an adjustment in "culture, mindset, organizational structure, service distribution, care management, resource allocation, technology support, partner relationships, and payor contracting" (Remington, 2014, p. 4). It will necessitate retooling of staff with the knowledge, skills, and attitudes required to facilitate patient engagement, manage chronic conditions, prevent ambulatory care-sensitive admissions (e.g., admissions related to diabetes and hypertension), manage populations longitudinally to facilitate wellness and prevention, provide effective care coordination, expand care/ case management, and integrate information technology driven by data analytics (Remington, 2014).

"The unprecedented spread of mobile technologies, as well as advancements in their innovative application to address health priorities" (World Health Organization, 2011, p. 5) has evolved into a new field of eHealth, known as mHealth and do-it-yourself medicine (DIYM). It is likely that mHealth will be a transformative force in the shift to an engaged, population-based approach to health care. Medical and public health practice is supported by mHealth through the use of mobile devices, such as mobile phones and their associated apps, patient-monitoring devices, personal digital assistants (PDAs), and other wireless devices. With the increasing availability and scope of apps and mobile devices to track health and illness metrics, greater self-regulation is achieved and the setting of care becomes a virtual house call rather than a hospital or primary care provider visit. The potential to change when, where, and how health care is provided is made possible by mHealth, which ensures that important social, behavioral, and environmental data are used to understand the determinants of health and to improve health outcomes.

A NEW CONTEXT: THE TIME IS NOW FOR NURSING AND NURSE LEADERS

Although the need for change has not been acknowledged by everyone in health care, the reality is that change is already happening. In fact, as such historic nurse leaders as Margaret Sanger clearly recognized, change is an inevitability, and it is well worth leading by *challenging the process*—even when this may involve breaking some rules. Today, CMS programs that pay for quality, not quantity, have galvanized people into action in challenging old processes, and change has begun. This offers many exciting opportunities in achieving the goals of transformation and requires a strong nursing voice—it is the time for nursing and nurse leaders! The context of factors driving this change have created the perfect storm for nursing and nurse leaders, a perfect storm in which the purpose and values fundamental to nursing align with the purpose and values of the transformation mandate. Nursing is being called to the table and nurse leaders are responding.

The change being called for is *not* for more interventions or treatments, which are the domain of medicine. It *is* for support with managing people's human responses to illness, to removing their barriers to health, and coordinating their health and illness so they can experience maximal wellness and quality of life; this is the domain of nursing. This is the time for nursing and nurse leaders! We need new, visionary, innovative nurse leaders in the tradition of Florence Nightingale to *model the way* and lead change.

The American Nurses Association (ANA) *Social Policy Statement: The Essence of the Profession* defines the practice of nursing as the protection, promotion, and optimization of health and abilities; prevention of illness and injury; alleviation of suffering through the diagnosis and treatment of human response, and advocacy in the care of individuals, families, communities, and populations (ANA, 2010). The *Code of Ethics for Nurses with Interpretive Statements* affirms that nurses act to change those aspects of social structures that detract from health and well-being (ANA, 2015). This is what is being called for in health care reform. Both the fundamental definition of nursing and the ethical imperatives demanded in the *Code of Ethics* clearly align with the mandates for health care reform. This is the time for nursing and nurse leaders! We need new, passionate, dynamic nurse leaders like Mother Mary Aikenhead and Clara Barton to *inspire a shared vision* of nursing and health care—nurse leaders capable of leading change so that we achieve our preferred future for nursing, health, health care, and society.

In pursuit of reform, we must make sure that the change is not simply to "rearrange the deck chairs on a sinking ship" in order to preserve the status quo. The revolution requires changing the power structure within organized health care from a physician-dominated system to a collaborative system that draws on the expertise of the entire team. It necessitates leaders with strong collaboration skills. This is the strength of nursing. Nursing has a core value of collaboration, recognizing that it is essential to address the complexity of health care issues of individual patients and the public effectively. This is the time for nursing and nurse leaders! We need new, committed, courageous nurse leaders like Margaret Sanger, Sister Elizabeth Kenny, and Clara Maass to *challenge the process* and lead in successfully achieving the changes that are needed.

Achieving the mandate to have coordinated, affordable, quality care that is safe, accessible to all, patient centered, evidence based, and leading to improved outcomes requires a strong nursing voice. Nurses are at the center of patient care. "Nurses are the professionals most likely to intercept errors and prevent harm to patients" (Hughes, 2008, p. iii). Nursing practice covers a broad continuum from acute restorative care to health promotion to disease prevention, to coordination of care, to cure when possible, and to palliative care when cure is not possible (IOM, 2012, p. 4). Nursing competencies of care management, coordination, and patient education are practiced across the continuum of settings from acute care, to home care, to communities, and are vital to the reenvisioned patient-centered, coordinated health care system. This breadth of knowledge and experience is the domain of nursing. This is the time for nursing and nurse leaders! We need new, energetic, determined nurse leaders like Dorothea Dix, Lillian Wald, and Mary Breckinridge to empower and *enable others to act* and strategically participate in the changes that are needed to improve nursing and health care.

The mandate calls for an accessible, affordable system with stronger primary care services that delivers wellness and prevention care and moves from care of individuals to care of populations. As described in this book, nursing's legacy is rich with leaders in public health nursing. Public health nurses partner with the community to promote health and health equity. Advanced practice registered nurses (APRNs) serve as primary care providers and are at the forefront of providing preventative care to the public. Many APRNs are now prepared with doctor of nursing practice (DNP) degrees and have an expanded skill set to provide leadership in community health centers, serve on interdisciplinary teams, and advocate for and direct future health and social policy initiatives. This is the time for nursing and nurse leaders! We need new, committed, even heroic nurse leaders like Edith Cavell to *encourage the heart* as they lead change in nursing, health care, and society.

The power to change conditions in order to deliver better care does not rest solely with nursing but requires collaboration and interaction with other health professional, business, social, and policy groups. What makes this a unique time for nursing is that barriers that have limited nurses' ability to generate widespread transformation are being addressed through a remarkable blueprint outlining how, by working together, we can strengthen our capacity in nursing so we are prepared to lead, partner, and assume roles in the transformed health care system.

THE FUTURE OF NURSING: LEADING CHANGE, ADVANCING HEALTH

In 2008, the Robert Wood Johnson Foundation (RWJF) and the IOM worked together on an extraordinary collaborative initiative to advance nursing and health care reform. Their work and the action that has followed is a shining exemplar of process leadership as described by Kouzes and Posner (2012). Their actions were grounded in a *shared vision and shared values* of health and quality health care for all Americans along with the belief that "high-quality care cannot be achieved without exceptional nursing care and leadership" and that "nurses have key roles to play as team members and leaders for a reformed and better-integrated, patient-centered health care system" (IOM, 2012, pp. ix, xii). These values were articulated and apparent and guided their actions and willingness to confront difficult issues and make recommendations, some of which would be upsetting to the status quo of traditional nursing and medicine. Their landmark report, *The Future of Nursing: Leading Change, Advancing Health* (IOM, 2011), is a compelling guide for change and leadership in nursing.

The IOM committee, a panel of distinguished leaders across a variety of disciplines, asked purposeful questions in their examination of the role of nursing in society within the context of health care reform. They asked, "What roles can nursing assume to address the increasing demand for safe, high-quality, and effective health care services?" (IOM, 2011, p. xi) and what was needed to strengthen the nursing workforce to be partners and lead in a transformed health care system. In the process of this work, the committee

> envisioned a future system that makes quality care accessible to the diverse populations of the United States, intentionally promotes wellness and disease prevention, reliably improves health outcomes, and provides compassionate care across the lifespan. In this future, primary care and prevention are central drivers of the healthcare system. Inter-professional collaboration and coordination are the norm. Payment for health care services rewards value, not volume of services, and quality of care is provided at a price that is affordable for both individuals and society. (IOM, 2011, p. 2)

The report provided rich examples of how nursing and nurse leaders are and can continue making an impact toward reform and how the work of nursing is inextricably intertwined with the work of health care reform. To reach the vision for a strengthened nursing workforce that can assume significant roles in the transformed health system, four key messages (domains) and eight recommendations with actions that could be taken in both the practice and policy arenas at local, state, and national levels were described (Table 12.1). To make this vision a reality, the report and its diverse and prestigious leadership called on all nurses, as well as other leaders and health care stakeholders, to find their common commitment to a reformed health care system and to take action on the recommendations in these four key areas. This was a vision that was inspiring. This was a vision that resonated with the nursing committee, and the report enabled people to act by providing a blueprint for action.

TABLE 12.1 • Nurses of the Future: Four Key Messages (Domains) and Eight Recommendations

Domains	Recommendations
1. Nurses should practice to the full extent of their education and training.	1. Remove scope-of-practice barriers. 2. Expand opportunities for nurses to lead and diffuse collaborative improvement efforts.
2. Nurses should achieve higher levels of education and training through an improved education system that promotes seamless academic progression.	3. Implement nurse residency programs. 4. Increase the proportion of nurses with a baccalaureate degree to 80% by 2020. 5. Double the number of nurses with a doctorate by 2020. 6. Ensure that nurses engage in lifelong learning.
3. Nurses should be full partners, with physicians and other health professionals, in redesigning health care in the United States.	7. Prepare and enable nurses to lead change to advance health.
4. Effective workforce planning and policy making require better data collection and an improved information infrastructure.	8. Build an infrastructure for the collection and analysis of interprofessional health care workforce data.

Source: Institute of Medicine (2011).

RWJF support did not end with the publication of the report. RWJF committed to making the report actionable and, under the leadership of senior nursing advisor Susan Hassmiller (who wrote the foreword for this book), partnered with the Center to Champion Nursing in America (CCNA), an initiative of the AARP, and launched the Campaign for Action. This campaign has brought together leaders in each state and the District of Columbia to build capacity and operationalize the recommendations from the report in their own states. It has brought about an unprecedented level of action by nurses in partnership with a wide range of health care providers; consumer advocates; policy makers; and business, academic, and philanthropic leaders. It has truly *enabled others to act*. The groundswell of activity from action coalitions and nursing organization task forces have been recognized and celebrated. The RWJF publications *Charting Nursing's Future* (RWJF, 2011) and the *Interdisciplinary Nursing Quality Research Initiative* (INQRI; RWJF, 2013) provide stories of success and research evidence demonstrating how nurses' practices, processes, and work environments impact quality patient care.

The exciting outcome is that the report has not been a tome sitting on a bookshelf accumulating dust. It has become the rallying cry for nurses, nurse leaders, and nursing groups to align, unite under their shared value of nursing and its contribution to patient-centered care and health, and to take action. At no other time in nursing's history has there been such a concerted effort of action. Nurse leaders are responding to the challenge, and the process of *modeling the way, inspiring a shared vision, challenging the process, enabling others to act,* and *encouraging the heart* is happening over and over again all across the country and the momentum continues to grow. The words of the report are being transformed into meaningful action and change is happening! Nurses have found their voice. They are becoming involved and are partners and leaders in the revolution.

PREPARING NURSE LEADERS FOR A NEW FUTURE

Nurses are at the policy table like never before and there is widespread recognition that if we are to meet the goals of a reformed health care system, then we will need a strong nursing workforce prepared to take on new ways of thinking and new roles. It is the time for all nurses to pick up the gauntlet and enact their professional responsibility to lead change in those aspects of organizational and social structures that detract from achieving quality care and health and well-being. Imagine . . . three million nurses from the bedside to the boardroom truly accepting accountability for being full partners in transforming the health care system, pushing beyond traditional structures and processes, and assuming accountability for quality. Nursing is being turned to for our knowledge and wisdom about nursing and patient care. It is time for passionate nurse leaders who will push the limits, envision a new future, and truly believe that there is nothing that can't be done.

New knowledge and skills and new ways of thinking will be needed. Nurses must reflect on what their own leadership development needs are while planning for developing the current health care workforce as well as the future workforce.

From the start, we must shift our paradigm of what it means to provide care. We must move beyond an episodic perspective and embrace ownership for the patient across the continuum of care while assuming accountability for safe transitions. We must reach outside of the confines of a single institution and form collaborative partnerships to improve health care across the continuum and to build communities that support health and well-being. We must cease practicing from a paternalistic, authority-based approach and actively engage patients and families and caregivers as full partners. We must have a consistent goal of achieving maximal health and functional status and must use outcomes as a measure of effectiveness, both at the individual patient level and at the population level. We must meet patients where they are and find out what matters to them, and they must be actively engaged so they, in time, become able to capably and confidently manage their care and achieve maximum levels of health and well-being. We must assume accountability for assuring safety and quality and take proactive measures to change the status quo that prevents excellence from being the norm. We must lead and function with exquisite teamwork.

In the tradition of Florence Nightingale and Clara Barton, nurse leaders of today and tomorrow can begin this process by creating a sense of understanding, urgency, and excitement. Nurse leaders must make sure everyone truly understands what is happening in health care with value-based reimbursement and growing demands for quality outcomes. With a sense of what is driving change, nurse leaders must continuously and consistently articulate the opportunities for nursing and the critical need for nursing knowledge in order to achieve quality outcomes. As Lillian Wald and Mary Breckinridge did decades ago, nurse leaders today must create excitement for the challenges that are before us and strive for an infrastructure in which nurses are expected—and supported within their roles—to contribute to improving health care quality and outcomes. We must celebrate movement toward quality and change. We must establish learning communities to create greater understanding and expertise in care coordination, motivational interviewing, self-management, team building, and leadership skills. These skills are needed across all settings of care but will be increasingly important in the ambulatory and community environments. It is in these settings that future health care will be provided and new opportunities for nurses in the roles of transitional and care coordinators and health coaches will exist. We must strive for transparency so that all team members have access to and understand the data on organization-, unit-, and even individual-level outcomes. With transparency and understanding, holding others accountable for outcomes is possible. We must activate highly effective interdisciplinary teams across the continuum of care to address barriers and facilitators to quality outcomes and form partnerships to make necessary changes. We need to make sure that these teams include patient and family representatives.

It has been easy to blame the system for problems in health care, but we must recognize that we *are* the system. The historic nurse leaders whose stories have been told throughout this book—Nightingale, Aikenhead, Barton, Sanger, Kenny, Maass, Dix, Wald, Breckinridge, and Cavell—never simply accepted the status quo—nor can we. The legacy of these exemplary nurse leaders inspires us to become activist agents of change. It is in the tradition of these historic nurse leaders that we recognize that the time has come for nursing, at the heart of patient care, to take the lead in the revolution to making health care more patient centered and quality driven. All nurses can and must be involved as activist agents of change. If all practicing nurses were given the expectation that they must be involved in at least one project to improve the experience and quality of care, the results would be phenomenal. As the life stories of these distinguished nurse leaders of the past teach us, the time for nursing and nurse leaders has always been now. There has been and will always be a need for nurses to lead change in nursing, health, health care, and society. Just as nurse leaders before us clearly understood, we must also recognize that the future is now.

QUESTIONS FOR DISCUSSION

1. Make a list of health-related issues that appear in your local news and in the international news. What health issues are people in your community and the people of the world concerned about? Share your thoughts about how you, as a nurse leader, might lead change regarding policy relevant to some of these issues. Emphasize the way in which research evidence can inform future policy making in these areas.
2. Share a few of your personal career goals. What position would you like to hold 10 to 15 years from now? What types of offices would you like to hold? What awards would you like to have received? What honors would you like to have had bestowed upon you? What articles/books would you have liked to publish? What would you like to be "known for" in nursing? Think big!
3. In the future, what will others say about your impact as a nurse leader on the nursing profession, health care, and society?

REFERENCES

American Academy of Ambulatory Care Nursing. (2011). *What is ambulatory care nursing? American Academy of Ambulatory Care Nursing, Viewpoint.* Retrieved from https://www.aaacn.org/what-ambulatory-care-nursing

American Nurses Association. (2010). *Nursing's social policy statement: The essence of the profession.* Silver Spring, MD: Author.

American Nurses Association. (2015). *Code of ethics for nurses with interpretive statements.* Silver Spring, MD: Author.

Berwick, D. (2011). Improving the rules for hospital participation in Medicare and Medicaid. *Journal of the American Medical Association, 306*(20), 2256–2257.

Blue Cross Blue Shield. (2015). *A study of cost variations for knee and hip replacement surgeries in the U.S. The Health of America Report.* Retrieved from http://www.bcbs.com/healthofamerica/BCBS_BHI_Report-Jan-_21_Final.pdf

Boccuti, C., & Casillas, G. (2015). *Aiming for fewer hospital U-turns: The Medicare hospital readmission reduction program. Jan 29, 2015.* The Kaiser Family Foundation Issues Briefing. Retrieved from http://kff.org/medicare/issue-brief/aiming-for-fewer-hospital-u-turns-the-medicare-hospital-readmission-reduction-program

Brownstein, R. (2014, March). U.S. health care is the best! And the worst. *National Journal Magazine.* Retrieved from http://www.nationaljournal.com/next-america/health/u-s-health-care-is-the-best-and-the-worst-20140313

Calsyn, M., & Lee, E. O. (2012). *Alternatives to fee-for-service payments in health care. Center for American progress.* Retrieved from https://www.americanprogress.org/wp-content/uploads/2012/09/FeeforService-1.pdf

Centers for Medicare & Medicaid Services (CMS). (2013). *CMS strategy: The road forward 2013–2017.* Retrieved from http://www.cms.gov/About-CMS/Agency-Information/CMS-Strategy/Downloads/CMS-Strategy.pdf

Centers for Medicare & Medicaid Services. (2015). *Better care, smarter spending, healthier people: Improving our health care delivery system.* Retrieved from http://www.cms.gov/Newsroom/MediaReleaseDatabase/Fact-sheets/2015-Fact-sheets-items/2015-01-26.html

The Commonwealth Fund. (2011, October). *Why not the best? Results from the national score card on U.S. health system performance.* New York, NY: Author.

Haas, S. A. (n.d.). *Prevention and early detection of "never events" within ambulatory settings to enhance quality and safety and prevent financial losses. American Academy of Ambulatory Care Nursing, Viewpoint.* Retrieved from https://www.aaacn.org/prevention-and-early-detection-never-events-within-ambulatory-settings-enhance-quality-and-safety

Herman, B. (2013, November). Chuck Lauer: The future of healthcare demands proactive leaders. *Becker's Hospital Review.* Retrieved June 30, 2015, from http://www.beckershospitalreview.com/hospital-management-administration/chuck-lauer-the-future-of-healthcare-demands-proactive-leaders.html

Hughes, R. G. (Ed.). (2008). *Patient safety and quality: An evidence-based handbook for nurses.* (Prepared with support from the Robert Wood Johnson Foundation). AHRQ Publication No. 08-0043. Rockville, MD: Agency for Healthcare Research and Quality.

Institute for Healthcare Improvement (IHI). (2015). *IHI triple aim initiative.* Retrieved June 30, 2015, from http://www.ihi.org/Engage/Initiatives/TripleAim/Pages/default.aspx

Institute of Medicine. (2001). *Crossing the quality chasm: A new health system for the 21st century.* Washington, DC: National Academies Press.

Institute of Medicine. (2011). *The future of nursing: Leading change, advancing health.* Washington, DC: National Academies Press.

Institute of Medicine. (2012). *Best care at lower cost: The path to continuously learning health care in America.* Washington, DC: National Academies Press.

Institute of Medicine. (2013). *U.S. health in international perspective: Shorter lives, poorer health.* Washington, DC: National Academies Press.

Kindig, D., & Stoddart, G. (2003). What is population health? *American Journal of Public Health, 93*(3), 380–383.

Kohn, L. T., Corrigan, J., & Donaldson, M. S. (2000). *To err is human: Building a safer health system.* Washington, DC: National Academies Press.

Kouzes, J. M., & Posner, B. Z. (2012). *The leadership challenge* (5th ed.). San Francisco, CA: Jossey-Bass.

Mechanic, D., & Reinhard, S. C. (2002). Contributions of nurses to health policy: Challenges and opportunities. *Nursing and Health Policy Review, 1*(1), 7–15.

Porter, M. E., & Lee, T. H. (2013, October). The strategy that will fix health care. *Harvard Business Review.* Retrieved from https://hbr.org/2013/10/the-strategy-that-will-fix-health-care

Porter, M. E., & Stern, S. (2015). *Social progress index 2015.* Washington, DC: Social Progress Imperative.

Prasad, V., & Cifu, A. (2011). Medical reversal: Why we must raise the bar before adopting new technologies. *Yale Journal of Biology and Medicine, 84*(4), 471–478.

Remington, L. (2014, July/August). New value equations between acute and post-acute stakeholders: The economic, financial and clinical impact of five disruptive trends. *Remington Report.* Retrieved from http://remingtonreport.com/images/Value_Equation_ja14.pdf

Robert Wood Johnson Foundation. (2011). *Charting nursing's future part I*. Princeton, NJ: Author. Retrieved from http://www.rwjf.org/en/about-rwjf/newsroom/series/charting-nursings-future.html

Robert Wood Johnson Foundation. (2013). *The Interdisciplinary Nursing Quality Research Initiative* (INQRI). Retrieved from http://www.rwjf.org/en/library/research/2013/04/the-interdisciplinary-nursing-quality-research-initiative.html

Salmond, S. W., & Atkins, R. (2015, May 23). Taking steps to keep up with nursing's changing role in health care. *Star-Ledger*. Retrieved from http://www.nj.com/opinion/index.ssf/2015/05/taking_steps_to_keep_up_with_nursings_changing_rol.html

Skinner, J., Fisher, E., & Weinstein, J. (2014, August 26). *The 125 percent solution: Fixing variations in health care prices* [Health Affairs blog]. Retrieved from http://healthaffairs.org/blog/2014/08/26/the-125-percent-solution-fixing-variations-in-health-care-prices/

Treas, J. (2010). The great American recessions: Sociologic insights on blame and pain. *Sociologic Perspectives, 53*(1), 3–18.

Wennberg, J. E. (1984). Dealing with medical practice variations: A proposal for action. *Health Affairs, 3*(2), 6–32.

World Health Organization (WHO). (2011). mHealth: New horizons for health through mobile technologies. In *Global observatory for ehealth series* (Vol. 3). Geneva, Switzerland: Author. Retrieved from http://whqlibdoc.who.int/publications/2011/9789241564250_eng.pdf

FURTHER READING

Dartmouth Atlas of Health Care. (2015). *Understanding of the efficiency and effectiveness of the health care system*. Retrieved from http://www.dartmouthatlas.org/

Lee, T. H., & Cosgrove, T. (2014). Engaging doctors in the health care revolution. *Harvard Business Review, 92*(6), 104–111, 138. Retrieved from https://hbr.org/2014/06/engaging-doctors-in-the-health-care-revolution

Index

accountable care organizations (ACOs), 275–276
Act for the Suppression of Trade in, and Circulation of, Obscene Literature and Articles of Immoral Use, 108
Advanced practice registered nurses (APRNs), 279
Affordable Care Act (ACA), 272–273
Aikenhead, Mary
  canonization, 66
  childhood
    Catholicism, 59
    family business and finances, 59–60
    Mammy Rorke's nursing care, 58–59
    parents, 58
  global legacy, 65–66
  health problems, 65
  hospice care, 64–65
  of hospitals and nursing, 63–64
  initiated hospice care, 10
  Irish Sisters of Charity, 62–63
  as a novitiate, 60
  visions and dreams, 60–62
American Civil War, 189–191
American Committee for Devastated France (CARD), 230, 231
American Moral Tales, for Young Persons, 180
American Nurses Association (ANA), 150, 278
American Public Health Association (APHA), 158
American Society of Superintendents of Training Schools for Nurses, 46
Antislavery movement, 73
Australian Army Nursing Service, 130

Barton, Clara
  antislavery movement, 73
  belief system, 72
  Civil War service
    Battle of Antietam, 74
    Battle of Cedar Mountain, 75
    Battle of Chantilly, 75
    Battle of Fredericksburg, 75
    Battle of Harpers Ferry, 75
    Bureau of Correspondence for Friends of Paroled Prisoners, 76
    humanitarianism, 75–76
    lecture circuit, 77
    Massachusetts Sixth Regiment, 73
    Massachusetts 54th Regiment, 75
    Red Cross movement (*see* Red Cross movement)
    "the search for the missing men" venture, 76
  family background, 72
  final years of life, 94–95
  Fowler's prediction, 72
  as a government patent clerk, 73
  inspiring a shared vision, 10–11
  relief effort, 92
  teaching career, 72, 73
  U.S. Sanitary Commission, 74
Best Care at Lower Cost: The Path to Continuously Learning Healthcare in America (2012), 271
birth control movement
  abortion consequences, 114–115
  Birth Control Review, The, 119
  Brownsville trial, 120
  cervical caps, 117
  condoms, 116–117
  contraceptive practices, 115–116
  diaphragms, 117

birth control movement (*cont.*)
English Malthusianism, 114
first birth control clinic, 118–120
health promotion items, 116
hormone ebbing and flowing, 116
pessary usage, 119
safe period/rhythm method, 116
vaginal douching, 116
Woman Rebel, The, 118
Blue Cross Blue Shield study, 272
Breckinridge, Mary
death of, 238–239
enabling others to act, 15, 237–238
family and early life
death of husband, 228
education, 227–228
journaling, 226–227
Moscow foundling asylum, 226
Russian method of childbirth, 226
honoring, 239–240
married life, second marriage,
229–230
Mary Breckinridge Hospital, 239
nurse and midwifery service
CARD, 230, 231
community health nursing
program, 230–231
contributions, 236–237
Frontier Nursing Service, 235, 238,
240–241
fund collection, 233
Hyden Hospital, 236
maternal–child care, 229, 234
nurse-midwife recruitment, 234
professional nurses' training
program, 231
public health nursing, 231
rural health care, 231–233
training, 228–229
Wendover home, 234–235
nursing leadership, 224–225
pregnancy and motherhood, 229–230

Cavell, Edith Louisa
Brown's altruistic courage, 257–258
challenges, 251
as a governess, 252
children's Christmas party, 256

Christian beliefs, 249
death, 260, 261
education
nurse training, 253
primary, 249
encouraging the heart, 16
François family, 249–250
moral obligation, 251–252
nursing career
in Brussels, during German
occupation, 256
social profile, 250
and probationer nurse, 253–256
public perception, 250–251, 253–254
setting of standards, 257
World War I, 258–260
teaching positions, 252
Centers for Medicare and Medicaid
Services (CMS)
fiscal and quality issues, 274
Hospital Readmissions Reduction
Program, 274–275
IMPACT Act, 275
prevention and population health,
275–276
value-based reimbursement
approaches, 273–274
*Code of Ethics for Nurses with Interpretive
Statements,* 278
Comstock Act, 108
Crimean War. *See* Nightingale, Florence

Dartmouth Atlas of Health Care,
271–272
Daughters of the American Revolution
(DAR), 150
diagnosis-related group (DRG)-based
operating payments, 274
Dix, Dorothea Lynde
adolescence, 177–178
American Civil War, 189–191
death of sister, 179
enabling others to act, 14–15
grandfather (Elijah Dix), 176–177
international leadership, 188–189
leadership development, 184–185
literary talents, 181
mentors of

Beecher, Catherine, 181
Emerson, George B., 181
Rathbones, 181–182
mother's poor health, 177
national leadership, 186–188
political leadership and moral movement
insane asylum reform movement, 182
Memorial to the Legislature of Massachusetts report, 183–184
moral treatment approach, 182
presidential campaign, 182–183
prisoners' letters and leadership expansion, 186
religious commitment, 180–181
social life, 179
teaching role
Boston Female Monitorial School, 179
publications, 179
Unitarianism, 178
doctor of nursing practice (DNP), 279

eHealth, 277
English Malthusianism, 114
Evening Hours, 180

Finlay's mosquito vector hypothesis, 159
Franco-Prussian War, 79
Frontier Nursing Service, 235, 238, 240–241
future of nursing leadership, 269–283

health care-acquired conditions (HCACs), 273
Henry Street Nurses Settlement
district nurses, 214
public education, 214
public health, 200–202, 212–213
Spanish flu, 211–213, 216
Hospital Consumer Assessment of Healthcare Providers and Systems (HCAHPS) survey, 274
Hospital Readmissions Reduction Program, 274

Hospital Value-Based Performance Program, 274

Improving Medicare Post-Acute Care Transformation Act of 2014 (IMPACT Act), 275
inpatient prospective payment system (IPPS), 274–275
insane asylum reform movement, 182
Institute of Medicine (IOM) report, 270–271
Institution for the Care of Sick Gentlewomen in Distressed Circumstances, 27
International Committee of the Red Cross (ICRC), 80, 81
Irish Sisters of Charity, congregation
convents, 62–63
ministries for prisons, schools, and orphanages, 63, 65

Kenny, Elizabeth
challenging the process, 12–13
family background, 129
health issues, 131
knowledge of human anatomy, 129–130
nursing
appendicitis treatment, 132
Australian Army Nursing Service, 130
cerebral palsy treatment, 131
dark ship assignment, 130
influenza epidemic treatment, 131
staff nurse, military, 130
polio treatment
acute polio cases, 137
in America, 138–140
in Australia, 136–138
challenges, 136–137
immobilization treatment, 135
mental awareness, 141
muscle reeducation, 140–141
muscle transplantation, 141
neuromuscular system functioning, 142

Kenny, Elizabeth
  polio treatment (*cont.*)
    patient and family involvement,
      142
    physical therapy, 142
    Salk and oral vaccine, 142
    splinting, 135
    success, 138
    symptoms, 135
    therapist training, 137
    viral transmission, 134–135
    politics of medicine, 131–132
    societal values, 133
    stretcher invention, 132–133

leadership
  characteristics, 6–7
  evidence-based practices
    challenging the process, 11–13
    enabling others to act, 13–15
    encouraging the heart, 15–16
    inspiring a shared vision, 9–11
    modeling the way, 7–9
  nursing history, 3–4
  nursing leadership *vs.* management,
    5–6

Maass, Clara Louise
  challenging the process, 13, 168
  childhood, 149
  death and human experimentation,
    162–164
  modeling the way, 167
  nursing
    American troops in the Philippine
      islands, 154–156
    contract annulment, 156–158
    training school, 149–150
  posthumous honors, 164–167
  Spanish–American War
    American Nurses Association, 150
    contract nurses, 151–152
    Daughters of the American
      Revolution, 150
    U.S. Army Medical Department,
      150–151

    yellow fever victims, 152–154,
      158–161
Medicare, 274
Meditations for Private Hours, 180
Memorial to the Legislature of
    Massachusetts report, 183
mHealth, 277

National Archives and Records
    Administration (NARA), 156
National Association for the
    Advancement of Colored People
    (NAACP), 203
National Consumers League (NCL), 206
National Negro Conference, 203
New South Wales Nurses and
    Midwives' Association
    (NSWNMA), 261
New York Call, the, 113
Nightingale, Florence
  administrative craftsmanship, 23
  British Army and military health
    system
    Egyptian-Sudan campaign, 40
    Government of India Act, 37
    Great Mutiny, 37
    India Sanitation Commission
      report findings, 37–38
    Nightingale's technocratic advice,
      39
  celebrity status, 23
  Crimean War
    army medical system changes,
      preliminary documents, 35
    data-based decision making, 30–31
    medical statistical report, 36
    Nightingale Fund, 33–34
    peacetime mortality of soldiers,
      35–36
    royal Commissariat Commission,
      33
    royal Sanitary Commission, 32–33
    Scutari experiences, 29–33
  demystification, 46–49
  health care administration and
    nursing, 26–27
  London's *The Times* report, 22
  male role models, 27

modeling the way, 8–9
nurse training programs
  British and American nurse
    leaders, 45–46
  district training programs, 45
  graduates, 41–42
  hospital design and construction,
    42–43
  nursing superintendent position,
    43
  sanitary reform interventions,
    40–44
  workhouse infirmaries, 44
nursing superintendent, 27–29
radicalization
  Christian spirituality, 24
  education, 24
  German experiences, 25–26
  influential thinkers and leaders,
    23–24
  nurse training, 26
  political influence, 25
  William Nightingale's support, 25
self-effacement technique, 28
social reform organizations, 27
nursing and nurse leaders
  ANA Social Policy Statement, 278
  APRNs, 279
  Clara Barton, 278
  domains and recommendations,
    281
  future aspects, 282–283
  Margaret Sanger, 277–278
  Mother Mary Aikenhead, 278
  RWJF and IOM support, 279–281
nursing leadership, future of
  a new context, 277–279
  nurses leading change, 269–283
  preparing nurse leaders, 282–283
  re-visioning health care
    The Future of Nursing, 279–282
    health care reform, 272–273
    new care models, 275–276
    new care settings and new
      technologies, 276–277
    volume- to value-based
      reimbursement, 273–275
  unsustainable U.S. health system,
    270–272

nursing management, 6

Our Ladies Hospice for the Dying, 65

patient-centered medical homes
  (PCMHs), 276
Physician Quality Reporting System
  (PQRS), 276
provider-preventable conditions
  (OPPCs), 273
public health nursing. See Lillian D. Wald

Red Cross
  American, 82–83
    accounting system, 93–94
    African American victims of storm,
      86
    first aid program, 94
    flood relief efforts, 84
    Michigan forest fires, disaster
      response in, 83
    New Orleans Red Cross, 85
    official federal charter, 92–93
    Philadelphia local Red Cross
      Auxiliary, 85
    Red Cross Auxiliary Society, 83
  Battle of El Caney, 90
  Battle of San Juan, 90–91
  Cuban peasants, 88–90
  European Societies, 82
  financial support, 80
  founder, 78
  Franco-Prussian War, 79
  ICRC, 80, 81
  International Conference of the Red
    Cross, 85
  international relief efforts, 86–88
  model of care, 79
  Spanish military forces, 91–92
  Treaty of Geneva, 78–79
  in United States, 80, 81
Remarks on Prisons and Prison Discipline
  in the United States, 186
reproductive health care movement.
  See Margaret Higgins Sanger
Robert Wood Johnson Foundation
  (RWJF), 279–281

Sanger, Margaret Higgins
  accomplishments, 120–122
  biography, 108–112
  birth control movement
    abortion consequences, 114–115
    cervical caps and diaphragms, 117
    condoms, 116–117
    contraceptive practices, 115–116
    English Malthusianism, 114
    health promotion items, 116
    hormone ebbing and flowing, 116
    public service and progress,
      118–120
    safe period/rhythm method, 116
    vaginal douching, 116
  challenging the process, 12
  education, 110–111
  marriage, 111–112
  motherhood and middle-class living
    period, 112
  nursing education, 111
  as a public health nurse, 114
  sex education, 113
  Socialist Party, 112–113
Social Progress Index, 271

The Pearl or Affection's Gift: A Christmas
    and New Year's Present, 181
To Err is Human: Building a Safer Health
    System, 270
Treaty of Geneva, 78

U.S. Army Medical Department, 150–151
U.S. health care system
  acute care model, 271
  Affordable Care Act, 272–273
  CMS (see Centers for Medicare and
    Medicaid Services)
  cost of, 271–272
  fee-for-service payment model, 273
  IMPACT Act, 275
  IOM report, 270, 271
  new care settings and technologies,
    276–277
U.S. Health in International Perspective:
    Shorter Lives, Poorer Health, 271
U.S. Sanitary Commission, 74

value-based reimbursement approaches,
    273–274
Visiting Nurse Service of New York
    (VNSNY), 215–219

Wald, Lillian D.
  age of transformation, 196–197
  early life
    childhood, 197
    classroom health educator, 198–199
    education, 197–198
    empathic competence, 199
    home nursing courses, 198
    patient and community
      empowerment model, 199
  empowering communities
    biopsychosocial model of health
      care, 203
    community-based nursing practice,
      205
    memorial service, 204
    neighborhood-based access, 204
    racial and ethnic groups, 203
    Sanger's autobiography, 205–206
  enabling others to act, 15
  philanthropy and business interests
    fund for visiting nurse services, 211
    neighborhood-based health,
      209–210
    story-telling ability, 210–211
    Wald's positive language and
      personal energy, 211
  public health and settlement
    movements
    Henry Street Settlement, 200–202
    mortality statistics, 200
    organization's activities, 201–202
    settlement houses, 200–201
    social justice, 199–200
  social institution mobilization
    advocacy, 208–209
    assertiveness and political acumen,
      207
    cooperation and collaboration,
      206–207
    federal agency, 207–208
  Spanish flu pandemic
    data-gathering effort, 214

Henry Street Settlement visiting
nurses, 212–213
New York City's public health
responses, 213–215
Nurses' Emergency Council, 214
public education, 214
VNSNY's response to Superstorm
Sandy, 216–219
*Wide Neighborhoods: A Story of the
Frontier Nursing Service*, 238
Woman Rebel, The, 118
Women's Central Association of Relief
(WCAR), 190

Yellow Fever Commission
American Public Health Association,
158
fever transmission, mosquitoes,
161–162
Finlay's mosquito vector hypothesis,
159
immunization, 160
Las Animas Hospital, 161
mosquito theory, 159
nonfatal cases, 159–160
surgeon members, 158
treatment, 161

Printed in the United States
By Bookmasters